Advancing the Knowledge and Application of Health Behavior Theories

Advancing the Knowledge and Application of Health Behavior Theories

Topic Editors

Yifei Liu

Dhananjay Nayakankuppam

MDPI

Basel • Beijing • Wuhan • Barcelona • Belgrade • Novi Sad • Cluj • Manchester

Topic Editors
Yifei Liu
Division of Pharmacy Practice and Administration
The University of Missouri
Kansas City, MO
USA

Dhananjay Nayakankuppam
Department of Marketing
The University of Iowa
Iowa City, IA
USA

Editorial Office
MDPI AG
Grosspeteranlage 5
4052 Basel, Switzerland

This is a reprint of the Topic, published open access by the journals *European Journal of Investigation in Health, Psychology and Education* (ISSN 2254-9625), *Healthcare* (ISSN 2227-9032), *Nursing Reports* (ISSN 2039-4403) and *Pharmacy* (ISSN 2226-4787), freely accessible at: https://www.mdpi.com/topics/health_behavior_theories.

For citation purposes, cite each article independently as indicated on the article page online and as indicated below:

Lastname, A.A.; Lastname, B.B. Article Title. *Journal Name* **Year**, *Volume Number*, Page Range.

ISBN 978-3-7258-8113-0 (Hbk)
ISBN 978-3-7258-8114-7 (PDF)
https://doi.org/10.3390/books978-3-7258-8114-7

Contents

About the Editors

Yifei Liu

Yifei Liu is a Fellow of the American Pharmacists Association and an Associate Professor at the University of Missouri—Kansas City School of Pharmacy. His research focuses on patient and provider behavior, the implementation and evaluation of healthcare services, and the determinants of healthcare utilization and disease risk, with additional emphasis on psychiatric pharmacy and the opioid epidemic. He has contributed extensively to interdisciplinary research that bridges pharmacy practice, health outcomes, and behavioral science. In addition, he has been actively engaged in academic publishing and editorial leadership, serving as associate editor, editorial board member, advisory board member, and co-editor for multiple journals and research topics.

Dhananjay Nayakankuppam

Dhananjay Nayakankuppam is a Professor and Henry B. Tippie Research Fellow at the Tippie College of Business at the University of Iowa. His research focuses on consumer judgment and decision making, social cognition, and the psychological processes that shape attitudes, preferences, and choice behavior. His work spans topics such as implicit theories, evaluative judgment, regulatory focus, and cognitive fluency to understand the mechanisms underlying how people form preferences and make decisions under uncertainty. In addition to consumer psychology research, he has engaged in interdisciplinary work applying behavioral theories to health-related contexts, including medication adherence, preventive health behaviors, and patient decision making.

European Journal of
Investigation in Health, Psychology and Education

MDPI

Editorial

Advancing Health Behavior Theories in Research and Practice

Yifei Liu [1,*] and Dhananjay Nayakankuppam [2]

[1] Division of Pharmacy Practice and Administration, University of Missouri-Kansas City School of Pharmacy, Kansas City, MO 64108, USA
[2] Department of Marketing, Tippie College of Business, University of Iowa, Iowa City, IA 52242, USA
* Correspondence: liuyif@umkc.edu

1. Overview of the Topic

Understanding health behaviors is fundamental to designing effective health interventions. Health behavior theories provide structured frameworks for explaining why individuals engage in specific health-related actions and how these actions may change over time. These theoretical perspectives guide not only the conceptual understanding of behavior but also the methodological design of research and interventions aimed at promoting better health outcomes. Over the past several decades, a range of theoretical frameworks has contributed to the development of behavior science, and these frameworks have informed numerous interventions across diverse contexts (Glanz et al., 2015). However, contemporary healthcare systems face complex challenges. Aging population, rising prevalence of chronic diseases, technological transformations in healthcare delivery, and health inequities have highlighted the need for continued refinement of health behavior theories. Behavioral research must therefore evolve to integrate interdisciplinary perspectives and generate insights that can translate effectively into clinical practice. This Topic brings together contributions that collectively aim to advance the understanding and application of health behavior theories. The intended audience for this Topic includes researchers, healthcare practitioners, and policymakers working at regional, national, and international levels.

2. Contributions to Literature

This Topic represents a collaborative effort across five participating journals to expand knowledge on the development, refinement, and application of health behavior theories. The collection comprises twelve empirical studies (including one study with a correction) and one systematic review, all grounded in theoretical frameworks and examining a range of health behaviors. The scope of the Topic encompasses multiple areas of health behavior research. One area involves the testing and refinement of theoretical models. As health contexts change and new evidence emerges, it becomes essential to evaluate existing frameworks and explore modifications or extensions that better capture the complexity of behavior change processes. Another area concerns the identification of predictors and determinants of health behaviors. By examining cognitive, social, and environmental influences on behavior, research can provide insights that guide the development of more effective interventions. Measurement and methodological development also play a role in advancing behavioral science. Valid and reliable measures of theoretical constructs are essential for testing models and evaluating interventions. In addition, the Topic emphasizes the translation of theoretical knowledge into practical applications. Health behavior theories are most valuable when they inform the design and implementation of interventions that improve health outcomes. Research addressing intervention development, health promotion strategies, and evaluation of healthcare services demonstrates how theoretical insights can be translated into practice (Glanz et al., 2015). The Topic also reflects the diversity of healthcare settings in which behavioral research is conducted. Studies span a wide range of contexts, which underscores the importance of applying behavioral theories across different levels of healthcare delivery and across patient populations.

3. Remaining Challenges

Despite the advances demonstrated in this Topic, several challenges remain in the study and application of health behavior theories. One challenge is the integration of individual-level theories with broader perspectives. Health behaviors are influenced not only by individual cognition and motivation but also by social networks, institutional structures, and policy environments. Expanding theoretical frameworks to incorporate these multi-level influences remains an important area for future research. Measurement challenges also persist. Accurately assessing psychological constructs such as attitudes and self-efficacy can be difficult, particularly when relying on self-reported data. Advances in digital technologies and data collection methods may offer opportunities to enhance measurement precision and capture behavioral processes in real time. Finally, translating theoretical insights into sustainable health interventions continues to be a complex task. Bridging the gap between theory and practice requires collaboration between researchers, practitioners, and policymakers to ensure that theoretical models inform practical decision-making in healthcare systems.

Looking ahead, a few directions for future research emerge from the themes of this Topic. First, interdisciplinary collaboration will remain essential for advancing behavioral science. Integrating perspectives from public health, behavioral psychology, sociology, and health services research can contribute to more comprehensive models that reflect the multifaceted nature of health behaviors. Second, methodological innovation should continue to be a priority. Emerging tools such as digital health platforms, wearable technologies, and real-time behavioral monitoring systems may provide new opportunities to study behavior dynamically and evaluate interventions more effectively.

4. Conclusions

The articles included in this Topic highlight the enduring importance of health behavior theories for understanding and improving health outcomes. By exploring theoretical constructs, examining behavioral determinants, and translating insights into practical applications, the Topic aims to advance health behavior research. At the same time, the collection underscores the need for continued theoretical refinement, methodological innovation, and interdisciplinary collaboration. Addressing these areas will help ensure that health behavior theories remain responsive to evolving healthcare challenges and capable of guiding effective interventions that promote health outcomes across patient populations.

Conflicts of Interest: The authors declare no conflict of interest.

Reference

Glanz, K., Rimer, B. K., & Viswanath, K. V. (Eds.). (2015). *Health behavior: Theory, research, and practice* (5th ed.). Jossey-Bass/Wiley.

https://doi.org/10.3390/ejihpe16040051

pharmacy

MDPI

Opinion

The Influence of Health Behavior Theory on Implementation Practice and Science: Brief Review and Commentary

Anne E. Sales [1,2,3,*], Stacy L. Farr [3,4,5] and John A. Spertus [3,4,5]

1 Sinclair School of Nursing, Department of Family and Community Medicine, School of Medicine, University of Missouri, Columbia, MO 65211, USA
2 Center for Clinical Management Research, VA Ann Arbor Healthcare System, Ann Arbor, MI 48105, USA
3 Healthcare Institute for Innovations in Quality, University of Missouri-Kansas City, Kansas City, MO 64110, USA
4 Saint Luke's Mid America Heart Institute, Kansas City, MO 64111, USA
5 Department of Biomedical and Health Informatics, UMKC School of Medicine, Kansas City, MO 64108, USA
* Correspondence: asales@missouri.edu

Abstract: As research defines new treatments and policies to improve the health of patients, an increasing challenge has been to translate these insights into routine clinical practice to benefit patients and society. An important exploration is how theories of human behavior change fit into the science of implementation and quality improvement. In this paper, we begin with a brief review of the intellectual roots of implementation science and quality improvement, followed by a discussion of how theories and principles of behavior change can inform both goals and challenges in using behavior change theories. The insights offered through health behavior change theory have led to changes in how we plan for implementation and select, develop, design and tailor implementation interventions and strategies. While the degree to which organizational and external contexts influence the behavior of providers in these organizations varies widely, some degree of context external to the individual is important and needs adequate consideration. In short, health behavior change theory is essential but not sufficient to integrate in most implementation efforts, where priority must be given to both individual factors and contexts in which individuals operate.

Keywords: implementation science; implementation research; implementation practice; quality improvement; health behavior change

1. Introduction

As research defines new treatments to improve the survival and health status of patients, an increasing challenge lies in how to translate these insights into routine clinical practice to benefit patients and society. Implementing change and improvement in healthcare is multi-faceted, but requires behavior change of many healthcare stakeholders. Healthcare providers, leaders, and administrators, as well as payers, patients, and other professionals, all have relevant roles and actions in translating evidence into care. This paper aims to describe how theories of human behavior change play a key role in the science of implementation and quality improvement.

2. Methods

We begin with a brief review of the intellectual roots of implementation science and quality improvement, followed by a discussion of how theories and principles of behavior change can inform both goals and challenges in applying behavior change theories. We use the term "implementation science" when referring to the underlying science of studying changes in healthcare delivery and "implementation practice and research" when referring more generally to work being conducted. We conducted the brief review by searching for papers that cite the Theoretical Domains Framework (TDF) (described in

Section 3.1) and focusing on papers that advanced the framework and created tools for use in implementation research and practice. The search was conducted by AES and covered the period from 2005, when the first TDF paper was published, through the first half of 2022. This was not intended as an exhaustive systematic review.

3. A Brief Review of Implementation Science and Practice

The term "implementation science" has been in general use since the mid-2000s, with more direct applicability to health care with the launch of the journal *Implementation Science* in 2006 [1]. Even though research related to implementation is conducted in many fields, including education, social services, construction, and others, in health care the term largely focuses on the implementation of evidence-based practices or policies into care.

Evidence-based practice has its roots in the evidence-based medicine movement, sparked by the work of Archie Cochrane in the 1950s [2,3]. Evidence-based medicine generally focuses on the *efficacy* of medical practice by testing the impact of a treatment when delivered with great reproducibility on an ideal population. However, when applied more broadly, outside of the setting of a randomized trial, the *effectiveness* of treatment is described by understanding the impact on outcomes in a more real-world setting with a more diverse population of patients. Differences between efficacy and effectiveness highlighted the need to select patients more reproducibly for treatment and to deliver the therapy more consistently. This sparked the movement to create and implement practice guidelines, in which the best available evidence is framed as recommendations for practice. Initial efforts at guideline implementation focused on teaching and the dissemination of the guidelines, which were often not very effective in inducing major changes in practice patterns.

Concurrent with the initial work to implement practice guidelines, research was conducted on small area variation, to understand how variable clinical practice is. This work, with a seminal paper published in 1973 in *Science* [4,5], sparked a movement within the field of health services research to better understand and explain how and why clinical practice varies as much as it does, even within relatively small geographic regions.

The field of implementation science largely grew from these two overlapping movements: one to define the appropriate practice of medicine through producing and synthesizing evidence, and the other to describe and understand how medicine is practiced, emphasizing practice variability. Through the 1990s, as the field of implementation science began to coalesce, these issues drove considerable health services research and highlighted the need for methodological rigor in learning how best to synthesize and appraise the empirical literature. This also created increasing pressure to understand how to implement practice change in health care.

The small area variation literature also prompted a separate stream of research innovation. In a widely cited paper, Donald Berwick described methods of continuous quality improvement in health care, contrasting methods used in manufacturing industries with the standards of the time in health care [6,7]. The application of quality improvement methods from manufacturing [8,9] has been widely accepted in health care organizations, as the tools are relatively easy to learn and apply. Lean methods [10,11] as well as a number of related approaches, such as Six Sigma [12] and Define, Measure, Analyze, Improve and Control (DMAIC) [13], have been applied throughout the health care industry.

Both implementation science and quality improvement practice focus on process and tool development. Implementation science has been more focused on using and developing theory than quality improvement practice, which has focused on practical applications of these methods to improve health care quality [14,15]. In implementation research, theoretical perspectives have been drawn from the social sciences, including sociology, anthropology, and economics, and more recently, from the organizational sciences and business. Increasingly, psychological theory has been incorporated into implementation research, particularly theory focused on human behavior change. Early papers from the late 1990s and early 2000s describe ways in which implementation research uses and tests these theories to effect successful implementation of evidence-based practices.

3.1. Behavior Change Theory in Implementation Research

The field of implementation science continues to evolve as experience and insights require more refined strategies for understanding and changing healthcare. A seminal work that brought human behavior change theory squarely into the forefront of implementation research was a 2005 publication by an influential group of implementation scientists, health psychologists, and health services researchers in the United Kingdom [16]. This paper described a lengthy process in which over 30 human behavior change theories were assembled by experts, reviewed by the interdisciplinary group of researchers, then deconstructed into specific constructs used in each of the underlying theories. These constructs were then reassembled into a "menu of constructs" or framework [17] called the Theoretical Domains Framework (TDF). Importantly, the TDF is intended to help in understanding behaviors from any of the potential adopters of behavior change, including patients, providers, or other healthcare stakeholders, both individually or as teams [18]. As a consolidated determinants framework [19], the TDF provides important information about factors that are theorized to influence the success or failure of implementation or behavior change. The TDF was refined in 2012 [20]. The motive for the TDF revisions [20] was to disperse some of the constructs in the original domains and to add new constructs. For example, the former domain "Motivation and Goals" was split into "Intentions" and "Goals" as separate domains.

In Table 1, we provide an overview comparing domains of the TDF with two other widely used determinants frameworks, the Consolidated Framework for Implementation Research (CFIR) [21] and the Tailored Implementation for Chronic Disease checklist (TICD) [22]. It is notable that the majority of domains in the TDF are included in just one domain in either the CFIR or the TICD. The number and type of constructs in the two domains in the CFIR (Characteristics of Individuals) and TICD (Individual Health Professional Factors) are different from each other, but neither include the depth or richness of the large number of constructs (over 50) in these ten or eleven domains of the TDF.

Table 1. Comparing Domains of the TDF, CFIR and TICD.

TDF Domain	CFIR Domain	TICD Domain
Knowledge	Characteristics of Individuals	Individual Health Professional Factors
Skills	Characteristics of Individuals	Individual Health Professional Factors
Social/Professional Role and Identity	Characteristics of Individuals	Individual Health Professional Factors
Beliefs about Capabilities	Characteristics of Individuals	Individual Health Professional Factors
Optimism	Characteristics of Individuals	Individual Health Professional Factors
Beliefs about Consequences	Characteristics of Individuals	Individual Health Professional Factors
Reinforcement	Characteristics of Individuals	Individual Health Professional Factors; Incentives and Resources
Intentions	Characteristics of Individuals	Individual Health Professional Factors
Goals	Characteristics of Individuals	Individual Health Professional Factors
Memory, Attention and Decision Processes	Characteristics of Individuals	Individual Health Professional Factors
Environmental Context and Resources	Outer Setting; Inner Setting	Professional Interactions; Capacity for Organizational Change; Patient Factors; Social, Political and Legal Factors
Social Influences	Inner Setting	Professional Interactions
Emotion	Characteristics of Individuals	Individual Health Professional Factors
Behavioral Regulation	Characteristics of Individuals; Inner Setting	Individual Health Professional Factors; Incentives and Resources; Professional Interactions

The decision to eliminate the domain "Nature of the Behaviors" from the TDF was an important change. This domain's constructs corresponded to important domains in the CFIR and TICD, not shown in Table 1 because the domain no longer exists in the TDF.

Much of the content of the former "Nature of the Behaviors" TDF domain is contained in the CFIR domain "Characteristics of the Intervention" and in the TICD domain "Guideline Factors". Excluding this content from the revised TDF, although justified because it pertains to the context of the actual innovation or change rather than to behavior specifically, means that using the TDF alone can miss important factors.

A large number of implementation practice and research studies have used and attempted to test specific components of underlying human behavior change theories [23–28]. The Theory of Planned Behavior [29] was initially widely used [26,30,31], but after the TDF was published, attention shifted to this more inclusive framework that allows the use of concepts beyond those in the Theory of Planned Behavior. Human behavior change theories have been applied to the use of certain implementation strategies in health care, notably audit with feedback [24,32–37].

Michie continued developing approaches using the material in the TDF, notably the Behavior Change Wheel (BCW) and the Capabilities-Opportunity-Motivation-Behavior framework (COM-B) [38]. Summarizing several existing frameworks, Michie and her colleagues describe nine different intervention functions and seven policy categories which might make those interventions possible. The interventions mostly function at the level of the individual, while policy interventions are typically at the larger societal level; a component not explicitly discussed in this approach is the organizational context within which the individual works.

3.2. *A Brief Note on the Use of Determinants Frameworks in Implementation Practice and Research*

An important problem in implementation research is defining what approaches or strategies/interventions to use in trying to implement a new evidence-based practice [39]. In the absence of determinants frameworks, which catalog the factors that have been demonstrated empirically or theoretically to affect whether implementation is successful in a specific instance [19], the usual practice has been to simply make as educated a guess as possible, often without systematic effort to understand the underlying reasons why that practice is not already being used [28,40,41]. Making efforts to understand the underlying or root causes of gaps in practice, then using a theory to select, design and tailor implementation interventions or strategies, has been argued both as a way of achieving more effective implementation more often, and to build and refine theory to understand how best to achieve effective implementation. Determinants frameworks are one component of the design process. Additional components include frameworks describing implementation strategies [42,43], which can be linked to key determinants that have been assessed as influential in a specific implementation problem using logic models [44], or other approaches [45]. Michie and colleagues' COM-B model and related approaches bundle key determinants with prescribed interventions to support implementation planning [38].

3.3. *Behavior Change Techniques and Their Taxonomy*

In further work, Michie and colleagues created the Behavior Change Technique Taxonomy (BCTT), which catalogs 93 evidence-based techniques for changing behavior, categorized into 19 hierarchically grouped domains. These can be mapped to the 14 domains of the TDF [46], enhancing the ease with which behavior change techniques can be used to design implementation strategies or interventions, although the mapping is complex.

Implementation strategies, described in both the Expert Recommendations for Implementation Change (ERIC) project [42,47] or the Effective Practice Organization Collaboration [43], are often fairly abstract and lack the detail required to deploy them operationally. One advantage of behavior change techniques is that they primarily operate at the level of the individual, or internally to the individual, offering the opportunity to specify and design strategies using behavioral techniques that can address specific, individual-level barriers.

A key advantage to behavior change techniques is the clear link to a theoretical basis for its effect, or its mechanism of action. This link has been developed further through systematic reviews and research exploring the evidence from empirical studies that have already been completed [48,49], which describe empirically derived links between behavior change techniques and the theoretical mechanisms underlying them. Recent work has focused on making a web-based tool available to assist intervention designers in developing theoretically based interventions to support behavior change, including implementation of evidence-based practices [50]. This begins to address a core problem in implementation research, which is how to find robust and accessible links between the determinant assessed as high priority, and strategies to address these determinants, particularly negative ones (barriers) [39]. Coupled with other research focused on mechanisms of action of implementation strategies [51], these efforts may help make implementation intervention design more robust, more replicable, more reliable, and ultimately more effective.

In Figure 1, we illustrate the relationships among determinants frameworks such as the TDF, strategies and behavior change techniques, and the tools that attempt to make this linkage more explicit.

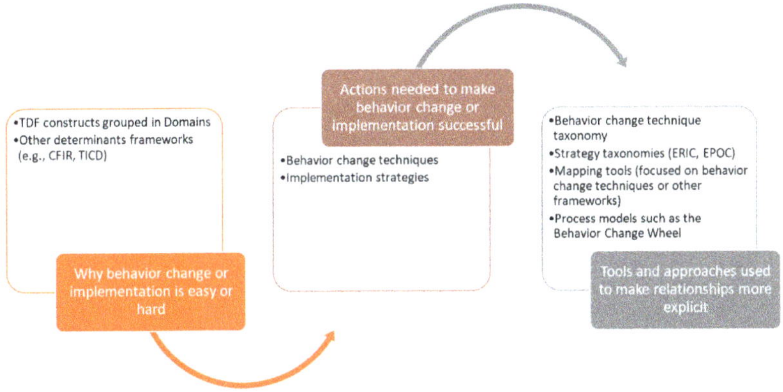

Figure 1. Relationships among determinants frameworks, strategies and tools.

3.4. Case Example: Audit with Feedback

Audit with feedback is a widely used strategy in implementation practice and research, which has been systematically reviewed, and its effectiveness—and the conditions under which it appears to be effective—has been assessed using meta-analysis [32]. It has been shown to be modestly effective in increasing the likelihood that a desired behavior change is achieved as part of implementation efforts. Theories underlying its use have been proposed [36,52], and theories used in designing audit with feedback interventions have been carefully studied [34,35]. Nonetheless, there has been little change in the effectiveness of audit with feedback interventions over the last decade [53], and we still have relatively little understanding of how these interventions work [54].

Part of the complexity is the multiple theories at different levels underpinning this seemingly simple intervention. We illustrate this in Figure 2, which shows how many factors in the context of a feedback intervention, in addition to the actual design of the feedback report itself, including its mode of delivery, can vary, and each of these theories requires design elements in the feedback intervention if they are assessed as important.

Specifically, the TDF and its constructs primarily apply to individual feedback, but multiple domains might pertain, including knowledge; possibly skills if skills are applicable to the specific feedback data; social/professional role and identity; beliefs about capabilities; beliefs about consequences; reinforcement; intentions; goals; memory, attention and decision processes; emotion; and behavioral regulation. The only TDF domains that explicitly include other contextual variables would be the environmental context and resources or social influences. While these constructs may be useful, there is a great deal not included in these that is included in both the CFIR and the TICD. In the CFIR, both the inner setting and outer setting domains would apply to both the internal organizational context, as well as the external context in which the organization operates. For TICD, the individual health professional factors domain (which includes multiple constructs from the TDF) would likely apply as well as: patient factors (depending on the nature of the feedback report data); professional interactions; incentives and resources; capacity for organizational change; and social, political and legal factors which primarily refer to external context.

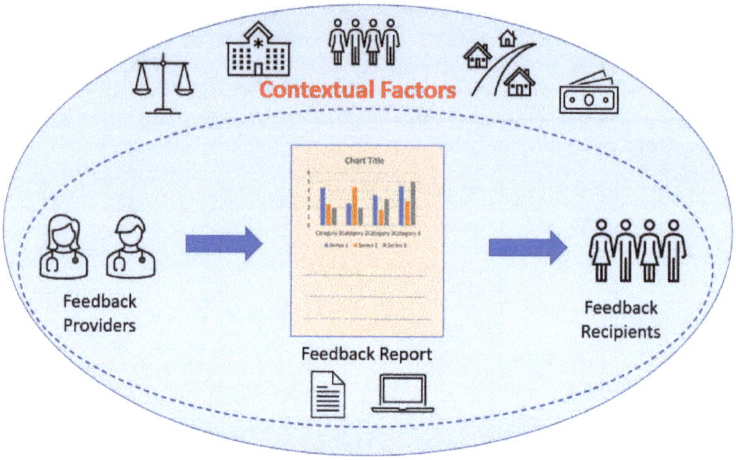

Figure 2. Multiple levels of elements affecting the effectiveness of a feedback report.

We note the complexity of the multiple domains and constructs within each domain. As we show in Figure 1, there are relationships, albeit complex, between the determinants in frameworks and decisions about selecting strategies and behavior change techniques. We strongly recommend working with an expert in implementation science or practice who has expertise in using determinants frameworks to design and deploy implementation strategies and interventions.

In addition to the domains of the CFIR and TICD, which provide more detailed coverage of the internal organizational context as well as the external environments, both the CFIR and the TICD include domains that focus on the specific attributes of the innovation/intervention being implemented. This reflects the decision to remove the "Nature of the Behaviors" domain from the TDF. While the principle of focusing on aspects of behavior, and the attributes of the innovation may not directly relate to the behavior of individuals, this remains an important omission for the TDF.

For example, in work conducted in Canadian long term care facilities [55,56], we found key differences between requirements for behavior change for pain assessment compared with depression screening and screening for pressure injuries. The actual behavior in each of these is different, requiring different timeframes, actions by different professionals, and different responses, all of which had impact on response to feedback.

For example, pain assessment should be done on at least a daily basis, if not every shift, because the experience of pain can change quite rapidly. Screening for depression may not need to be done as frequently, as depression symptoms are usually relatively stable over time, and weekly or even monthly assessment may be more appropriate than daily. Assessment for signs of pressure injury should be done very frequently, generally on an hourly basis for people at high risk. The difference in cadence or timing for each of these assessments affects the likelihood of changing behavior, because there are more opportunities for behavior change and rapid assessment of change in behaviors that occur more frequently.

4. Discussion: Current State of the Science and Practice

Health behavior change theory has had a marked impact on implementation research and practice. It has contributed particularly to an understanding of how individuals process information, make decisions, and act on cues to change behavior. The insights offered through health behavior change theory have led to changes in how we plan for implementation and select, develop, design and tailor implementation interventions and strategies. An especially promising area is the development of online tools that summarize a huge amount of prior research in health behavior change and enable implementation practitioners and researchers to readily access recommendations about which behavior change techniques to include in implementation interventions, once determinants have been assessed. We note that discussion of conducting determinant assessment is outside the scope of this article. A good overview of one of these tools is given in Johnston et al., 2021 [50].

However, we have also pointed out some limitations in the current tools and approaches used in health behavior change when they are applied to implementation research. In particular, implementation practice and research in health care often takes place within the context of organizations whose mission is to deliver health care services, or to enhance health and wellbeing through programs such as well child immunization or other activities (e.g., gyms and other community-based organizations). While the degree to which organizational and external contexts influence the behavior of providers in these organizations varies widely, some degree of context external to the individual is important and needs adequate consideration. Some of this is included in the External Context and Resources and Social Influence domains of the TDF, but this content is limited in its granularity and nuance. We recommend that use of a consolidated determinants framework like the TICD, which includes key constructs from the TDF as well as the CFIR, can address this limitation. In short, while a focus on the individual is essential in most implementation efforts, it is equally important to focus on and understand the context in which the individual operates.

5. Conclusions

Implementing evidence into clinical practice and society is multi-faceted and requires behavior change from multiple healthcare stakeholders. These behaviors influence how we plan, design, and customize interventions and implementation strategies and overcome barriers. While quality improvement also exists within organizational contexts and priorities outside of individual behavior change, health behavior change theory is a critical underpinning to implementation science.

Author Contributions: Conceptualization, A.E.S., S.L.F. and J.A.S.; conceptualizing, A.E.S., S.L.F. and J.A.S.; writing—review and editing, A.E.S., S.L.F. and J.A.S. All authors have read and agreed to the published version of the manuscript.

Funding: This work received no external funding.

Institutional Review Board Statement: Not applicable.

Informed Consent Statement: Not applicable.

Data Availability Statement: Not applicable.

Conflicts of Interest: AES declares no conflicts of interest related to this article. SLF is a consultant to Novartis and owns Zena Healthcare Group, LLC. JAS is the principal investigator of grants from the National Institutes of Health, Abbott Vascular and the American College of Cardiology Foundation; is a consultant to Janssen, Novartis, Terumo, Myokardia/Bristol Myers Squibb, AstraZeneca, Bayer and Merck; serves on the Scientific Advisory Board of United Healthcare and the Board of Directors for Blue Cross Blue Shield of Kansas Cit; and owns the copyright to the KCCQ, SAQ, and PAQ.

References

1. Eccles, M.P.; Mittman, B.S. Welcome to Implementation Science. *Implement. Sci.* **2006**, *1*, 1. [CrossRef]
2. Stavrou, A.; Challoumas, D.; Dimitrakakis, G. Archibald Cochrane (1909–1988): The father of evidence-based medicine. *Interact. Cardiovasc. Thorac. Surg.* **2013**, *18*, 121–124. [CrossRef]
3. Davidoff, F.; Haynes, B.; Sackett, D.; Smith, R. Evidence based medicine. *BMJ* **1995**, *310*, 1085–1086. [CrossRef]
4. Wennberg, J.; Gittelsohn, A. Small Area Variations in Health Care Delivery. *Science* **1973**, *182*, 1102–1108. [CrossRef] [PubMed]
5. Wennberg, J.; Gittelsohn, A. Variations in medical care among small areas. *Sci. Am.* **1982**, *246*, 120–134. [CrossRef] [PubMed]
6. Berwick, D.M. Continuous improvement as an ideal in health care. *N. Engl. J. Med.* **1989**, *320*, 53–56. [CrossRef]
7. Berwick, D.M. The science of improvement. *JAMA J. Am. Med. Assoc.* **2008**, *299*, 1182–1184. [CrossRef] [PubMed]
8. Perla, R.J.; Provost, L.P.; Parry, G.J. Seven propositions of the science of improvement: Exploring foundations. *Qual. Manag. Healthc.* **2013**, *22*, 170–186. [CrossRef] [PubMed]
9. Quality Improvement Essentials Toolkit. Available online: http://www.ihi.org/resources/Pages/Tools/Quality-Improvement-Essentials-Toolkit.aspx (accessed on 21 April 2021).
10. DelliFraine, J.L.; Langabeer, J.R., II; Nembhard, I.M. Assessing the Evidence of Six Sigma and Lean in the Health Care Industry. *Qual. Manag. Healthc.* **2010**, *19*, 211. [CrossRef]
11. Standiford, T.; Conte, M.L.; Billi, J.E.; Sales, A.; Barnes, G.D. Integrating Lean Thinking and Implementation Science Determinants Checklists for Quality Improvement: A Scoping Review. *Am. J. Med. Qual.* **2020**, *35*, 330–340. [CrossRef] [PubMed]
12. Schweikhart, S.A.; Dembe, A.E. The Applicability of Lean and Six Sigma Techniques to Clinical and Translational Research. *J. Investig. Med.* **2009**, *7*, 748–755. [CrossRef] [PubMed]
13. Taner, M. An application of Six Sigma methodology to turnover intentions in health care. *Int. J. Healthc. Qual. Assur.* **2009**, *22*, 252–265. [CrossRef] [PubMed]
14. Batalden, P.B.; Davidoff, F. What is "quality improvement" and how can it transform healthcare? *Qual. Saf. Healthc.* **2007**, *16*, 2–3. [CrossRef] [PubMed]
15. Batalden, P.; Davidoff, F.; Marshall, M.; Bibby, J.; Pink, C. So what? Now what? Exploring, understanding and using the epistemologies that inform the improvement of healthcare. *Health Policy* **2011**, *20* (Supp. 1), 99–106. [CrossRef] [PubMed]
16. Michie, S.; Johnston, M.; Abraham, C.; Lawton, R.; Parker, D.; Walker, A. Making psychological theory useful for implementing evidence based practice: A consensus approach. *Qual. Saf. Healthc.* **2005**, *14*, 26–33. [CrossRef]
17. Brehaut, J.C.; Eva, K.W. Building theories of knowledge translation interventions: Use the entire menu of constructs. *Implement. Sci.* **2012**, *7*, 114. [CrossRef] [PubMed]
18. Atkins, L.; Francis, J.; Islam, R.; O'Connor, D.; Patey, A.; Ivers, N.; Foy, R.; Duncan, E.M.; Colquhoun, H.; Grimshaw, J.M.; et al. A guide to using the Theoretical Domains Framework of behaviour change to investigate implementation problems. *Implement. Sci.* **2017**, *12*, 77. [CrossRef]
19. Nilsen, P. Making Sense of Implementation Theories, Models and Frameworks. *Implement. Sci.* **2015**, *10*, 53–79. Available online: https://www.scopus.com/inward/record.uri?eid=2-s2.0-84928389723&doi=10.1186%2Fs13012-015-0242-0&partnerID=40&md5=987200423c4b15f7807c0cad8865228c (accessed on 1 September 2022). [CrossRef] [PubMed]
20. Cane, J.; O'Connor, D.; Michie, S. Validation of the theoretical domains framework for use in behaviour change and implementation research. *Implement. Sci.* **2012**, *7*, 37. [CrossRef] [PubMed]
21. Damschroder, L.J.; Aron, D.C.; Keith, R.E.; Kirsh, S.R.; Alexander, J.A.; Lowery, J.C. Fostering implementation of health services research findings into practice: A consolidated framework for advancing implementation science. *Implement. Sci.* **2009**, *4*, 50. [CrossRef] [PubMed]
22. Flottorp, S.A.; Oxman, A.D.; Krause, J.; Musila, N.R.; Wensing, M.; Godycki-Cwirko, M.; Baker, R.; Eccles, M.P. A checklist for identifying determinants of practice: A systematic review and synthesis of frameworks and taxonomies of factors that prevent or enable improvements in healthcare professional practice. *Implement. Sci. BioMed. Cent.* **2013**, *8*, 1–11. [CrossRef] [PubMed]
23. Grimshaw, J.M.; Eccles, M.P.; Steen, N.; Johnston, M.; Pitts, N.B.; Glidewell, L.; Maclennan, G.; Thomas, R.; Bonetti, D.; Walker, A. Applying psychological theories to evidence-based clinical practice: Identifying factors predictive of lumbar spine x-ray for low back pain in UK primary care practice. *Implement. Sci. BioMed. Cent.* **2011**, *6*, 1–13. [CrossRef]
24. Gardner, B.; Whittington, C.; McAteer, J.; Eccles, M.P.; Michie, S. Using theory to synthesise evidence from behaviour change interventions: The example of audit and feedback. *Soc. Sci. Med.* **2010**, *70*, 1618–1625. [CrossRef] [PubMed]
25. Sanson-fisher, R.W.; Grimshaw, J.M.; Eccles, M.P. The science of changing providers' behaviour: The missing link in evidence-based practice. *Med. J. Aust.* **2004**, *180*, 205–206. [CrossRef] [PubMed]
26. Eccles, M.; Grimshaw, J.; Walker, A.; Johnston, M.; Pitts, N. Changing the behavior of healthcare professionals: The use of theory in promoting the uptake of research findings. *J. Clin. Epidemiol.* **2005**, *58*, 107–112. [CrossRef]
27. Michie, S.; Johnston, M.; Francis, J.; Hardeman, W.; Eccles, M. From Theory to Intervention: Mapping Theoretically Derived Behavioural Determinants to Behaviour Change Techniques. *Appl. Psychol.* **2008**, *57*, 660–680. [CrossRef]
28. The Improved Clinical Effectiveness through Behavioural Research Group (ICEBeRG). Designing theoretically-informed implementation interventions. *Implement. Sci.* **2006**, *1*, 4. [CrossRef] [PubMed]
29. Ajzen, I.; Manstead, A.S.R. Changing health-related behaviours: An approach based on the theory of planned behaviour. In *The Scope of Social Psychology Theory and Applications*; Hewstone, M., Schut, H., de Wit, J.B.F., van den Bos, K., Stroebe, M.S., Eds.; Psychology Press: London, UK, 2007; pp. 43–63.

30. Francis, J.J.; Eccles, M.P.; Johnston, M.; Whitty, P.; Grimshaw, J.M.; Kaner, E.F.S.; Smith, L.; Walker, A. Explaining the effects of an intervention designed to promote evidence-based diabetes care: A theory-based process evaluation of a pragmatic cluster randomised controlled trial. *Implement. Sci.* **2008**, *3*, 50. [CrossRef] [PubMed]
31. Eccles, M.P.; Grimshaw, J.M.; MacLennan, G.; Bonetti, D.; Glidewell, L.; Pitts, N.B.; Steen, N.; Thomas, R.; Walker, A.; Johnston, M. Explaining Clinical Behaviors Using Multiple Theoretical Models. *Implement. Sci.* **2012**, *7*, 1–13. Available online: https://www.scopus.com/inward/record.uri?eid=2-s2.0-84867453413&doi=10.1186%2F1748-5908-7-99&partnerID=40&md5=7701c8b0906a5a9dc50125b06b4298a6 (accessed on 1 September 2022). [CrossRef]
32. Ivers, N.; Jamtvedt, G.; Flottorp, S.; Young, J.M.; Odgaard-Jensen, J.; French, S.D.; O'Brien, M.A.; Johansen, M.; Grimshaw, J.; Oxman, A.D. Audit and feedback: Effects on professional practice and healthcare outcomes. *Cochrane Database Syst. Rev.* **2012**, *6*, CD000259. [CrossRef] [PubMed]
33. Brehaut, J.C.; Colquhoun, H.L.; Eva, K.W.; Carroll, K.; Sales, A.; Michie, S.; Ivers, N.; Grimshaw, J.M. Practice Feedback Interventions: 15 Suggestions for Optimizing Effectiveness. *Ann. Intern. Med.* **2016**, *164*, 435–441. [CrossRef]
34. Colquhoun, H.L.; Brehaut, J.C.; Sales, A.; Ivers, N.; Grimshaw, J.; Michie, S.; Carroll, K.; Chalifoux, M.; Eva, K.W. A Systematic Review of the Use of Theory in Randomized Controlled Trials of Audit and Feedback. *Implement. Sci.* **2013**, *8*, 1–8. Available online: https://www.scopus.com/inward/record.uri?eid=2-s2.0-84878728562&doi=10.1186%2F1748-5908-8-66&partnerID=40&md5=828636d20ad9b296d42388fb97db2352 (accessed on 1 September 2022). [CrossRef] [PubMed]
35. Colquhoun, H.L.; Carroll, K.; Eva, K.W.; Grimshaw, J.M.; Ivers, N.; Michie, S.; Sales, A.; Brehaut, J.C. Advancing the literature on designing audit and feedback interventions: Identifying theory-informed hypotheses. *Implement. Sci.* **2017**, *12*, 117. [CrossRef] [PubMed]
36. Kluger, A.N.; DeNisi, A. The effects of feedback interventions on performance: A historical review, a meta-analysis, and a preliminary feedback intervention theory. *Psychol. Bull.* **1996**, *119*, 254–284. [CrossRef]
37. Hysong, S.J. Audit and Feedback Features Impact Effectiveness on Care Quality. *Med. Care* **2009**, *47*, 356–363. [CrossRef] [PubMed]
38. Michie, S.; van Stralen, M.M.; West, R. The behaviour change wheel: A new method for characterising and designing behaviour change interventions. *Implement. Sci.* **2011**, *6*, 42. [CrossRef]
39. Powell, B.J.; Beidas, R.S.; Lewis, C.C.; Aarons, G.A.; McMillen, J.C.; Proctor, E.K.; Mandell, D.S. Methods to Improve the Selection and Tailoring of Implementation Strategies. *J. Behav. Health Serv. Res.* **2017**, *44*, 177–194. [CrossRef] [PubMed]
40. Davies, P.; Walker, A.E.; Grimshaw, J.M. A systematic review of the use of theory in the design of guideline dissemination and implementation strategies and interpretation of the results of rigorous evaluations. *Implement. Sci.* **2010**, *5*, 14. [CrossRef] [PubMed]
41. Grol, R.P.T.M.; Bosch, M.C.; Hulscher, M.E.J.L.; Eccles, M.P.; Wensing, M. Planning and studying improvement in patient care: The use of theoretical perspectives. *Milbank Q.* **2007**, *85*, 93–138. [CrossRef]
42. Powell, B.J.; Waltz, T.J.; Chinman, M.J.; Damschroder, L.J.; Smith, J.L.; Matthieu, M.M.; Proctor, E.K.; Kirchner, J.E. A refined compilation of implementation strategies: Results from the Expert Recommendations for Implementing Change (ERIC) project. *Implement. Sci.* **2015**, *10*, 21. [CrossRef] [PubMed]
43. Effective Practice and Organisation of Care (EPOC). *EPOC Taxon.* **2021**, *v*. Available online: https://zenodo.org/record/5105851 (accessed on 1 September 2022).
44. Smith, J.D.; Li, D.H.; Rafferty, M.R. The Implementation Research Logic Model: A method for planning, executing, reporting, and synthesizing implementation projects. *Implement. Sci.* **2020**, *15*, 84. [CrossRef]
45. Fernandez, M.E.; ten Hoor, G.A.; van Lieshout, S.; Rodriguez, S.A.; Beidas, R.S.; Parcel, G.; Ruiter, R.A.C.; Markham, C.M.; Kok, G. Implementation Mapping: Using Intervention Mapping to Develop Implementation Strategies. *Front. Public Health* **2019**, *7*, 158. [CrossRef] [PubMed]
46. Cane, J.; Richardson, M.; Johnston, M.; Ladha, R.; Michie, S. From lists of behaviour change techniques (BCTs) to structured hierarchies: Comparison of two methods of developing a hierarchy of BCTs. *Br. J. Health Psychol.* **2015**, *20*, 130–150. [CrossRef] [PubMed]
47. Waltz, T.J.; Powell, B.J.; Matthieu, M.M.; Damschroder, L.J.; Chinman, M.J.; Smith, J.L.; Proctor, E.K.; Kirchner, J.E. Use of concept mapping to characterize relationships among implementation strategies and assess their feasibility and importance: Results from the Expert Recommendations for Implementing Change (ERIC) study. *Implement. Sci.* **2015**, *10*, 109. [CrossRef] [PubMed]
48. Carey, R.N.; Connell, L.E.; Johnston, M.; Rothman, A.J.; de Bruin, M.; Kelly, M.P.; Michie, S. Behavior Change Techniques and Their Mechanisms of Action: A Synthesis of Links Described in Published Intervention Literature. *Ann. Behav. Med.* **2019**, *53*, 693–707. [CrossRef] [PubMed]
49. Michie, S.; Carey, R.N.; Johnston, M.; Rothman, A.J.; de Bruin, M.; Kelly, M.P.; Connell, L.E. From Theory-Inspired to Theory-Based Interventions: A Protocol for Developing and Testing a Methodology for Linking Behaviour Change Techniques to Theoretical. *Ann. Behav. Med.* **2018**, *52*, 501–512. Available online: https://academic.oup.com/abm/article-abstract/52/6/501/4737217 (accessed on 1 September 2022). [CrossRef] [PubMed]
50. Johnston, M.; Carey, R.N.; Bohlen, L.E.C.; Johnston, D.W.; Rothman, A.J.; de Bruin, M.; Kelly, M.P.; Groarke, H.; Michie, S. Development of an Online Tool for Linking Behavior Change Techniques and Mechanisms of Action Based on Triangulation of Findings from Literature Synthesis and Expert. *J. Integr. Nephrol. Androl.* **2021**, *11*, 1049–1065. Available online: https://academic.oup.com/tbm/article-abstract/11/5/1049/5880520 (accessed on 1 September 2022). [CrossRef]

51. Powell, B.J.; Fernandez, M.E.; Williams, N.J.; Aarons, G.A.; Beidas, R.S.; Lewis, C.C.; McHugh, S.M.; Weiner, B.J. Enhancing the Impact of Implementation Strategies in Healthcare: A Research Agenda. *Front. Public Health* **2019**, *7*, 3. [CrossRef]
52. Hollenbeck, J.R.; Ilgen, D.R.; LePine, J.A.; Colquitt, J.A.; Hedlund, J. Extending the multilevel theory of team decision making: Effects of feedback and experience in hierarchical teams. *Acad. Manag. J.* **1998**, *41*, 269–282. [CrossRef]
53. Ivers, N.M.; Grimshaw, J.M.; Jamtvedt, G.; Flottorp, S.; O'Brien, M.A.; French, S.D.; Young, J.; Odgaard-Jensen, J. Growing Literature, Stagnant Science? Systematic Review, Meta-Regression and Cumulative Analysis of Audit and Feedback Interventions in Health Care. *J. Gen. Intern. Med.* **2014**, *29*, 1534–1541. [CrossRef]
54. Foy, R.; Eccles, M.P.; Jamtvedt, G.; Young, J.; Grimshaw, J.M.; Baker, R. What do we know about how to do audit and feedback? Pitfalls in applying evidence from a systematic review. *BMC Health Serv. Res.* **2005**, *5*, 50. [CrossRef] [PubMed]
55. Sales, A.E.; Schalm, C.; Baylon, M.B.; Fraser, K.D. Data for Improvement and Clinical Excellence: Report of an Interrupted Time Series Trial of Feedback in Long-Term Care. *Implement. Sci.* **2014**, *9*, 1–10. Available online: https://www.scopus.com/inward/record.uri?eid=2-s2.0-84920821620&doi=10.1186%2Fs13012-014-0161-5&partnerID=40&md5=1a65bff3d6c28591c620437997f842bb (accessed on 1 September 2022). [CrossRef] [PubMed]
56. Sales, A.E.; Fraser, K.; Baylon, M.A.B.; O'Rourke, H.M.; Gao, G.; Bucknall, T.; Maisey, S. Understanding feedback report uptake: Process evaluation findings from a 13-month feedback intervention in long-term care settings. *Implement. Sci.* **2015**, *10*, 1–14. [CrossRef] [PubMed]

pharmacy MDPI

Review

The Moderating Power of Impulsivity: A Systematic Literature Review Examining the Theory of Planned Behavior

Lindsey A. Hohmann [1] and Kimberly B. Garza [2,*]

[1] Department of Pharmacy Practice, Harrison College of Pharmacy, Auburn University, 1330J Walker Building, Auburn, AL 36849, USA; lah0036@auburn.edu
[2] Department of Health Outcomes Research and Policy, Harrison College of Pharmacy, Auburn University, 4306B Walker Building, Auburn, AL 36849, USA
* Correspondence: kbl0005@auburn.edu; Tel.: +1-334-844-8360

Abstract: The theory of planned behavior (TPB) states that behavioral intention is the best predictor of actual behavior change. However, intention explains only a portion of the variance in behavior. Of specific interest is the question of which moderating or mediating variables can be leveraged to aid health promotion interventions utilizing the tenets of behavioral economics (delay discounting and commitment contracts) in the intention–behavior pathway. Impulsivity has been postulated to fill this role and may be applied to multiple behaviors. We aim to determine if impulsivity moderates the association between intention and actual behavior in the TPB, to discover what other variables may moderate or mediate this association, and to apply the findings to future studies in the field of behavioral economics. To this end, a systematic review was conducted using the PubMed, PsychINFO, and Embase online databases. Eligible studies in peer-reviewed journals published prior to November 2021 were selected. Thirty-three studies were included in the final review, examining physical activity, diet, preventive health, mental health, addiction, and medication adherence behaviors. Three main concepts emerged: (1) impulsivity moderates the association between intention and behavior change; (2) self-efficacy moderates the association between intention and behavior change; and (3) planning and self-efficacy contribute to moderated mediation. This review demonstrates a gap in the literature regarding the application of the TPB to the intention–behavior pathway for health behaviors. Future studies in behavioral economics may leverage the variables of impulsivity, self-efficacy, and planning to predict follow-through in this area and to develop targeted change initiatives.

Keywords: theory of planned behavior; impulsivity; behavioral economics; health behaviors; systematic review; intention–behavior gap; health behavior theories

1. Introduction

The classic theory of planned behavior (TPB) states that behavioral intentions are the best predictors of actual behavior change [1–3]. Support for the traditional TPB is found throughout the literature, most often using cross-sectional surveys, pre-post surveys, or small timeseries [4–8]. The bulk of the research has been within the psychology of eating and drinking behavior, as well as physical and sexual activity, gambling, and smoking, where intention has been shown to mediate the association between behavioral perceptions and behavior change [5,6,9–13]. Variables of behavioral perception, including attitude towards behavior, subjective norms, and perceived behavioral control, have accounted for a range of 40 to 77% of the variance in subjects' intentions to change behavior [10,14–16]. Attitude towards behavior is defined as a positive or negative individual view of that behavior, while subjective norms are defined as views or behaviors that are generally accepted or expected in the community or by personally important individuals [14]. Similarly, perceived behavioral control is defined as an individual's belief regarding their ability to change a particular behavior [14]. Furthermore, behavioral intention has been shown to account for 15 to 39% of the variance in actual behavior change [9,15]. This fluctuation may be partially explained by variation in the topic of study (smoking, condom use, etc.) [10,15], but this does not answer the question of what accounts for the remaining variance in actual behavior change. Is intention to change behavior the only mediator between perceptions and behavior change, and is intention alone really a good predictor of behavior change? Is intention itself dependent on some other variable?

This question leads us to consider factors that may influence the relationship between intention to change behavior and actual behavior change. It seems likely that there is some additional variable that mediates (is in the causal pathway between intention and behavior change) or moderates (influences the direction and strength of the intention–behavior relationship) this process [17], especially as we take into consideration the concept of behavioral economics, which combines principles of economics and cognitive psychology and states that people do not always behave rationally [18]. Furthermore, based on the authors' previous research [19,20], it also seems likely that this intention–behavior pathway is moderated by a level of impulsivity, where impulsivity is a broad concept containing four general domains: urgency, lack of premeditation, sensation seeking, and lack of perseverance [21]. In the realm of behavioral economics, impulsivity is defined as the tendency to place a much higher value on immediate rewards compared to rewards received in the future and is commonly operationalized using various binary, choice-discounting tasks [22]. One might imagine that, even with a strong intention to change behavior, the powerful influence of impulsive choice (or difficulty delaying gratification) can undermine attempts at actual behavior change. One might intend to go to the gym regularly, but when tempted by the prospect of sleeping in or engaging in more pleasurable sedentary behaviors, that intention may not result in frequent gym attendance. Outside of the behavioral economics literature, impulsivity has also been found to moderate the relationship between eating traits and body mass index [23], as well as between negative life events and suicidal behavior [24]. Although impulsivity, thus, seems a likely culprit, the influences of other variables cannot be discounted.

Investigating moderators and mediators of the intention–behavior pathway is, thus, critical in informing future interventions to promote beneficial health behavior and improve health outcomes. With this belief in mind, we begin to pursue leads on potential mediators and moderators of the intention–behavior gap by conducting a short literature review across a wide variety of health behaviors with the goal of informing future studies in the field of behavioral economics.

2. Methods

A systematic literature review was performed using the PubMed, PsychINFO, and Embase online databases according to the Preferred Reporting Items for Systematic Reviews and Meta-Analyses (PRISMA) guidelines [25]. The searches were conducted in October 2021, and entries began broadly with "theory of planned behavior", then were progressively narrowed by adding or modifying terms, with search strings combined using the Boolean operator "OR". The search strings included "'Theory of planned behavior' and intention and behavior and (moderator or mediator)", "(Impulse or impulsiv*) and mediator and intention", "(Impulse or impulsiv*) and behavior and moderator and intention", "Intention and behavior and (Impulse or impulsiv*) AND 'theory of planned behavior'." The database hits were then combed through by title and abstract for the most relevant studies, with those mentioning novel mediators and moderators selected for full-text review. Google Scholar was also used with a "snowballing" method, in which additional papers were identified from manually searching the text and reference sections of papers selected from database hits.

Eligibility was determined by two reviewers (LAH and KBG) in an unblinded and standardized manner. The primary author (LH) conducted title and abstract reviews, followed by full-text reviews. Full-text reviews were then independently conducted by a second reviewer (KBG), and discrepancies were resolved via discourse and consensus.

Studies written in English and utilizing an experimental, quasi-experimental, or observational design in peer-reviewed journals published prior to November 2021 were included in this review. The variables sought included novel, participant-level moderators or mediators between intention and behavior change in the theory of planned behavior. In order to provide a foundation for future interventions across a variety of disciplines within behavioral economics, studies examining a broad range of health behaviors were eligible for this review. Studies were excluded if they were: unclear whether moderation or mediation was being tested (not explicitly stated by the authors or unable to distinguish by methods); not examining the theory of planned behavior; or not testing the moderation or mediation of variables between intention and a health behavior change. Moderating or mediating variables controlling for study procedures were not of interest. EndNote version X9 (ClarivateTM, Philadelphia, PA, USA) citation management software was used as a data organization tool and to assist with removal of duplicate articles.

The data were extracted by one investigator (LH) using a standardized template, including study design, intervention setting and population, study period, health behavior, measure scales used, statistical significance (yes or no), and risk of bias. Risk of bias (ROB) was assessed within each study using the mixed methods appraisal tool (MMAT) version 2018 [26]. This tool is suitable for a wide variety of study designs and consists of a 5-item measure of methodological quality (e.g., *"Is the sample representative of the target population?"*) rated as "Yes" (quality criteria are met), "No" (quality criteria are not met), or "Can't Tell" (not enough information to determine whether quality criteria are met). The quality scores were calculated based on the number of items rated "Yes", with a score of 0–1 being low quality (high risk of bias), 2–3 being moderate quality (moderate risk of bias), and 4–5 being high quality (low risk of bias) [27]. The findings were independently confirmed by a second reviewer (KBG), with discrepancies resolved via discourse and consensus. Due to the heterogeneous nature of behavioral intervention studies, the results were not pooled, nor were meta-analytic methods used. No registration was filed for this protocol.

3. Results

3.1. Database Hits

The initial search yielded 822 hits, with 698 after the removal of duplicates (Figure 1). After title and abstract review, 41 full-text articles were assessed for eligibility, and 33 studies met the inclusion criteria and were retained in the final review [16,21,28–58]. The majority of the studies utilized a noncontrolled timeseries or pre-post design, with follow-up periods ranging from 1 week to 6 months (Table 1). No significant conflicts of interest were noted amongst the studies, with the risks of bias rated as low (n = 22) or moderate (n = 11) (Figure 2a,b). The behaviors of interest included physical activity (n = 17), diet (n = 9), preventive health behaviors (e.g., condom use or sun protection; n = 7), addiction (n = 6), mental health (n = 3), and medication adherence (n = 1) (Table 2a). Most articles reported moderation analyses (n = 30), followed by mediation (n = 5), moderated mediation (n = 4), and moderated moderation (n = 3), with more than one type of analysis or variable of interest per study in some cases (Table 2b). The specific moderating and mediating variables surrounding the intention–behavior gap are presented below.

3.2. Moderators and Mediators with a High Level of Support

Sixteen articles assessing moderators and mediators of the intention–behavior gap contributed to a straightforward picture of variables' effects, with the majority of these studies (n = 12) reporting statistically significant findings and limited contradictory findings (Table 2c and Figure 3).

3.2.1. Impulsivity Moderates the Association between Intention and Behavior Change

Six studies showed that impulsivity moderates the relationship between behavioral intention and actual behavior change (Tables 1 and 2c, and Figure 3) [21,28–32]. These results spanned several disciplines, most notably substance misuse and addiction, diet, and physical activity. The common theme of these studies was that the intention to change behavior leads to an actual behavior change, but the magnitude of this change depends on the level of impulsivity in the individual. Specifically, Moshier and colleagues studied the effect of impulsivity on illicit drug use and found that premeditation and sensation seeking were moderator variables affecting the pathway between the intention to stop drug use and actual drug use in the previous month [21]. Similarly, Mullan et al. found that higher inhibitory control and planning ability, two elements implicit in the concept of impulsivity, resulted in less binge drinking in college students with the intention to drink [30], and Wang [32] found that lower problem-gambling severity (a proxy for impulsivity) led to less unintended sports-gambling behavior. This moderation was echoed by the findings of Churchill [28,29], who demonstrated greater decreases in unintended snacking [28] and increases in intended fruit and vegetable consumption [29] when urgency (or impulsivity) was lower. Furthermore, Pfeffer and colleagues [31] found that self-control moderated the path between intentions and physical activity, such that higher self-control resulted in increased physical activity in those intending to exercise.

Although the majority of the articles demonstrated support for impulsivity as a moderator, three studies assessed the moderating role of impulsivity in the intention–behavior gap but found no statistical significance [33–35]. Specifically, Chevance and colleagues' [33] investigation of physical activity, Crandall's [34] assessment of mindfulness mobile app usage, and Stevens' [35] evaluation of alcohol consumption did not demonstrate a significant association.

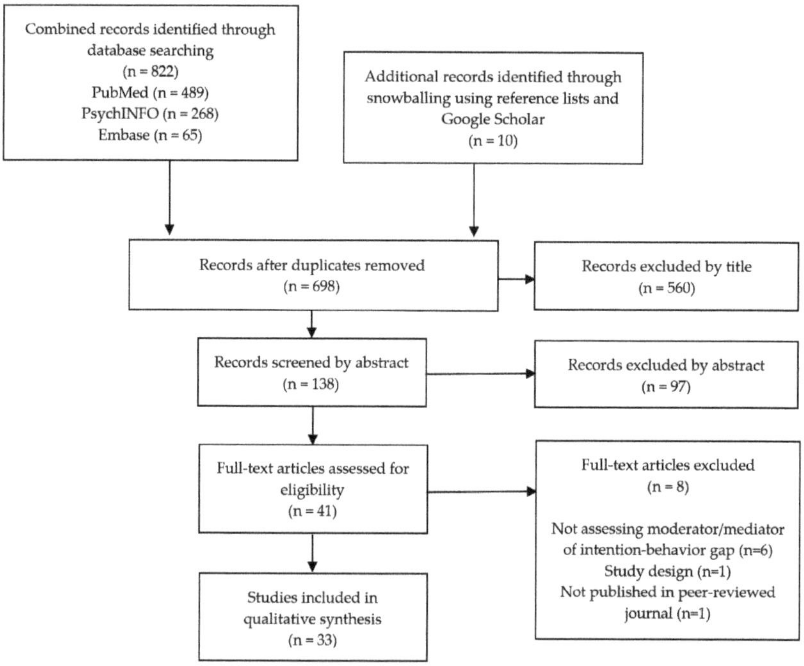

Figure 1. PRISMA Diagram. Database hits and stepwise inclusion or exclusion of studies.

Table 1. Final study characteristics.

Article Author, Year	Study Design	Intervention Population	Follow-Up Period	Behavior of Interest	Moderating or Mediating Variables (Scales)	Statistical Significance (p-Value)
Allom, 2016 [42]	Noncontrolled timeseries (pre-post)—T1, T2	n = 101 Australian college students Mean age: 19.60 yrs Female: 81.40%	1 week	Physical activity	Moderation • Habit strength (12-item Self-Report Habit Index)	No
Baumann, 2015 [57]	Noncontrolled timeseries (pre-post)—T1, T2	n = 433 German adult job agency clients Mean age: 30.6 yrs Female: 36%	3 months	At-risk alcohol use	Moderation • Belief incongruence ○ Normative belief incongruence (4-item measure) ○ Behavioral belief incongruence (6-item measure) ○ Control belief incongruence (4-item measure)	 Yes (<0.05) No No
Cao, 2021 [49]	Noncontrolled timeseries (pre-post)—T1, T2	n = 591 Chinese college students Mean age: not reported (range 19–24 yrs) Female: 57.53%; and n = 285 Chinese adult wage earners Mean age: not reported (range 27–58 yrs) Female: 44.56%	1 week	Physical activity	Moderation • Mental toughness (8-item Mental Toughness Inventory (MTI)) ○ Among college students ○ Among wage earners	 Yes (<0.01) No
Chevance, 2018 [33]	Noncontrolled timeseries (pre-post)—T1, T2	n = 76 French adults Mean age: 56 yrs Female: not reported	4 months	Physical activity	Moderation • Trait impulsivity (20-item UPPS-P Impulsive Behavior Scale) ○ Lack of conscientiousness • Executive functions (Computerized Wisconsin Card-Sorting Test)	 No No No
Churchill, 2010 [28]	Noncontrolled timeseries (pre-post)—T1, T2	n = 256 UK adults Mean age: 33.05 yrs Female: 79.36%	2 weeks	Avoidance of snacking	Moderation • Impulsivity at T2 (45-item UPPS Impulsive Behavior Scale) ○ Urgency ○ Lack of premeditation ○ Lack of perseverance ○ Sensation seeking	 Yes (<0.05) No No No
Churchill, 2011 [29]	Controlled timeseries—T1, T2, T3	n = 323 UK adults Mean age: 32.8 yrs Female: 81.42% Students: 52.94%	2 weeks (1-week intervals)	Fruit and vegetable consumption	Moderation • Impulsivity at T1 (45-item UPPS Impulsive Behavior Scale) ○ Urgency ○ Lack of premeditation ○ Lack of perseverance ○ Sensation seeking	 Yes (<0.05) No No No
Crandall, 2019 [34]	Noncontrolled timeseries (pre-post)—T1, T2	n = 85 Undergraduate college students in Utah, US Mean age: 21.81 yrs Female: 53%	2 weeks	Mindfulness meditation mobile app use	Moderation • Executive functioning (three tasks from the NIH Toolbox (NIH-TB) ○ Cognitive shifting (NIH-TB Dimensional Change Card-Sort Test) ○ Inhibitory control and attention (NIH-TB Flanker Inhibitory Control and Attention Test) ○ Working memory (NIH-TB List-Sorting Working Memory Test)	 No No No No

Table 1. *Cont.*

Article Author, Year	Study Design	Intervention Population	Follow-Up Period	Behavior of Interest	Moderating or Mediating Variables (Scales)	Statistical Significance (p-Value)
De Bruijn, 2009 [46]	Cross-sectional interviewer-administered survey	$n = 405$ Dutch adults Mean age: 60.25 yrs Female: 57.53%	No follow-up	Fruit consumption	Moderation • Five-Factor Model of Personality (FFM) ○ Neuroticism (6-item measure) ○ Conscientiousness (6-item measure)	 Yes (<0.001) No
Gaum, 2019 [56]	Cross-sectional survey	$n = 112$ German adults with history of depression Mean age: 42.3 yrs Female: 75%	No follow-up	Implementation of depression prevention strategies at work	Moderation • Anticipated stigmatization (2-item German Inventory of Subjective Stigma Experience) • Experienced stigmatization (2-item German Inventory of Subjective Stigma Experience)	 Yes (0.003) No
Gibson, 2021 [53]	Noncontrolled timeseries (pre-post)—T1, T2	$n = 507$ US adults Mean age: 50.39 yrs Female: 50.9%	3 months	Social distancing during COVID-19	Moderation • Age • Race • Intention stability over time	 Yes (<0.001) Yes (0.002) Yes (<0.001)
Gourlan, 2019 [58]	Noncontrolled timeseries (pre-post)—T1, T2	$n = 219$ French adults Mean age: 41.28 Female: 52.51%	3 months	Physical activity	Moderation • Planning (5-item French Action-Planning Scale) • Perceived built environment (3-item measure) Moderated Moderation • Planning*Environment	 No No Yes (0.02)
Gucciardi, 2016 [45]	Noncontrolled timeseries (pre-post)—T1, T2	$n = 193$ Australian adults Mean age: 30.79 yrs Female: 55.44%	2 weeks	Rehabilitation exercises for knee pain	Moderation • Mental toughness (8-item index)	 Yes (0.013)
Hannan, 2015 [50]	Noncontrolled timeseries (pre-post)—T1, T2	$n = 117$ Australian adults and undergraduate students Mean age: 28.29 yrs Female: 73.50%	1 week	Physical activity	Moderation • Mental toughness (8-item Mental Toughness Index (MTI))	 No
Hartson, 2020 [51]	Noncontrolled timeseries (pre-post)—T1, T2	$n = 232$ US Hispanic adolescents Mean age: 15.23 yrs Female: 51.3%	2 weeks	Physical activity	Moderation • Mindfulness (10-item Child and Adolescent Mindfulness Measure)	 No
Koring, 2012 [37]	Noncontrolled timeseries—T1, T2, T3	$n = 290$ German adults Mean age: 41.9 yrs Female: 77%	6 weeks	Physical activity	Moderation • Self-efficacy (2-item measure) Mediation • Planning (2-item measure) Moderated Mediation • Planning*Self-efficacy	 Yes (<0.05) Yes (<0.05) Yes (<0.05)

Table 1. *Cont.*

Article Author, Year	Study Design	Intervention Population	Follow-Up Period	Behavior of Interest	Moderating or Mediating Variables (Scales)	Statistical Significance (*p*-Value)
Kothe, 2015 [40]	Cross-sectional survey	*n* = 228 Australian adults with Celiac disease Mean age: 45.2 yrs Female: 89.5%	No follow-up	Gluten-free diet adherence	Moderation • Perceived behavioral control (PBC) (17-item TPB Celiac Disease Questionnaire) • Habit (12-item Self-Reported Habit Index) Moderated Moderation • PBC*Habit	No Yes (0.013) Yes (<0.001)
Lange, 2018 [55]	Study I. Noncontrolled timeseries—T1, T2, T3	*n* = 461 German adults Mean age: 38.2 yrs Female: 81.6%	4 months	Fruit and vegetable intake	Moderated Mediation • Planning*Sex (3-item planning measure)	Yes (0.040)
	Study II. Noncontrolled timeseries—T1, T2, T3	*n* = 193 German university students Mean age: 24.5 yrs Female: 80.8%	2 weeks	Physical activity	• Planning*Sex (4-item planning measure)	Yes (0.022)
	Study III. Noncontrolled timeseries (pre-post)—T1, T2	*n* = 166 German adults Mean age: 37.6 yrs Female: 49.3%	2 weeks	Sun protection	• Planning*Sex (2-item planning measure)	Yes (0.014)
Lin, 2018 [43]	Noncontrolled timeseries (pre-post)—T1, T2	*n* = 535 Iranian women with high-risk pregnancies Mean age: 32.29 yrs Female: 100%	8 weeks	Medication adherence (aspirin)	Mediation • Planning ○ Action planning (4-item measure) ○ Coping planning (5-item measure)	Yes (<0.01) Yes (<0.01)
Lippke, 2009 [38]	Noncontrolled timeseries (pre-post)—T1, T2	*n* = 812 German adults Mean age: 36.69 yrs Female: 74.4%	4 weeks	Physical activity	Moderation • Self-efficacy (3-item measure) Mediation • Action planning (3-item measure) Moderated Mediation • Action planning*Self-efficacy	Yes (<0.01) Yes (<0.01) Yes (<0.01)
Luszczynska, 2010 [16]	Study I. Noncontrolled timeseries (pre-post)—T1, T2	*n* = 534 Chinese adolescents, grades 7–12 Mean age: 13.8 yrs Female: 54%	4 weeks	Physical activity	Moderation • Self-efficacy (3-item scale) Mediation • Coping planning (4-item measure) Moderated Mediation • Coping planning*Self-efficacy	Yes (<0.01) Yes (<0.01) Yes (<0.01)

Table 1. *Cont.*

Article Author, Year	Study Design	Intervention Population	Follow-Up Period	Behavior of Interest	Moderating or Mediating Variables (Scales)	Statistical Significance (*p*-Value)
	Study II. Noncontrolled timeseries (pre-post)—T1, T2	*n* = 620 Polish high school adolescents Mean age: 16.46 yrs Female: 62%	10 weeks	Physical activity	Moderation • Maintenance of self-efficacy (7-item measure developed via elicitation study) Mediation • Action planning (5-item measure) Moderated Mediation • Action planning*Self-efficacy	 Yes (<0.05) Yes (<0.05) Yes (<0.05)
MacCann, 2015 [47]	Cross-sectional survey	*n* = 1017 US college students Mean age: 23.1 yrs Female: 63.9%	No follow-up	Physical activity	Moderation • Personality (6 HEXACO personality domains measured via 96-item International Personality Item Pool (IPIP)) ○ Honesty and humility (16 items) ○ Emotionality (16 items) ○ Extraversion (16 items) ○ Agreeableness (16 items) ○ Conscientiousness (16 items) ○ Openness to Experience (16 items)	 No No No No No No
Monds, 2016 [48]	Cross-sectional survey	*n* = 1036 US college students Mean age: 23.08 yrs Female: 63.9%	No follow-up	Fruit and vegetable consumption	Moderation • Personality (6 HEXACO personality domains measured via 96-item International Personality Item Pool (IPIP)) ○ Honesty and humility (16 items) ○ Emotionality (16 items) ○ Extraversion (16 items) ○ Agreeableness (16 items) ○ Conscientiousness (16 items) ○ Openness to Experience (16 items)	 No No No No No No
Moshier, 2013 [21]	Cross-sectional survey	*n* = 84 Adults receiving methadone maintenance treatment from 2 outpatient clinics in Boston, US Mean age: 40 yrs Female: 56%	No follow-up	Illicit drug use	Moderation • Impulsivity (44-item UPPS Impulsivity Scale) ○ Urgency ○ Lack of premeditation ○ Lack of perseverance ○ Sensation seeking	 No Yes (0.015) No Yes (0.007)
Mullan, 2011 [30]	Noncontrolled timeseries (pre-post)—T1, T2	*n* = 153 Australian university students Mean age: 20.1 yrs Female: 73.86%	1 week	Binge drinking of alcohol	Moderation • Impulsivity and Self-Regulation (Executive Function measures) ○ Planning ability (the Tower of Hanoi task) ○ Inhibitory control (the Stroop Task) ○ Decision making (the Iowa Gambling Task) ○ Cognitive flexibility (the Wisconsin Card-Sorting Task)	 Yes (0.03) Yes (0.035) No No

Table 1. *Cont.*

Article Author, Year	Study Design	Intervention Population	Follow-Up Period	Behavior of Interest	Moderating or Mediating Variables (Scales)	Statistical Significance (p-Value)
Packel, 2015 [44]	Cross-sectional survey	$n = 96$ Adults with colorectal cancer in Pennsylvania, US Mean age: 65.6 yrs Female: % not reported	No follow-up	Physical activity	Mediation • Planning ○ Action planning (4-item Action-Planning and Coping-Planning Scale—Physical Exercise) ○ Coping planning (5-item Action-Planning and Coping-Planning Scale—Physical Exercise)	 Yes (0.007) Yes (0.001)
Pfeffer, 2020 [31]	Noncontrolled timeseries (pre-post)—T1, T2	$n = 118$ University students Mean age: 24.74 yrs Female: 70.3%	4 weeks	Physical activity	Moderation • Trait self-control (13-item Brief Self-Control Scale)	 Yes (0.033)
Rhodes, 2021 [52]	2-arm parallel randomized trial (groups collapsed)—T1, T2, T3, T4	$n = 254$ Canadian adults who were new parents Mean age: 31.94 yrs Female: 50%	Baseline, 6 weeks, 12 weeks, 6 months	Physical activity	Moderation • Gender Moderated Moderation • Gender*Action control (M-PAC model) ○ Gender*Affective attitude ○ Gender*Perceived opportunity ○ Gender*Planning ○ Gender*Habit ○ Gender*Identity	 Yes (<0.01) No Yes (<0.05) No No No
Schutz, 2011 [36]	Noncontrolled timeseries (pre-post)—T1, T2	$n = 237$ HIV-positive men who have sex with men in Montreal, Canada Mean age: 42.5 yrs	6 months	Condom use	Moderation • Self-efficacy (11-item interview measure) • Perceived behavioral control (3-item interview measure) • Past behavior (3-item interview measure) • Moral norm (3-item interview measure) • Anticipated regret (3-item interview measure) • Role beliefs (3-item interview measure) • Sociodemographics • Context • Life experience	 Yes [a] No No No No No No No No
Schüz, 2020 [54]	Study I. Cross-sectional survey	$n = 1005$ US adults Mean age: 33.6 yrs Female: 47.1%	No follow-up	1. Fruit and vegetable consumption 2. Physical activity 3. Low-fat diet 4. Alcohol consumption 5. Flossing daily 6. Testicular or breast self-exams	Moderation • Socioeconomic status (SES) ○ Education level (categorical multiple choice based on the US Census Current Population Survey and International Standard Classification of Education (ISCED)) ○ Income (categorical multiple choice) ○ Occupation status (percentage unemployment level matched to zip code based on American Community Survey; area-level SES measure) ○ Zip code (text entry; area-level SES measure) ○ Subjective SES (10-point ladder subjective SES scale)	 Yes (<0.05) No No No No

Table 1. *Cont.*

Article Author, Year	Study Design	Intervention Population	Follow-Up Period	Behavior of Interest	Moderating or Mediating Variables (Scales)	Statistical Significance (*p*-Value)
	Study II. Noncontrolled timeseries (pre-post)—T1, T2	*n* = 1273 International adults Mean age: 31.57 yrs Female: 50.5%	4 weeks	1. Fruit and vegetable consumption 2. Physical activity 3. Alcohol consumption 4. Flossing daily 5. Not sitting for extended periods 6. Healthy snack consumption	Moderation • Socioeconomic status (SES) ○ Education level (categorical multiple choice based on the US Census Current Population Survey and International Standard Classification of Education (ISCED)) ○ Income (categorical multiple choice) ○ Occupation status (personal employment) ○ Subjective SES (10-point ladder subjective SES scale)	 Yes (<0.01) No No Yes (<0.05)
Stevens, 2017 [35]	Noncontrolled timeseries (pre-post)—T1, T2	*n* = 77 US young adults Mean age: 20.8 yrs Female: 60.5%	10 days	Alcohol consumption	Moderation • Impulsivity ○ Lack of planning (59-item UPPS-P Impulsive Behavior Scale) ○ Lack of perseverance (59-item UPPS-P) ○ Negative urgency (59-item UPPS-P) ○ Positive urgency (59-item UPPS-P) ○ Sensation seeking (59-item UPPS-P) ○ Response inhibition (Go-Stop Impulsivity Paradigm) ○ Response initiation (Immediate memory Task (IMT)) ○ Delay discounting (27-item Monetary Choice Questionnaire (MCQ) and Two-Choice Impulsivity Paradigm (TCIP))	 No No No No No No No No
Wang, 2021 [32]	Cross-sectional survey	*n* = 334 US college students. Mean age: 21 yrs Female: 32.3%	No follow-up	Sports gambling	Moderation • Problem-gambling severity (4-item scale)	 Yes (0.003)
Zhang C.Q., 2020 [41]	Noncontrolled timeseries—T1, T2, T3	*n* = 297 College students in China Mean age: not reported (range: 18-35 yrs) Female: 82.49%	2 months	Hand washing and sleep hygiene	Moderation (intention—hand washing) • Action planning (3-item scale) • Coping planning (3-item scale) • Action self-efficacy (3-item scale) • Maintenance self-efficacy (3-item scale) Moderation (intention—sleep hygiene) • Action planning (3-item scale) • Coping planning (3-item scale) • Action self-efficacy (3-item scale) • Maintenance self-efficacy (3-item scale)	 Yes (<0.001) No No No No No No No
Zhang R., 2019 [39]	Noncontrolled timeseries (pre-post)—T1, T2	*n* = 157 Office employees in China Mean age: 33.26 yrs Female: 64.97%	1 month	Transport-related walking	Moderation • Worksite neighborhood walkability index (abbreviated Neighborhood Environment Walkability Scale (Chinese NEWS-A))	 No

[a] *p*-value not reported. * Variables interact within moderated mediation or moderated moderation analyses.

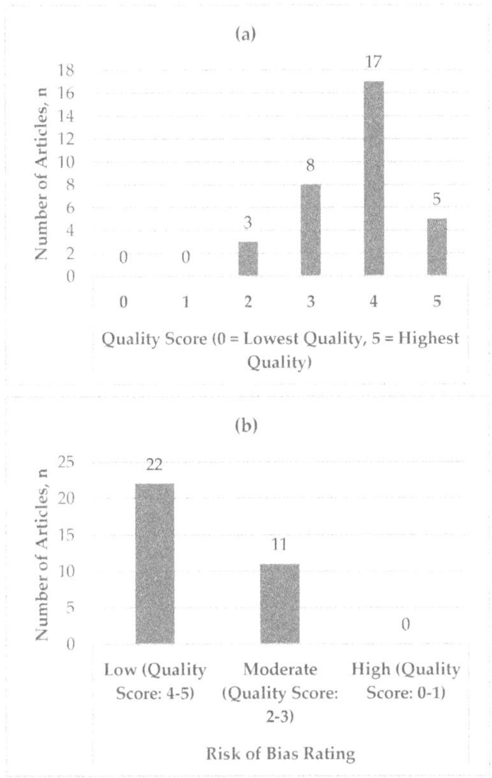

Figure 2. (**a**,**b**) Risk of bias assessment using mixed methods appraisal tool (MMAT): (**a**) frequency of article quality scores in risk of bias assessment (n = 33) and (**b**) frequency of article risk of bias ratings (n = 33).

Table 2. (**a**) Number of articles describing a particular behavior, (**b**) number of articles describing moderation or mediation analyses within the intention–behavior gap, and (**c**) number of articles describing a particular moderator or mediator within the intention–behavior gap.

(a)		
Behavior Category	**Specific Behaviors Included in Category**	n
Physical Activity	General physical activity, transport-related walking, and knee pain rehabilitation exercises	17
Diet	Fruit and vegetable consumption, snacking, low-fat diet, and gluten-free diet	9
Preventive Health Behaviors	Flossing, hand washing, social distancing, limited sitting, condom use, breast or testicular self-exam, and sun protection	7
Addiction	Alcohol use, illicit drug use, and sports gambling	6
Mental Health	Mindfulness meditation app, depression prevention strategies, and sleep hygiene	3
Medication Adherence	Aspirin adherence	1

Table 2. *Cont.*

(b)

Type of Analysis	*n*		
	Statistically Significant	**Not Statistically Significant**	**Total**
Moderation	19	11	30
Mediation	5	0	5
Moderated Mediation	4	0	4
Moderated Moderation	3	0	3

(c)

Moderator or Mediator Category	Moderator and Mediator Variables	*n*		
		Statistically Significant	**Not Statistically Significant**	**Total**
More Support	Impulsivity Moderation	6	3	9
	Self-Efficacy Moderation	4	1	5
	Planning Mediation	5	0	5
	Planning*Self-Efficacy-Moderated Mediation	3	0	3
Less Support	Personality Moderation	2	5	7
	Socioeconomics Moderation	4	0	4
	Perceptions and Beliefs Moderation	2	0	2
	Environment Moderation	1	1	2
	Habit Moderation	1	1	2

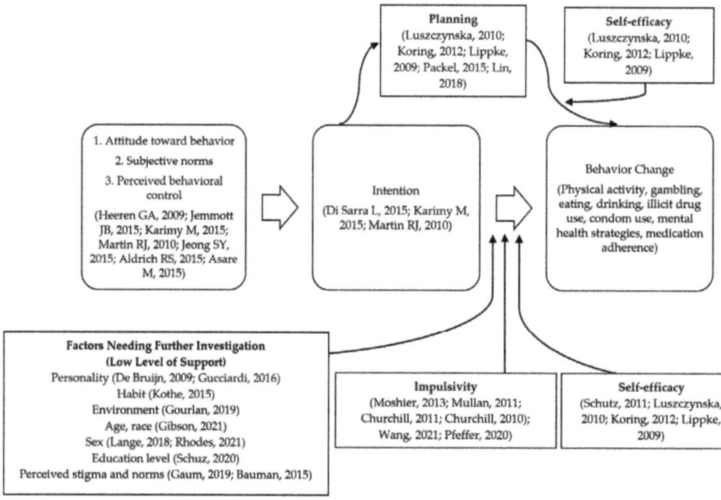

Figure 3. Summary of statistically significant literature review findings as applied to an extended view of the theory of planned behavior [5,6,9–12,14–16,21,29–32,36–40,43–45,52–54,57].

3.2.2. Self-Efficacy Moderates the Association between Intention and Behavior Change

Moderation was not only shown to occur via impulsivity, but self-efficacy demonstrated a moderation effect as well ($n = 4$; Tables 1 and 2c, and Figure 3) [16,36–38]. Schutz and colleagues showed that HIV-positive men who have sex with men were approximately 21 times more likely to act on their intentions to use condoms when they had higher self-efficacy [36]. Self-efficacy was defined in this case as the perceived ability to surmount barriers that impede the fulfillment of a particular behavior [36,59]. In this way, self-efficacy is related to the concept of perceived behavioral control, or one's belief in the ability to affect change in a particular behavior [14,60]. Similarly, Koring [37], Lippke [38], and Luszczynska [16] all found that intentions to be physically active were put into practice more often in those with higher versus lower self-efficacy. On the other hand, C.Q. Zhang and colleagues [41] assessed the moderating roles of action self-efficacy (perceived ability to start a behavior) and maintenance self-efficacy (perceived ability to continue a behavior in the face of barriers) [61] on hand-washing and sleep hygiene behaviors, but no statistically significant moderating effects were found. Further pursuit of this thread led to a more complex view of self-efficacy as a part of moderated mediation in the context of an additional variable: planning.

3.2.3. Planning Mediates the Association between Intention and Behavior Change

Five studies demonstrated a statistically significant mediating effect of planning in the intention–behavior pathway (Tables 1 and 2c, and Figure 3) [16,37,38,43,44]. Four of these studies focused on behaviors related to physical activity [16,37,38,44]. Koring [37], Luszczynska [16], Lippke [38], and Packel [44] found that the intention to exercise translated into actual physical activity indirectly via planning. While Koring [37] assessed planning in general, other studies have broken planning down into its constituent parts of action planning (making plans to act on intentions) and coping planning (making plans to overcome expected barriers) [61]. Specifically, Luszczynska [16] and Packel [44] found that both action planning and coping planning filled this mediating role, while Lippke [38] found statistical significance for action planning alone. In terms of behaviors other than physical activity, Lin and colleagues [43] found that the intention to adhere to a medication influenced actual medication adherence (to aspirin) indirectly via both action planning and coping planning. However, when planning was viewed in combination with self-efficacy, a more complicated picture of moderated mediation emerged.

3.2.4. Planning and Self-Efficacy Contribute to Moderated Mediation

Moderated mediation between intentions and behavior change was demonstrated via planning and self-efficacy in several studies (n = 3; Tables 1 and 2c, and Figure 3) [16,37,38]. Moderated mediation occurs when a variable mediates the relationship between the behavioral intention and the behavior change, and an additional variable acts as the moderator of this process. Koring [37], Luszczynska [16], and Lippke [38] and colleagues independently found that planning mediated the pathway from intentions to actual changes in physical activity. Individuals' levels of self-efficacy moderated this relationship; in other words, higher self-efficacy increased the likelihood of plans being realized as actual changes in physical activity behavior [16,37,38]. This was a more complicated process than noted by Schutz's [36], Lin [43], and Packel [44] and opened the consideration of additional moderators and mediators within the theory of planned behavior and the intention–behavior gap, specifically.

3.3. *Moderators and Mediators with Less Support*

Seventeen articles reported moderators and mediators of the intention–behavior gap that were less clear, with fewer statistically significant findings (n = 10) or mixed findings, which warrant additional investigation in future studies (Table 2c and Figure 3).

3.3.1. Personality Moderates the Association between Intention and Behavior Change

Of seven studies assessing personality traits as moderators in the intention–behavior pathway, two studies found statistically significant moderators [45,46], while five studies did not [47–51] (Tables 1 and 2c, and Figure 3). De Bruijn et al. [46] assessed neuroticism and conscientiousness, which are two traits from the Five-Factor Model of Personality (FFM), and found that neuroticism moderated the intention–fruit consumption gap, such that lower neuroticism led to a stronger relationship between intention and behavior. Additionally, Gucciardi [45] found mental toughness to be a statistically significant moderator, resulting in increased translation of exercise intentions into actual exercise performance. On the other hand, MacCann [47] and Monds [48] assessed the moderating effect of the HEXACO personality domains (honesty and humility, emotionality, extraversion, agreeableness, conscientiousness, and openness to experience) on the intention–physical activity and intention–fruit and vegetable consumption pathways, respectively, and found no statistically significant moderators. Similarly, Hannan [50] and Hartson [51] found no moderating roles for mental toughness or mindfulness, respectively, between intention and physical activity, while Cao [49] found that mental toughness served as a moderator in the intention–physical activity gap in Chinese college students but not in adult wage earners.

3.3.2. Socioeconomic Factors Moderate the Association between Intention and Behavior Change

Four studies assessed moderation by socioeconomic factors ($n = 4$ statistically significant), with a wide variety of factors assessed, including age, race, sex, and education level (Tables 1 and 2c, and Figure 3) [52–55]. Gibson [53] found that age and race moderated between the intention to social distance and actual social distancing behavior during the COVID-19 pandemic, such that intentions were translated into practice more often in older adults and those identifying as White. Additionally, Schuz [54] found that a higher education level resulted in a greater influence of intention on multiple different behaviors, including fruit and vegetable consumption, physical activity, alcohol consumption, flossing, healthy snack consumption, limiting the amount of time spent sitting daily, low-fat diet, and breast or testicular self-exams. Lange and colleagues [55] examined the role of sex in a moderated mediation model and found that sex moderated the effect of planning in the intention–behavior gap in cases of fruit and vegetable consumption, physical activity, and sun protection behaviors, with planning mediating the intention–behavior pathway for men but not women. On the other hand, Rhodes [52] found a moderating effect of sex within the intention–physical activity pathway, such that intention was successfully translated into physical activity for women but not men. However, when the perceived opportunity for exercise was added to the model, physical activity intentions were successfully realized for men more than women (moderated moderation). With the limited number of studies focused on each socioeconomic factor, it was difficult to draw conclusions about any particular factor.

3.3.3. Perceptions and Beliefs Regarding Stigma and Norms Moderate the Association between Intention and Behavior Change

Two studies found particular perceptions or beliefs that moderated the intention–behavior gap (Tables 1 and 2c, and Figure 3) [56,57]. Specifically, Gaum and colleagues [56] found that lower anticipated stigma resulted in the increased implementation of depression prevention strategies in the workplace. Likewise, Bauman [57] demonstrated that those with higher normative belief incongruence (changes in normative beliefs over time) were more likely to consume alcohol despite the opposite intention. However, multiple studies assessing perceived stigma or belief incongruence are necessary in order to come to a more firm conclusion regarding their roles as moderators.

3.3.4. Environment Moderates the Association between Intention and Behavior Change

The evidence was mixed concerning the moderating effect of environment on the intention–behavior gap, with one study finding a statistically significant effect [58] and one study finding no effect [39] (Tables 1 and 2c, and Figure 3). Gourlan and colleagues [58] found that built environment, when combined with planning, contributed to moderated moderation of the intention–physical activity gap, such that those with a greater level of planning and living closer to exercise facilities were more likely to follow through with intentions to exercise. However, R. Zhang [39] found that perceived worksite neighborhood walkability had no moderating role between the intention to walk and actual physical activity.

3.3.5. Habit Moderates the Association between Intention and Behavior Change

Evidence was also mixed for the moderating role of habit (Tables 1 and 2c, and Figure 3) [40,42]. Specifically, Kothe [40] found that self-reported habit strength increased follow-through on the intention to adhere to a gluten-free diet. On the other hand, Allom et al. [42] found that habit strength did not serve to moderate the intention–physical activity gap.

4. Discussion

The bulk of our findings regarding additional variables in an extended version of the theory of planned behavior suggested the moderation of the intention–behavior pathway by impulsivity [21,28–31] or self-efficacy [16,36–38], mediation by planning [16,37,38,43,44], and some evidence for moderated mediation via planning and self-efficacy [16,37,38]. However, the evidence for moderation by other personality and demographic traits, such as neuroticism, age, and gender, was sparse [46,48,53], with a lack of consistent measurement instruments or definitions for personality traits. Furthermore, there was a paucity of research investigating habit, built environment, and stigmatizing and normative beliefs within the intention–behavior gap, as well as research evaluating the interactions of these variables with impulsivity. These findings align with previous systematic reviews focused solely on physical activity and sun protection behaviors, which have found some evidence for the moderation of the intention–behavior gap by self-efficacy but have shown mixed evidence for sociodemographic variables [62,63]. Future studies assessing the moderators and mediators between intention and behavior should focus on the aforementioned variables, which have a current low level of support in the literature.

When taken as a whole, these studies showed the broad application of the theory of planned behavior throughout various disciplines. Studies investigating physical activity and dietary behaviors were most prominent, as well as substance misuse, mental health, condom use, and other preventive health behaviors. However, using our protocol and inclusion criteria, only one study was found that addressed patient medication adherence. One can imagine that medication-taking behavior is highly related to the level of impulsivity, given that many medications for chronic diseases have immediate costs, including adverse effects, while the benefits of taking them are often not apparent until sometime in the future. Indeed, studies have shown that certain character traits, including impulsivity, predict low medication adherence [64]. However, patient medication adherence remains low despite educational interventions targeting patients and providers [65]. Thus, this is a critical area for future study.

4.1. Implications

This review has implications for future studies in the field of behavioral economics and health outcomes. The concepts of impulsivity and planning are especially relevant to this field, as the theoretical framework of the discipline relies on these individual characteristics. Commitment contracts (financial or social incentives to perform a behavior to which individuals agree ahead of time) in behavioral economics are particularly relevant to the role of planning as a mediational variable. Studies have shown that the use of financial commitment contracts, where participants' previously deposited money is deducted for not meeting a behavioral goal, are able to overcome high levels of impulsivity to increase follow-through in the desired behavior [66]. Reward substitution, or the provision of short-term financial or social incentives to avoid engaging in an undesirable behavior, has also been used successfully to overcome difficulty in delaying gratification [67]. Future studies may include pre-post or small timeseries surveys examining the role of impulsivity as a moderator between patient intentions and health behaviors. Follow-up studies may use commitment contracts, incentives, or decision aids as a means to investigate behavior follow-through in highly impulsive participants. Further investigation also needs to be conducted on the effects of age and gender in the intention–behavior pathway; if effects are found, this may be significant for the development of targeted and tailored health behavior tools or interventions. The pursuit of such studies can help to fill the knowledge gap demonstrated by this review and may have implications for patient and prescriber incentives in the increasingly outcome-oriented United States healthcare system.

4.2. Limitations

Although this systematic review was performed following the PRISMA guidelines [25], the results must be interpreted with caution in light of several limitations. First, the majority of the studies exploring this topic utilized cross-sectional, pre-post, or small timeseries designs with no more than 6 months of follow up, which may not be sufficient time to effect or maintain a behavioral change, limiting the validity of the findings. However, given the psychological nature of many of these studies, these designs were the most ethical and feasible.

Second, the heterogeneity of the study designs and behaviors studied limited the ability to pool the findings. This precludes the use of meta-analytic methods. However, the findings may still be clinically valuable and informative for behavioral interventions.

Third, studies using the theory of reasoned action (TRA) were not included in this review. The TRA is closely related to the TBP, but the TPB includes one additional construct-perceived behavioral control. In order to focus the review effort, only studies examining the TPB were included; however, the inclusion of "TRA" in the search parameters may have yielded additional studies in other areas of health behavior. This may be included in future studies. However, a preliminary search did not yield appreciably different results.

Fourth, varying definitions and measurements of impulsivity were found amongst the studies. Where the definitions were unclear, the reviewers' judgement was used; however, this may limit the replicability of the search. Furthermore, planning was found to be a mediational variable in several studies, yet planning may also be related to the concept of impulsivity or self-regulation [30], making this association unclear. Additionally, in some cases, it was difficult to determine whether moderation or mediation was being tested if it was not explicitly stated by the authors.

5. Conclusions

The bulk of the evidence from this review pointed to impulsivity as a moderator between intention and behavior change, with a possible moderating role of self-efficacy. Furthermore, planning, which has been defined in several studies as a composite of both action planning and coping planning [68,69], may play a mediational role between behavioral intention and actual behavior change. However, despite the breadth of the application in topics of psychology, this review demonstrated a gap in the literature regarding the study of moderators and mediators in the theory of planned behavior as it applies to behavioral economics and health outcomes. Future studies assessing moderators and mediators between intentions and health behavior should focus on personality, habit, built environment, stigmatizing and normative beliefs, and sociodemographic variables, which have a current low level of support in the literature.

Author Contributions: Conceptualization, L.A.H. and K.B.G.; Methodology, L.A.H. and K.B.G.; Validation, L.A.H. and K.B.G.; Investigation, L.A.H.; Formal Analysis, L.A.H.; Data Interpretation, L.A.H. and K.B.G.; Data Curation, L.A.H.; Writing—Original Draft Preparation, L.A.H..; Writing—Review and Editing, L.A.H. and K.B.G.; Visualization, L.A.H.; Supervision, K.B.G.; Project Administration, L.A.H. and K.B.G. All authors have read and agreed to the published version of the manuscript.

Funding: This research received no external funding.

Institutional Review Board Statement: Not applicable.

Informed Consent Statement: Not applicable.

Data Availability Statement: Not applicable.

Conflicts of Interest: The authors declare no conflict of interest.

References

1. Ajzen, I. Theories of Cognitive Self-Regulation, the Theory of Planned Behavior. *Organ. Behav. Hum. Decis. Processes* **1991**, *50*, 179–211. [CrossRef]
2. Conner, M.; Armitage, C.J. Extending the theory of planned behavior: A review and avenues for further research. *J. Appl. Soc. Psychol.* **1998**, *28*, 1429–1464. [CrossRef]
3. Ajzen, I. The theory of planned behavior: Frequently asked questions. *Hum. Behav. Emerg. Technol.* **2020**, *2*, 314–324. [CrossRef]
4. Pearson, M.R.; Henson, J.M. Unplanned drinking and alcohol-related problems: A preliminary test of the model of unplanned drinking behavior. *Psychol. Addict. Behav.* **2013**, *27*, 584–595. [CrossRef] [PubMed]
5. Heeren, G.A.; Jemmott, J.B., 3rd; Mandeya, A.; Tyler, J.C. Sub-Saharan African university students' beliefs about condoms, condom-use intention, and subsequent condom use: A prospective study. *AIDS Behav.* **2009**, *13*, 268–276. [CrossRef] [PubMed]
6. Jemmott, J.B., 3rd; Stephens-Shields, A.; O'Leary, A.; Jemmott, L.S.; Teitelman, A.; Ngwane, Z.; Mtose, X. Mediation of effects of a theory-based behavioral intervention on self-reported physical activity in South African men. *Prev. Med.* **2015**, *72*, 1–7. [CrossRef] [PubMed]
7. Reyes Fernandez, B.; Warner, L.M.; Knoll, N.; Montenegro Montenegro, E.; Schwarzer, R. Synergistic effects of social support and self-efficacy on dietary motivation predicting fruit and vegetable intake. *Appetite* **2015**, *87*, 330–335. [CrossRef]
8. McDermott, M.S.; Oliver, M.; Simnadis, T.; Beck, E.J.; Coltman, T.; Iverson, D.; Caputi, P.; Sharma, R. The Theory of Planned Behaviour and dietary patterns: A systematic review and meta-analysis. *Prev. Med.* **2015**, *81*, 150–156. [CrossRef]
9. Di Sarra, L.; Ghezzi, V.; Eastland, T.Y.; Antonini, F.; Scialo, G.; Zega, M.; Alvaro, R. Applying the Theory of Planned Behavior to Explain Women's Role in Prostate Cancer Screening. *Res. Theory Nurs. Pract.* **2015**, *29*, 200–213. [CrossRef]
10. Karimy, M.; Zareban, I.; Araban, M.; Montazeri, A. An Extended Theory of Planned Behavior (TPB) Used to Predict Smoking Behavior Among a Sample of Iranian Medical Students. *Int. J. High Risk Behav. Addict.* **2015**, *4*, e24715. [CrossRef]
11. Martin, R.J.; Usdan, S.; Nelson, S.; Umstattd, M.R.; Laplante, D.; Perko, M.; Shaffer, H. Using the theory of planned behavior to predict gambling behavior. *Psychol. Addict. Behav.* **2010**, *24*, 89–97. [CrossRef] [PubMed]
12. Jeong, S.Y.; Kim, K.M. Influencing factors on hand hygiene behavior of nursing students based on theory of planned behavior: A descriptive survey study. *Nurse Educ. Today* **2016**, *36*, 159–164. [CrossRef] [PubMed]
13. Godin, G.; Gagnon, H.; Lambert, L.-D.; Conner, M. Determinants of condom use among a random sample of single heterosexual adults. *Br. J. Health Psychol.* **2005**, *10*, 85–100. [CrossRef] [PubMed]
14. Aldrich, R.S. Using the Theory of Planned Behavior to Predict College Students' Intention to Intervene with a Suicidal Individual. *Crisis* **2015**, *36*, 332–337. [CrossRef]
15. Asare, M. Using the Theory of Planned Behavior to Determine the Condom Use Behavior Among College Students. *Am. J. Health Stud.* **2015**, *30*, 43–50. [CrossRef]
16. Luszczynska, A.; Sheng Cao, D.; Mallach, N.; Pietron, K.; Mazurkiewicz, M.; Schwarzer, R. Intentions, planning, and self-efficacy predict physical activity in Chinese and Polish adolescents: Two moderated mediation analyses. *Int. J. Clin. Health Psychol.* **2010**, *10*, 265–278.
17. Scribbr. Mediator vs. Moderator Variables. 2021. Available online: https://www.scribbr.com/methodology/mediator-vs-moderator/ (accessed on 10 June 2022).
18. Rice, T. The Behavioral Economics of Health and Health Care. *Annu. Rev. Public Health* **2013**, *34*, 431–447. [CrossRef]
19. Messina, B.G.; Silvestri, M.M.; Diulio, A.R.; Murphy, J.G.; Garza, K.B.; Correia, C.J. Alcohol use, impulsivity, and the non-medical use of prescription stimulants among college students. *Addict. Behav.* **2014**, *39*, 1798–1803. [CrossRef]
20. Garza, K.B.; Harris, C.V.; Bolding, M.S. Examination of value of the future and health beliefs to explain dietary and physical activity behaviors. *Res. Soc. Adm. Pharm.* **2013**, *9*, 851–862. [CrossRef]
21. Moshier, S.J.; Ewen, M.; Otto, M.W. Impulsivity as a moderator of the intention-behavior relationship for illicit drug use in patients undergoing treatment. *Addict. Behav.* **2013**, *38*, 1651–1655. [CrossRef]
22. Chapman, G.B.; Elstein, A.S. Valuing the future: Temporal discounting of health and money. *Med. Decis. Mak. Int. J. Soc. Med. Decis. Mak.* **1995**, *15*, 373–386. [CrossRef]
23. Price, M.; Higgs, S.; Lee, M. Self-reported eating traits: Underlying components of food responsivity and dietary restriction are positively related to BMI. *Appetite* **2015**, *95*, 203–210. [CrossRef] [PubMed]
24. Zhang, J.; Lin, L. The moderating effects of impulsivity on Chinese rural young suicide. *J. Clin. Psychol.* **2014**, *70*, 579–588. [CrossRef] [PubMed]
25. Moher, D.; Liberati, A.; Tetzlaff, J.; Altman, D.G. Preferred reporting items for systematic reviews and meta-analyses: The PRISMA statement. *Ann. Intern. Med.* **2009**, *151*, 264–269. [CrossRef] [PubMed]
26. Hong, Q.N.; Fàbregues, S.; Bartlett, G.; Boardman, F.; Cargo, M.; Dagenais, P.; Gagnon, M.-P.; Griffiths, F.; Nicolau, B.; O'Cathain, A.; et al. The Mixed Methods Appraisal Tool (MMAT) version 2018 for information professionals and researchers. *Educ. Inf.* **2018**, *34*, 285–291. [CrossRef]
27. Hohmann, N.S.; McDaniel, C.C.; Mason, S.W.; Cheung, W.Y.; Williams, M.S.; Salvador, C.; Graves, E.K.; Camp, C.N.; Chou, C. Healthcare providers' perspectives on care coordination for adults with cancer and multiple chronic conditions: A systematic review. *J. Pharm. Health Serv. Res.* **2020**, *11*, 97–116. [CrossRef]
28. Churchill, S.; Jessop, D. Spontaneous implementation intentions and impulsivity: Can impulsivity moderate the effectiveness of planning strategies? *Br. J. Health Psychol.* **2010**, *15*, 529–541. [CrossRef]

29. Churchill, S.; Jessop, D.C. Too impulsive for implementation intentions? Evidence that impulsivity moderates the effectiveness of an implementation intention intervention. *Psychol. Health* **2011**, *26*, 517–530. [CrossRef]
30. Mullan, B.; Wong, C.; Allom, V.; Pack, S.L. The role of executive function in bridging the intention-behaviour gap for binge-drinking in university students. *Addict. Behav.* **2011**, *36*, 1023–1026. [CrossRef]
31. Pfeffer, I.; Strobach, T. Physical activity automaticity, intention, and trait self-control as predictors of physical activity behavior—A dual-process perspective. *Psychol. Health Med.* **2022**, *27*, 1021–1034. [CrossRef]
32. Wang, X.; Won, D.; Jeon, H.S. Predictors of Sports Gambling among College Students: The Role of the Theory of Planned Behavior and Problem Gambling Severity. *Int. J. Environ. Res. Public Health* **2021**, *18*, 1803. [CrossRef]
33. Chevance, G.; Stephan, Y.; Héraud, N.; Boiché, J. Interaction between self-regulation, intentions and implicit attitudes in the prediction of physical activity among persons with obesity. *Health Psychol. Off. J. Div. Health Psychol. Am. Psychol. Assoc.* **2018**, *37*, 257–261. [CrossRef] [PubMed]
34. Crandall, A.; Cheung, A.; Young, A.; Hooper, A.P. Theory-Based Predictors of Mindfulness Meditation Mobile App Usage: A Survey and Cohort Study. *JMIR Mhealth Uhealth* **2019**, *7*, e10794. [CrossRef]
35. Stevens, A.K.; Littlefield, A.K.; Talley, A.E.; Brown, J.L. Do individuals higher in impulsivity drink more impulsively? A pilot study within a high risk sample of young adults. *Addict. Behav.* **2017**, *65*, 147–153. [CrossRef] [PubMed]
36. Schutz, M.; Godin, G.; Kok, G.; Vézina-Im, L.-A.; Naccache, H.; Otis, J.; MAYA Study Group. Determinants of condom use among HIV-positive men who have sex with men. *Int. J. STD AIDS* **2011**, *22*, 391–397. [CrossRef] [PubMed]
37. Koring, M.; Richert, J.; Lippke, S.; Parschau, L.; Reuter, T.; Schwarzer, R. Synergistic effects of planning and self-efficacy on physical activity. *Health Educ. Behav. Off. Publ. Soc. Public Health Educ.* **2012**, *39*, 152–158. [CrossRef]
38. Lippke, S.; Wiedemann, A.U.; Ziegelmann, J.P.; Reuter, T.; Schwarzer, R. Self-efficacy moderates the mediation of intentions into behavior via plans. *Am. J. Health Behav.* **2009**, *33*, 521–529. [CrossRef]
39. Zhang, R.; Zhang, C.Q.; Gan, Y.; Li, D.; Rhodes, R.E. Predicting Transport-Related Walking in Chinese Employees by Integrating Worksite Neighbourhood Walkability and Social Cognition. *Appl. Psychol. Health Well-Being* **2019**, *11*, 484–498. [CrossRef]
40. Kothe, E.J.; Sainsbury, K.; Smith, L.; Mullan, B.A. Explaining the intention–behaviour gap in gluten-free diet adherence: The moderating roles of habit and perceived behavioural control. *J. Health Psychol.* **2015**, *20*, 580–591. [CrossRef]
41. Zhang, C.Q.; Fang, R.; Zhang, R.; Hagger, M.S.; Hamilton, K. Predicting Hand Washing and Sleep Hygiene Behaviors among College Students: Test of an Integrated Social-Cognition Model. *Int. J. Environ. Res. Public Health* **2020**, *17*, 1209. [CrossRef]
42. Allom, V.; Mullan, B.; Cowie, E.; Hamilton, K. Physical Activity and Transitioning to College: The Importance of Intentions and Habits. *Am. J. Health Behav.* **2016**, *40*, 280–290. [CrossRef] [PubMed]
43. Lin, C.Y.; Broström, A.; Nilsen, P.; Pakpour, A.H. Using extended theory of planned behavior to understand aspirin adherence in pregnant women. *Pregnancy Hypertens.* **2018**, *12*, 84–89. [CrossRef] [PubMed]
44. Packel, L.B.; Prehn, A.W.; Anderson, C.L.; Fisher, P.L. Factors influencing physical activity behaviors in colorectal cancer survivors. *Am. J. Health Promot. AJHP* **2015**, *30*, 85–92. [CrossRef] [PubMed]
45. Gucciardi, D.F. Mental toughness as a moderator of the intention-behaviour gap in the rehabilitation of knee pain. *J. Sci. Med. Sport* **2016**, *19*, 454–458. [CrossRef] [PubMed]
46. de Bruijn, G.-J.; Brug, J.; Van Lenthe, F.J. Neuroticism, conscientiousness and fruit consumption: Exploring mediator and moderator effects in the theory of planned behaviour. *Psychol. Health* **2009**, *24*, 1051–1069. [CrossRef]
47. MacCann, C.; Todd, J.; Mullan, B.A.; Roberts, R.D. Can personality bridge the intention-behavior gap to predict who will exercise? *Am. J. Health Behav.* **2015**, *39*, 140–147. [CrossRef]
48. Monds, L.A.; MacCann, C.; Mullan, B.A.; Wong, C.; Todd, J.; Roberts, R.D. Can personality close the intention-behavior gap for healthy eating? An examination with the HEXACO personality traits. *Psychol. Health Med.* **2016**, *21*, 845–855. [CrossRef]
49. Cao, Z.; Yang, Y.; Ding, W.; Huang, Z. From Physical Activity Intention to Behavior: The Moderation Role of Mental Toughness Among College Students and Wage Earners. *Front. Psychol.* **2021**, *12*, 584760. [CrossRef]
50. Hannan, T.E.; Moffitt, R.L.; Neumann, D.L.; Thomas, P.R. Applying the Theory of Planned Behavior to Physical Activity: The Moderating Role of Mental Toughness. *J. Sport Exerc. Psychol.* **2015**, *37*, 514–522. [CrossRef]
51. Hartson, K.R.; Avila, M.; Gance-Cleveland, B.; Harpin, S.B.; Tigges, B.; Cook, P.F. Predictors of Physical Activity in a Predominantly Hispanic Sample of Adolescents. *West. J. Nurs. Res.* **2020**, *42*, 514–523. [CrossRef]
52. Rhodes, R.E.; Beauchamp, M.R.; Quinlan, A.; Symons Downs, D.; Warburton, D.E.R.; Blanchard, C.M. Predicting the physical activity of new parents who participated in a physical activity intervention. *Soc. Sci. Med.* **2021**, *284*, 114221. [CrossRef] [PubMed]
53. Gibson, L.P.; Magnan, R.E.; Kramer, E.B.; Bryan, A.D. Theory of Planned Behavior Analysis of Social Distancing During the COVID-19 Pandemic: Focusing on the Intention-Behavior Gap. *Ann. Behav. Med. A Publ. Soc. Behav. Med.* **2021**, *55*, 805–812. [CrossRef] [PubMed]
54. Schüz, B.; Brick, C.; Wilding, S.; Conner, M. Socioeconomic Status Moderates the Effects of Health Cognitions on Health Behaviors within Participants: Two Multibehavior Studies. *Ann. Behav. Med. A Publ. Soc. Behav. Med.* **2020**, *54*, 36–48. [CrossRef] [PubMed]
55. Lange, D.; Barz, M.; Baldensperger, L.; Lippke, S.; Knoll, N.; Schwarzer, R. Sex differential mediation effects of planning within the health behavior change process. *Soc. Sci. Med.* **2018**, *211*, 137–146. [CrossRef]
56. Gaum, P.M.; Brey, F.; Kraus, T.; Lang, J. Does stigmatization moderate the association between intention and implementation of learned prevention-strategies at work after a depressive episode?—A cross-sectional pilot study. *J. Occup. Med. Toxicol.* **2019**, *14*, 26. [CrossRef]

57. Baumann, S.; Gaertner, B.; Schnuerer, I.; Haberecht, K.; John, U.; Freyer-Adam, J. Belief incongruence and the intention-behavior gap in persons with at-risk alcohol use. *Addict. Behav.* **2015**, *48*, 5–11. [CrossRef]
58. Gourlan, M.; Bord, A.; Cousson-Gélie, F. From intentions formation to their translation into behavior: An extended model of theory of planned behavior in the exercise domain. *Sport Exerc. Perform. Psychol.* **2019**, *8*, 317–333. [CrossRef]
59. Bandura, A. Self-efficacy: Toward a unifying theory of behavioral change. *Psychol. Rev.* **1977**, *84*, 191. [CrossRef]
60. St-Pierre, R.A.; Temcheff, C.E.; Derevensky, J.L.; Gupta, R. Theory of Planned Behavior in School-Based Adolescent Problem Gambling Prevention: A Conceptual Framework. *J. Prim. Prev.* **2015**, *36*, 361–385. [CrossRef]
61. Norman, P.; Conner, M. Health Behavior. In *Reference Module in Neuroscience and Biobehavioral Psychology*; Elsevier: Amsterdam, The Netherlands, 2017. [CrossRef]
62. Rhodes, R.E.; Dickau, L. Moderators of the intention-behaviour relationship in the physical activity domain: A systematic review. *Br. J. Sports Med.* **2013**, *47*, 215–225. [CrossRef]
63. Starfelt Sutton, L.C.; White, K.M. Predicting sun-protective intentions and behaviours using the theory of planned behaviour: A systematic review and meta-analysis. *Psychol. Health* **2016**, *31*, 1272–1292. [CrossRef] [PubMed]
64. Verdoux, H.; Lengronne, J.; Liraud, F.; Gonzales, B.; Assens, F.; Abalan, F.; Os, J.V. Medication adherence in psychosis: Predictors and impact on outcome. A 2-year follow-up of first-admitted subjects. *Acta Psychiatr. Scand.* **2000**, *102*, 203–210. [CrossRef] [PubMed]
65. Viswanathan, M.; Golin, C.E.; Jones, C.D.; Ashok, M.; Blalock, S.J.; Wines, R.C.; Coker-Schwimmer, E.J.; Rosen, D.L.; Sista, P.; Lohr, K.N. Interventions to improve adherence to self-administered medications for chronic diseases in the United States: A systematic review. *Ann. Intern. Med.* **2012**, *157*, 785–795. [CrossRef] [PubMed]
66. Halpern, S.D.; Asch, D.A.; Volpp, K.G. Commitment contracts as a way to health. *BMJ* **2012**, *344*, e522. [CrossRef]
67. Reimann, M.; Bechara, A.; MacInnis, D. Leveraging the happy meal effect: Substituting food with modest nonfood incentives decreases portion size choice. *J. Exp. Psychol. Appl.* **2015**, *21*, 276–286. [CrossRef]
68. Scholz, U.; Schuz, B.; Ziegelmann, J.P.; Lippke, S.; Schwarzer, R. Beyond behavioural intentions: Planning mediates between intentions and physical activity. *Br. J. Health Psychol.* **2008**, *13*, 479–494. [CrossRef]
69. Caudroit, J.; Boiche, J.; Stephan, Y. The role of action and coping planning in the relationship between intention and physical activity: A moderated mediation analysis. *Psychol. Health* **2014**, *29*, 768–780. [CrossRef]

pharmacy

MDPI

Article

Establishing the Approach of Norm Balance toward Intention Prediction across Six Behaviors under the Theory of Planned Behavior

Yifei Liu [1,*], Karen B. Farris [2], Dhananjay Nayakankuppam [3] and William R. Doucette [4]

1 Division of Pharmacy Practice and Administration, University of Missouri–Kansas City School of Pharmacy, Kansas City, MO 64108, USA
2 Department of Clinical Pharmacy, College of Pharmacy, University of Michigan, Ann Arbor, MI 48109, USA
3 Department of Marketing, Tippie College of Business, University of Iowa, Iowa City, IA 52242, USA
4 Department of Pharmacy Practice and Science, College of Pharmacy, University of Iowa, Iowa City, IA 52242, USA
* Correspondence: liuyif@umkc.edu

Abstract: *Background*: An innovative approach of Norm Balance is proposed under the Theory of Planned Behavior (TPB). In this approach, the measurement score of subjective norm is weighted by the relative importance of others, and the measurement score of self-identity is weighted by the relative importance of self. The study objective was to examine the effect of Norm Balance to predict behavioral intentions in two groups of college students. *Methods*: Cross-sectional surveys were used in two studies. For 153 business undergraduates, Study 1 examined three common intentions: eating a low-fat diet, exercising regularly, and dressing business-like. For 176 PharmD students, Study 2 examined three pharmacy-related intentions: informing relatives about counterfeit medications, buying prescription medications online, and completing a pharmacy residency. The relative importance of others vs. self was measured by asking study subjects to allocate 10 points between important others and oneself. Two sets of regressions were conducted and compared across six intentions using the traditional model and the Norm Balance model. *Results*: The 12 regressions explained 59–77% of intention variance. The variance explained by the two models was similar. When subjective norm or self-identity was non-significant in the traditional model, the corresponding Norm Balance component was significant in the Norm Balance model, except for eating a low-fat diet. When both subjective norm and self-identity were significant in the traditional model, the two Norm Balance components were significant in the Norm Balance model with increased coefficients. *Conclusions*: The proposed approach of Norm Balance provides a different view about the significance and coefficients of subjective norm and self-identity toward intention prediction.

Keywords: The Theory of Planned Behavior; intention; subjective norm; self-identify; Norm Balance

1. Introduction

1.1. Background

The Theory of Planned Behavior (TPB) is an essential framework to examine behaviors. According to the TPB, the principal determinant of behavior is behavioral intention, and behavioral intention is determined by attitude toward behavior, subjective norm, and perceived behavioral control [1,2]. However, the current TPB constructs may not be sufficient causes of intention or behavior, suggesting the addition of other variables to explain variance in intention or behavior [2,3]. Self-identity is a concept from identity theory and reflects the extent to which individuals perceive themselves as taking on a particular role in society [4,5]. The more a person perceives oneself as performing a particular role, the more self-identity will affect behavioral intention [6]. Self-identity has been shown to be a significant predictor of intention in the TPB for a variety of behaviors [6–19].

Subjective norm is a normative concept—the assessment of social pressures placed on an individual to perform a behavior [20]. There are two ways to measure the TPB constructs including subjective norm—indirect measures and direct measures [21]. Using indirect measures, a person's subjective norm is represented by normative beliefs weighted by the motivation to comply with the referent [20]. Using direct measures, subjective norm is determined by single items, such as "most people important to me think I should perform the behavior" [6,12,13,21]. Direct measures of the TPB constructs appear to be more strongly associated with intention than indirect measures and have been used in studies incorporating self-identity into the TPB [6–8,10,12–14,16,21].

Self-identity is also a normative construct which influences intention [6,22], but it differs from subjective norm. Self-identity is usually measured by single items, such as "I think of myself as someone as a behavior performer" [6,12,13]. Self-identity represents the social context on an actor, namely the category of an actor with identifiable social characteristics [7]. In contrast, subjective norm represents the pressure from an actor's reference groups on the behavioral performance [20]. In other words, the focus of self-identity is on oneself (personal norm), "whether I think I should perform a behavior", but the emphasis of subjective norm is one's reference group (referent norm), "whether my important others think I should perform a behavior".

1.2. Theorization

We proposed an innovative approach of Norm Balance in which self-identity and subjective norm need two parameters to be fully measured. Norm Balance is a theoretical approach rather than a construct. In this approach, subjective norm and self-identity are theorized under an overall domain of "norm", and each has a strength and proportion within the domain of "norm". The strength is represented by the measurement scores of subjective norm and self-identity. The proportion indicates the share each construct occupies in the domain of "norm", which is represented by the relative importance of others vs. self. Under this approach, for an individual, the measurement score of subjective norm should be weighted by the relative importance of others, and the measurement score of self-identity should be weighted be the relative importance of the self (Figure 1). For instance, one's important others think the individual should perform a behavior but the individual does not think so. If the person regards oneself as a more important source impacting the behavioral decision, the person may not intend to perform the behavior. To the contrary, if the person considers important others to be a more influential source impacting the behavioral decision, the person may intend to perform the behavior.

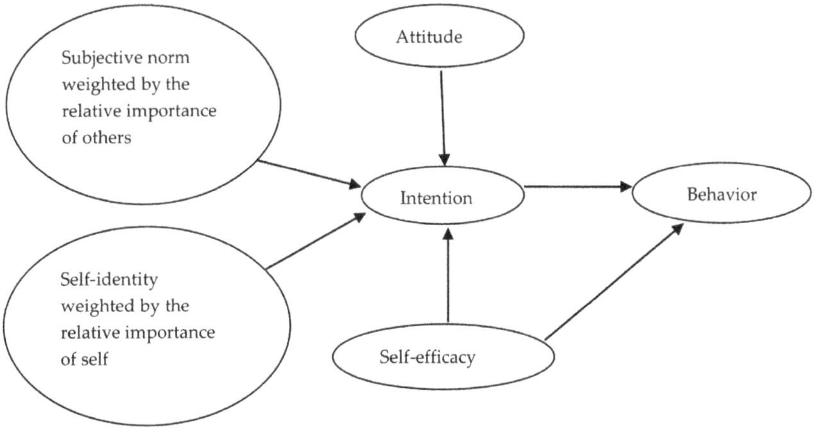

Figure 1. The proposed approach of Norm Balance under the TPB.

In addition, Ajzen theorized a hierarchical model of perceived behavioral control where perceived behavioral control is represented by two subcomponents: self-efficacy and controllability [23]. Self-efficacy has been consistently shown to be a stronger predictor of both intention and behavior than controllability [6,12,13,24]. Therefore, we used self-efficacy to represent perceived behavioral control.

1.3. Objective

The objective of this research was to examine the effect of Norm Balance to predict behavioral intentions in two groups of college students. If Norm Balance is a valid approach for intention prediction, the TPB could be modified to improve its predictive utility regarding intention. This research only examined intention prediction in Figure 1.

2. Methods

2.1. Design and Samples

Cross-sectional surveys were employed in two studies using convenience samples. Inclusion criteria of Study 1 were 153 undergraduates who took a course at a college of business. Inclusion criteria of Study 2 were 102 second-year PharmD students who took a course, and 74 third-year PharmD students who took one of two courses at a college of pharmacy. Hard copies of the instrument (Appendix A) were distributed to the students and collected from them while they were in class. There was no incentive to fill out the survey and the participation was voluntary.

In a regression analysis, as a rule-of-thumb, the sample size should be equal to or greater than "50 + 8 × m for the multiple correlation", or "104 + m for the partial correlation", where "m" is the number of predictors [25]. We expected to have nine independent variables in a regression model, so we needed a minimum of $50 + 8 \times 9 = 122$ subjects in either study. This estimated sample size of 122 was also sufficient ($>104 + 9 = 113$) to test individual predictors.

Study 1 examined three common behavior intentions: (1) eating a low-fat diet during the next week; (2) exercising for at least 20 min, three times during the next week; and (3) dressing in a business manner in school during the next week. Study 2 examined three pharmacy-related behavioral intentions: (1) informing relatives about the risk of counterfeit medications when they consider buying prescription medications on the internet; (2) buying prescription medications on the internet when having a prescription; and (3) completing a pharmacy practice residency in the future. The robustness of Norm Balance could be demonstrated by choosing different behavioral intentions in the two studies.

The number of intentions were limited to three for each study to reduce the response burden on participants. In Study 1, eating a low-fat diet and regular exercising are behaviors well examined under the TPB with addition of self-identity [9,11–13,16,17]. Then the social situations of the other intentions were altered, since Norm Balance may vary across different social contexts. For example, dressing in a business manner in school (Study 1) is relatively public, while buying prescription medications online (Study 2) is relatively private, though the two study samples were different. In addition, informing relatives about the counterfeit risk of prescription medications purchased online (Study 2) is in a family setting, while completing a pharmacy practice residency (Study 2) is in a professional setting. Furthermore, the intentions in Study 1 were for the shorter term, whereas the intentions in Study 2 were for the longer term.

2.2. Measures

Both studies assessed attitude toward behavior, subjective norm, self-efficacy, self-identity, and intention for each behavior. They also assessed the relative importance of others vs. self and control variables. Measures of attitude toward behavior, subjective norm, self-efficacy, self-identity, and intention were included in Appendix A. They were derived from reliable and valid multi-item instruments with 7-point response scales from the studies of Armitage and Connor by changing the context of the behavior [12,13]. The phrase "If I wanted to" was added to self-efficacy measures according to the suggestion of Rhodes and Courneya to assume motivation and to "reduce inadvertent tautological theorizing" [26].

The relative importance of others vs. self was measured by the following item:

> "Please allocate 10 points between the two sources below to indicate the extent of their impact on your decision to ... Please use whole numbers.
>
> People who are important to you____; Yourself____".

Control variables included age, gender, race, marital status, and whether having children. Based on the openness of the TPB to include additional variables, control variables were used to account for intention variance due to differences in demographic and other characteristics [2].

2.3. Data Analyses

For each behavior, overall measures of attitude toward behavior, subjective norm, self-efficacy, self-identity, and intention were calculated for each person by taking the mean of the corresponding items. The frequency, means, standard deviations, and bivariate correlations for the measured variables were calculated. Reliability analyses were performed for the multiple-item measurements. We hypothesized that the approach of Norm Balance would explain intention differently than simply using the measurement scores of subjective norm and self-identity. The following two multiple regression models across six behavioral intentions were conducted and compared. Both studies were approved by the Institutional Review Board of the University of Iowa.

The traditional model: Intention was regressed on attitude, subjective norm (measurement score), self-efficacy, self-identity (measurement score), and control variables.

The Norm Balance model: Intention was regressed on attitude, the relative importance of others × measurement score of subjective norm, self-efficacy, the relative importance of self × measurement score of self-identity, and control variables.

3. Results

The response rate of Study 1 was 98% (150 students out of 153), and the response rate of Study 2 was 93% (157 students out of 169). For both studies, the average respondent was in their 20s, white, single, and had no children (Table 1). The variables had high reliability (Cronbach's alpha > 0.7), except for subjective norm (measurement score) for informing relatives about the risk of counterfeit drugs, and self-identity (measurement score) for informing relatives about the risk of counterfeit drugs and buying prescription drugs online (Table 2).

Table 1. Characteristics of the study subjects.

Variable	Business Undergraduates	PharmD Students
Age, years		
Mean (SD)	21.3 (1.9)	23.9 (2.8)
Range	18–33	21–36
Total N	150	152
Gender, no. (%)		
Female	59 (39.3)	110 (71.4)
Male	91 (60.7)	44 (28.6)
Total N	150 (100)	154 (100)
Ethnicity, no. (%)		
White	136 (90.7)	138 (90.2)
Non-White	14 (9.3)	15 (9.8)
Total N	150 (100)	153 (100)

Table 1. *Cont.*

Variable	Business Undergraduates	PharmD Students
Marital status, no. (%)		
Single (never married)	145 (96.7)	118 (76.8)
Non-single	5 (3.3)	36 (23.4)
Total N	150 (100)	154 (100)
Having children, no. (%)		
Yes	4 (2.7)	10 (6.5)
No	146 (97.3)	144 (93.5)
Total N	150 (100)	154 (100)

Note: N varies for the PharmD students due to missing values.

Table 2. Reliability Analyses of Multiple-item Construct Measurements.

Construct Variable	Business Undergraduates (Cronbach' α)			PharmD Students (Cronbach' α)		
	Eating a Low-Fat Diet	Exercising Regularly	Dressing Business-Like	Informing Relatives	Buying Rx Drugs	Completing Residency
Intention (3-item)	0.942 (n = 150)	0.912 (n = 150)	0.912 (n = 150)	0.875 (n = 155)	0.944 (n = 157)	0.972 (n = 155)
Attitude toward behavior (3-item)	0.799 (n = 150)	0.720 (n = 150)	0.829 (n = 150)	0.732 (n = 152)	0.884 (n = 152)	0.923 (n = 154)
Subjective norm (3-item, measurement score)	0.806 (n = 150)	0.800 (n = 149)	0.754 (n = 149)	0.680 (n = 153)	0.843 (n = 157)	0.802 (n = 151)
Self-efficacy (3-item)	0.850 (n = 150)	0.887 (n = 150)	0.877 (n = 150)	0.890 (n = 154)	0.845 (n = 154)	0.795 (n = 155)
Self-identity (3-item, measurement score)	0.883 (n = 150)	0.861 (n = 150)	0.884 (n = 150)	0.681 (n = 155)	0.514 (n = 157)	0.884 (n = 155)

Note: (1) N varies for the PharmD students due to missing values; (2) Values are in bold when Cronbach' α < 0.7.

Across five intentions, the average relative importance of others vs. self was about 3 vs. 7, given 10 points to allocate; for the intention to inform relatives about counterfeit medications, the average relative importance of others vs. self was 4.5 vs. 5.5 (Table 3). In general, the subjects perceived themselves as having more influence than their important others on behavioral decisions (Tables 3 and 4). For each intention, there were subjects who did not care at all about the opinions of their important others (Table 4). For example, 19.5% of the PharmD students did not believe that their important others would impact their behavioral decision to purchase prescription drugs online. Additionally, the relative importance of others or self had low and non-significant correlations with the TPB constructs, which ranged from −0.27 to 0.27.

The regressions using the traditional model accounted for 60–77% of intention variance (Table 5). The regressions of Norm Balance model explained 59–77% of intention variance (Table 6). The variance explained by the two models was similar (difference $\leq$ 1%), except for the intention of purchasing prescription drugs online (the Norm Balance model explained 3% more). When subjective norm or self-identity was non-significant in the traditional model, the corresponding Norm Balance component was significant in the Norm Balance model, except for the intention of eating a low-fat diet (Table 7). When both subjective norm and self-identity were significant in the traditional model, two Norm Balance components were significant in the Norm Balance model with increased coefficients.

Table 3. Means and Standard Deviations of Construct Variables.

Construct Variable	Business Undergraduates Means (Std)			PharmD Students Means (Std)		
	Eating a Low-Fat Diet	**Exercising Regularly**	**Dressing Business-Like**	**Informing Relatives**	**Buying Rx Drugs**	**Completing Residency**
Intention (3-item) [a]	4.28 (1.69) (n = 150)	5.96 (1.29) (n = 150)	2.95 (1.58) (n = 150)	6.08 (0.99) (n = 155)	1.31 (0.95) (n = 157)	4.23 (1.83) (n = 155)
Attitude toward behavior (3-item) [a]	4.88 (1.26) (n = 150)	6.20 (1.00) (n = 150)	4.19 (1.36) (n = 150)	5.59 (1.03) (n = 152)	1.61 (1.10) (n = 152)	5.18 (1.61) (n = 154)
Subjective norm (3-item, measurement score) [a]	4.72 (1.33) (n = 150)	5.70 (1.08) (n = 149)	3.94 (1.17) (n = 149)	5.86 (0.96) (n = 153)	1.83 (1.07) (n = 157)	4.73 (1.31) (n = 151)
Self-efficacy (3-item) [a]	5.44 (1.26) (n = 150)	6.31 (1.08) (n = 150)	5.80 (1.32) (n = 150)	5.61 (1.24) (n = 154)	4.50 (2.04) (n = 154)	6.17 (1.01) (n = 155)
Self-identity (3-item, measurement score) [a]	4.73 (1.36) (n = 150)	5.39 (1.36) (n = 150)	3.76 (1.42) (n = 150)	5.59 (1.10) (n = 155)	1.97 (1.21) (n = 157)	5.97 (1.07) (n = 155)
Relative importance of others [b]	3.19 (1.63) (n = 150)	2.80 (1.50) (n = 150)	3.65 (1.99) (n = 150)	4.53 (2.07) (n = 146)	3.11 (2.20) (n = 149)	3.10 (1.92) (n = 149)
Relative importance of self [b]	6.81 (1.63) (n = 150)	7.20 (1.50) (n = 150)	6.35 (1.99) (n = 150)	5.47 (2.07) (n = 146)	6.89 (2.20) (n = 149)	6.90 (1.92) (n = 149)

Note: (1) N varies for the PharmD students due to missing values. (2) [a] 1–7 scale, and [b] 10 points to allocate.

Table 4. Frequency of Relative Importance of Others vs. Self.

Frequency (%)	Business Undergraduates			PharmD Students		
Relative Importance of Others vs. Self	**Eating Low-Fat Diet**	**Exercising Regularly**	**Dressing Business-Like**	**Informing Relatives**	**Buying Rx Drugs**	**Completing Residency**
0/10	4 (2.7)	6 (4.0)	7 (4.7)	6 (4.1)	29 (19.5)	9 (6.0)
1/9	15 (10.0)	22 (14.7)	19 (12.7)	2 (1.3)	14 (9.4)	30 (20.1)
2/8	36 (24.0)	43 (28.7)	22 (14.7)	18 (12.3)	22 (14.8)	28 (18.8)
3/7	40 (26.7)	33 (22.0)	22 (14.7)	22 (15.1)	13 (8.7)	19 (12.8)
4/6	25 (16.7)	26 (17.3)	21 (14.0)	18 (12.3)	13 (8.7)	15 (10.1)
5/5	15 (10.0)	14 (9.3)	36 (24.0)	38 (26.0)	42 (28.2)	36 (24.2)
6/4	9 (6.0)	3 (2.0)	10 (6.7)	11 (7.5)	8 (5.4)	5 (3.4)
7/3	5 (3.3)	3 (2.0)	10 (6.7)	20 (13.7)	8 (5.4)	7 (4.7)
8/2	1 (0.7)	0	3 (2.0)	9 (6.2)	0	0
9/1	0	0	0	2 (1.3)	0	0
10/0	0	0	0	0	0	0
Total N	150 (100)	150 (100)	150 (100)	146 (100)	149 (100)	149 (100)

Note: N varies for PharmD students due to missing values.

Table 5. Prediction of Intention Using TPB with Addition of Self-identity (the Traditional Model).

Dependent Variable	**Business Undergraduates**			**PharmD Students**		
Intention	**Eating a Low-Fat Diet (n = 150)**	**Exercising Regularly (n = 149)**	**Dressing Business-Like (n = 149)**	**Informing Relatives (n = 146)**	**Buying Rx Drugs (n = 146)**	**Completing Residency (n = 146)**
Regression model						
Adjusted R square	0.65	0.77	0.60	0.66	0.68	0.68
Df	9	9	9	9	9	9
F	31.19 **	56.46 **	25.67 **	32.81 **	35.25 **	36.21 **
Standardized Beta						
Construct measurements						
Attitude toward behavior	0.64 **	0.25 **	0.33 **	0.26 **	0.78 **	0.67 **
Subjective norm (measurement score)	0.04	0.09 *	0.11	0.25 **	−0.01	0.19 **
Self-efficacy	0.05	0.36 **	−0.06	0.19 **	−0.09	0.00
Self-identity (measurement score)	0.13 *	0.36 **	0.40 **	0.32 **	0.17 **	0.08
Control variables						
Age	0.05	−0.02	−0.10	0.06	−0.04	0.00
Gender (male)	−0.19 **	−0.15 **	0.06	0.01	0.05	−0.01
Ethnicity (White)	0.05	0.03	−0.05	0.05	0.03	−0.01
Marital status (single)	−0.03	0.00	−0.14 *	0.09	0.02	−0.04
Having children	−0.06	0.04	0.08	−0.05	−0.07	−0.02

** significant at 0.01; * significant at 0.05. Note: The number of cases varied due to missing data.

Table 6. Prediction of Intention Using Norm Balance (the Norm Balance Model).

Dependent Variable	**Business Undergraduates**			**PharmD Students**		
Intention	**Eating a Low-Fat Diet (n = 150)**	**Exercising Regularly (n = 149)**	**Dressing Business-Like (n = 149)**	**Informing Relatives (n = 141)**	**Buying Rx Drugs (n = 142)**	**Completing Residency (n = 141)**
Regression model						
Adjusted R square	0.64	0.77	0.59	0.67	0.71	0.68
Df	9	9	9	9	9	9
F	30.74 **	54.92 **	24.62 **	33.17 **	39.92 **	33.83 **
Standardized Beta						
Construct measurements						
Attitude toward behavior	0.67 **	0.26 **	0.35 **	0.31 **	0.75 **	0.75 **
Relative importance of others × measurement score of subjective norm	0.03	0.27 **	0.27 **	0.66 **	0.14 **	0.15 *
Self-efficacy	0.06	0.38 **	−0.06	0.21 **	−0.09	−0.03
Relative importance of self × measurement score of self-identity	0.11	0.47 **	0.42 **	0.70 **	0.15 **	0.22 **
Control variables						
Age	0.04	−0.02	−0.11	0.06	−0.02	−0.03
Gender (male)	−0.19 **	−0.16 **	0.06	0.03	−0.01	−0.01
Ethnicity (White)	0.06	0.04	−0.06	0.05	0.02	−0.03
Marital status (single)	−0.04	−0.01	−0.14 *	0.06	0.04	−0.02
Having children	−0.05	0.03	0.08	−0.05	−0.08	0.01

** significant at 0.01; * significant at 0.05. Note: The number of cases varied due to missing data.

Table 7. Comparison of Regression Coefficients of Subjective Norm and Self-identity between Two Models.

Dependent Variable	Business Undergraduates			PharmD Students		
Intention	Eating a Low-Fat Diet (n = 150)	Exercising Regularly (n = 149)	Dressing Business-Like (n = 149)	Informing Relatives (n = 146)	Buying Rx Drugs (n = 146)	Completing Residency (n = 146)
Standardized Beta of the traditional model						
Subjective norm (measurement score)	0.04	0.09 *	0.11	0.25 **	−0.01	0.19 **
Self-identity (measurement score)	0.13 *	0.36 **	0.40 **	0.32 **	0.17 **	0.08
Standardized Beta of the Norm Balance model						
Relative importance of others × measurement score of subjective norm	0.03	0.27 **	0.27 **	0.66 **	0.14 **	0.15 *
Relative importance of self × measurement score of self-identity	0.11	0.47 **	0.42 **	0.70 **	0.15 **	0.22 **

** significant at 0.01; * significant at 0.05. Note: The number of cases varied due to missing data.

4. Discussion

4.1. Predictive Utility of the Approach of Norm Balance

The regression results indicate that the Norm Balance components have a similar overall effect as using unweighted measurement scores of subjective norm and self-identity to explain intention variance. However, the proposed approach of Norm Balance provides a different view about the significance or coefficients of subjective norm and self-identity, because there were clear changes from the traditional model (Table 7). For example, for the intention to complete a pharmacy residency in Study 2, the traditional model showed that subjective norm (measurement score) was the second strongest intention predictor, while self-identity (measurement score) was non-significant. However, after considering the relative importance, self-identity became the second strongest intention predictor. That is, with more variation added to measurement scores using the relative importance of others vs. self, self-identity became a more powerful predictor for an intention than subjective norm. Another example is the intention to buy prescription medications on the internet in Study 2. After considering the relative importance, subjective norm changed from a non-significant predictor to a significant predictor. The low and non-significant correlations between the relative importance of others vs. self and intention indicate that the relative importance does not independently explain intention. This is consistent with the theorization of the relative importance, namely using it to weigh measurement scores rather than using it as an intention predictor. The low correlations between the relative importance and the measurement score of subjective norm or self-identity suggest that the relative importance is not another way to measure subjective norm or self-identity.

4.2. The Relative Importance of Others vs. Self

An interesting finding was that the average relative importance of others vs. self was around 3 vs. 7 (given 10 points to allocate) across five intentions (Table 3). In other words, the subjects tended to regard themselves as being over two times more important than their important others for most behavioral decisions. Even for a behavior which may be related to important others (e.g., informing relatives about counterfeit medications), the subjects still valued their own opinions more. Cultural variation in the self-concept also supports the existence of the relative importance of others vs. self in the proposed approach of Norm Balance. Western culture tends to be independent, where behaviors are associated with personal values; whereas eastern culture is more interdependent, where behaviors are made meaningful when using others' values for reference [27]. "Independence vs.

interdependence" is also the basis for other differences between western and eastern cultures, such as opinions toward achievement, self-criticism, equality, and so on [28]. The framework of individualism vs. collectivism provides an alternate view about cultural variation in the self-concept. For example, individualists are independent, prioritize their personal goals over collective goals, base their behaviors on attitudes and hedonism, and calculate the profit and cost of relationships [29]. Collectivists, on the other hand, are interdependent, subdue their personal goals in favor of collective goals, base their behaviors on norms and duties, and consider others' needs in social exchange. Individualism is common in Western Europe and North America, whereas collectivism is common in Asia and Africa [30]. Not measuring the relative importance of others vs. self may lead to the misinterpretation of results or ineffective interventions.

4.3. Limitations

There were three limitations in the studies. First, the reliability of self-identity (measurement score) for buying prescription drugs online was low (Cronbach's alpha = 0.514). The three self-identity items (measurement score) were: (1) "I think of myself as an internet shopper of prescription medication"; (2) "I think of myself as someone who is concerned with getting prescription medication on the internet for a low price"; and (3) "I think of myself as someone who is concerned with the convenience of internet purchase of prescription medication". These items may measure the different societal roles associated with internet shopping. For example, item (1) measured the role of "internet shopper", but item (2) might measure the role of "price grabber". Thus, the reliability was low. Second, the study subjects were college students with homogeneous demographics, such as age, education, ethnicity, and marital status. Therefore, the results may not be generalizable to other populations. Third, although the approach of Norm Balance accounted for 59–77% of the intention variance (Table 6), compared with the traditional model, it did not further improve the variance explanation. However, no improvement in explaining intention variance does not necessarily mean that this approach is invalid. It does offer another perspective to examine the significance or coefficients of subjective norm or self-identify (Table 7).

4.4. Future Research

Three directions exist for further efforts exploring the approach of Norm Balance. First, the development of other measures to capture the relative importance of others vs. self. Second, the use of this approach to assess the same behavior intention for oneself vs. others, or across different cultures, and then a comparison of the results. For instance, how parents' intention regarding the same health behavior varies for themselves vs. their children. Third, an examination of factors affecting this approach. According to the study results, it seems that behavior type or timeframe may have some influence.

5. Conclusions

In conclusion, the proposed approach of Norm Balance under the TPB explained similar intention variance to a traditional TPB model. However, it provides a different view about the significance or coefficients of subjective norm and self-identity.

Author Contributions: Conceptualization, Y.L.; methodology, Y.L.; validation, Y.L., K.B.F. and W.R.D.; formal analysis, Y.L.; investigation, Y.L.; resources, D.N. and W.R.D.; data curation, Y.L.; writing—original draft preparation, Y.L.; writing—review and editing, Y.L., K.B.F., D.N. and W.R.D.; supervision, K.B.F. and W.R.D.; project administration, Y.L. All authors have read and agreed to the published version of the manuscript.

Funding: This research received no external funding.

Institutional Review Board Statement: Two studies in this paper were approved by the Institutional Review Board (IRB) of the University of Iowa. IRB ID for Study 1: 200512762; and IRB ID for Study 2: 200512755.

Informed Consent Statement: Informed consent was obtained from all the subjects involved in Study 1, and cover letters rather than informed consent forms were used in Study 2.

Data Availability Statement: Data sharing is not applicable to this article.

Conflicts of Interest: The authors declare no conflict of interest.

Appendix A. Survey Items

Survey items for the intention of eating a low-fat diet in Study 1*

Attitude toward behavior

(1) "For me, eating a low-fat diet during the next week is" ("1 = unpleasant" and "7 = pleasant");
(2) "For me, eating a low-fat diet during the next week is" ("1 = negative" and "7 = positive");
(3) "For me, eating a low-fat diet during the next week is" ("1 = bad" and "7 = good").

Subjective norm

(1) "People who are important to me would disapprove/approve of my eating a low-fat diet during the next week" ("1 = disapprove" and "7 = approve");
(2) "People who are important to me think I should not/should eat a low-fat diet during the next week" ("1 = should not" and "7 = should");
(3) "People who are important to me want me to eat a low-fat diet during the next week" ("1 = strongly disagree" and "7 = strongly agree").

Self-efficacy

(1) "If you wanted to, how confident are you that you will be able to eat a low-fat diet during the next week?" ("1 = not very confident" and "7 = very confident");
(2) "If you wanted to, to what extent do you see yourself as being capable of eating a low-fat diet during the next week?" ("1 = very incapable" and "7 = very capable");
(3) "If I wanted to, I believe I am able to eat a low-fat diet during the next week" ("1 = definitely do not" and "7 = definitely do").

Self-identity

(1) "I think of myself as a healthy eater" ("1 = strongly disagree" and "7 = strongly agree");
(2) "I think of myself as someone who is concerned with healthy eating" ("1 = strongly disagree" and "7 = strongly agree");
(3) "I think of myself as someone who is concerned with health consequences of what I eat. ("1 = strongly disagree" and "7 = strongly agree").

Intention

(1) "I intend to eat a low-fat diet during the next week" ("1 = definitely do not" and "7 = definitely do");
(2) "I plan to eat a low-fat diet during the next week" ("1 = definitely do not" and "7 = definitely do");
(3) "I want to eat a low-fat diet during the next week" ("1 = definitely do not" and "7 = definitely do").

Relative importance of others vs. self

"Please allocate 10 points between the two sources below to indicate the extent of their impact on your decision to eat a low-fat during the next week. Please use whole numbers. People who are important to you____; Yourself____"

Note: * Survey items for the other intentions in both studies are similar to the items used for the intention of eating a low-fat diet, except for the context of the intention.

References

1. Ajzen, I. *Attitudes, Personality, and Behavior*; Dorsey Press: Chicago, IL, USA, 1988.
2. Ajzen, I. The theory of planned behavior. *Organ. Behav. Hum. Decis. Process.* **1991**, *50*, 179–211. [CrossRef]
3. Sutton, S. Predicting and explaining intentions and behavior: How well are we doing? *J. Appl. Soc. Psychol.* **1998**, *28*, 1317–1338. [CrossRef]
4. Stryker, S. Identity, salience and role performance: The relevance of symbolic interaction theory for family research. *J. Marriage Fam.* **1968**, *30*, 558–564. [CrossRef]
5. Stryker, S.; Serpe, R.T. Commitment, identity salience, and role behaviour. In *Personality, Roles, and Social Behaviour*; Ickers, W., Knowles, E.S., Eds.; Springer: New York, NY, USA, 1982; pp. 199–218.
6. Armitage, C.J.; Conner, M. Social cognitive determinants of blood donation. *J. Appl. Soc. Psychol.* **2001**, *31*, 1431–1457. [CrossRef]
7. Charng, H.W.; Piliavin, J.A.; Callero, P.L. Role identity and reasoned action in the prediction of repeated behavior. *Soc. Psychol. Q.* **1988**, *51*, 303–317. [CrossRef]
8. Sparks, P.; Shepherd, R. Self-identity and the theory of planned behavior: Assessing the role of identification with green consumerism. *Soc. Psychol. Q.* **1992**, *55*, 388–399. [CrossRef]
9. Sparks, P.; Shepherd, R.; Wieringa, N.; Zimmermanns, N. Perceived behavioural control, unrealistic optimism and dietary change: An exploratory study. *Appetite* **1995**, *24*, 243–255. [CrossRef]
10. Theodorakis, Y.; Bagiatis, K.; Goudas, M. Attitudes toward teaching individuals with disabilities: Application of planned behavior theory. *Adapt. Phys. Act. Q.* **1995**, *12*, 151–160. [CrossRef]
11. Sparks, P.; Guthrie, C.A. Self-identity in the theory of planned behavior: A useful addition or an unhelpful artifice? *J. Appl. Soc. Psychol.* **1998**, *28*, 1393–1410. [CrossRef]
12. Armitage, C.J.; Conner, M. The theory of planned behaviour: Assessment of predictive validity and "perceived control". *Br. J. Soc. Psychol.* **1999**, *38*, 35–54. [CrossRef]
13. Armitage, C.J.; Conner, M. Distinguishing perceptions of control from self-efficacy: Predicting consumption of a low-fat diet using the theory of planned behavior. *J. Appl. Soc. Psychol.* **1999**, *29*, 72–90. [CrossRef]
14. Terry, D.J.; Hogg, M.A.; White, K.M. The theory of planned behaviour: Self-Identity, social identity and group norms. *Br. J. Soc. Psychol.* **1999**, *38*, 225–244. [CrossRef] [PubMed]
15. Pierro, A.; Mannetti, L.; Livi, S. Self-identity and the theory of planned behavior in the prediction of health behavior and leisure activity. *Self Identity* **2003**, *2*, 47–61. [CrossRef]
16. Jackson, C.; Smith, R.A.; Conner, M. Applying an extended version of the theory of planned behaviour to physical activity. *J. Sport. Sci.* **2003**, *21*, 119–133. [CrossRef] [PubMed]
17. Ries, F.; Hein, V.; Pihu, M.; Armenta, J.M.S. Self-identity as a component of the Theory of Planned Behaviour in predicting physical activity. *Eur. Phys. Educ. Rev.* **2012**, *18*, 322–334. [CrossRef]
18. Dean, M.; Raats, M.M.; Shepherd, R. The role of self-identity, past behavior, and their interaction in predicting intention to purchase fresh and processed organic food. *J. Appl. Soc. Psychol.* **2012**, *42*, 669–688. [CrossRef]
19. De Maria, A.L.; Sundstrom, B.; Faria, A.A.; Moxley Saxon, G.; Ramos-Ortiz, J. Using the theory of planned behavior and self-identity to explore women's decision-making and intention to switch from combined oral contraceptive pill (COC) to long-acting reversible contraceptive (LARC). *BMC Womens Health* **2019**, *19*, 82.
20. Fishbein, M.; Ajzen, I. *Belief, Attitude, Intention, and Behavior: An Introduction to Theory and Research*; Addison—Wesley: Reading, MA, USA, 1975.
21. Montano, D.E.; Kasprzyk, D. Chapter 4, The theory of reasoned action and the theory of planned behavior. In *Health Behavior and Health Education: Theory, Research and Practice*, 3rd ed.; Glanz, K., Rimer, B.K., Lewis, F.M., Eds.; Jossey-Bass Publishers: San Francisco, NC, USA, 2002; pp. 69–76.
22. Conner, M.; Armitage, C.J. Extending the theory of planned behavior: A review and avenues for future research. *J. Appl. Soc. Psychol.* **1998**, *28*, 1429–1464. [CrossRef]
23. Ajzen, I. Perceived behavioral control, self-efficacy, locus of control, and the theory of planned behavior. *J. Appl. Soc. Psychol.* **2002**, *32*, 665–683. [CrossRef]
24. Manstead, A.S.R.; van Eekelen, S.A.M. Distinguishing between perceived behavioral control and self-efficacy in the domain of academic intentions and behaviors. *J. Appl. Soc. Psychol.* **1998**, *28*, 1375–1392. [CrossRef]
25. Green, S.B. How many subjects does it take to do a regression analysis? *Multivar. Behav. Res.* **1991**, *26*, 499–510. [CrossRef] [PubMed]
26. Rhodes, R.E.; Courneya, K.S. Self-efficacy, controllability and intention in the theory of planned behavior: Measurement redundancy or causal independence? *Psychol. Health* **2003**, *18*, 79–91. [CrossRef]
27. Markus, H.; Kitayama, S. Culture and self: Implication for cognition, emotion, and motivation. *Psychol. Rev.* **1991**, *98*, 224–253. [CrossRef]
28. Nisbett, R.E. *The Geography of Thought: How Asians and Westerners Think Differently and Why*; Simon & Schuster Inc.: New York, NY, USA, 2003.

29. Triandis, H.C. *Individualism and Collectivism*; Westview Press: Boulder, CO, USA, 1995.
30. Triandis, H.C. The psychological measurement of cultural syndromes. *Am. Psychol.* **1996**, *51*, 407–415. [CrossRef]

European Journal of
Investigation in Health, Psychology and Education

MDPI

Article

How Valid Is Bandura's Social Cognitive Theory to Explain Physical Activity Behavior?

Viktoria Sophie Egele *, Eric Klopp and Robin Stark

Department of Education, Saarland University, 66123 Saarbrücken, Germany; e.klopp@mx.uni-saarland.de (E.K.); r.stark@mx.uni-saarland.de (R.S.)

* Correspondence: viktoria.egele@uni-saarland.de

Abstract: (1) Background: Although social cognitive theory (SCT) has been widely tested and applied in numerous interventions aimed at optimizing physical activity behavior, the complete theory has rarely been tested in its entirety. Only selected elements have been tested, and specific samples, some of them pathological, have been studied rather than the general population, for whom a lack of physical activity is a huge problem. The present study addresses these two research gaps and tests the tenability of the theoretical assumptions of SCT to explain physical activity behavior in the general population. (2) Methods: A total of 194 German adults (109 male, 85 female) with a mean age of 26.03 years (SD = 10.33) completed two validated questionnaires concerning their expressions on SCT components (t1) and their physical activity (t2). SCT was modeled using a structural equation model with latent variables. (3) Results: The results showed the very good fit of the structural model, indicating that the theoretically stated relations between the constructs in SCT seem to be corroborated, despite some paths seeming to be more important than others. (4) Conclusions: The use of SCT to explain and predict behavior can be seen as justified, even though it once again appears that some aspects (i.e., self-efficacy) are more crucial than others.

Keywords: health behavior; validity; self-efficacy; outcome expectations; structural equation model

1. Introduction

Insufficient physical activity is a main cause of non-communicable diseases (e.g., coronary heart diseases and cancer), poor psychological well-being, and premature death (Miko et al., 2020; World Health Organization, 2018). The WHO recommends 150 min of moderate physical activity or 75 min of vigorous physical activity per week, alongside two sessions of additional muscle-strengthening exercise, for adults to achieve considerable health benefits (World Health Organization, 2018). Yet, in a recent long-term study including data from nearly two million people in 168 countries, it was evident that 31.3 percent of adults worldwide do not reach the recommended level of physical activity, and consequently are at increased health risk (Strain et al., 2024). Therefore, it is crucial to understand why individuals engage in physical activity.

Numerous studies have provided evidence that social cognitive theory (SCT) (Bandura, 1986) is suitable for explaining or predicting physical activity behavior (Auster-Gussman et al., 2022; Baird et al., 2021; Heiss & Petosa, 2016; Sebastian et al., 2021; Silveira & Motl, 2019; Stacey et al., 2015; Taylor et al., 2016; Zechner & Gill, 2016). SCT proposes that individuals' behaviors are influenced by a reciprocal interaction between personal, behavioral, and environmental factors. SCT emphasizes the following key components: perceived self-efficacy (the belief in one's ability to engage in physical activity successfully, even in the face of challenges), outcome expectations (the anticipated positive and negative consequences of engaging in physical activity), goal-setting (specific and achievable objectives for physical activity behavior), and sociocultural factors (environmental influences that support or hinder physical activity, such as access to facilities, social support, and time constraints) (Bandura, 2004).

Bandura (2000) suggests that self-efficacy is the most critical determinant of physical activity behavior. High self-efficacy leads to stronger outcome expectations, more concrete goals, and greater engagement in physical activity. Individuals with high self-efficacy are more likely to persist in physical activity despite obstacles and setbacks. The theoretical model is shown in Figure 1.

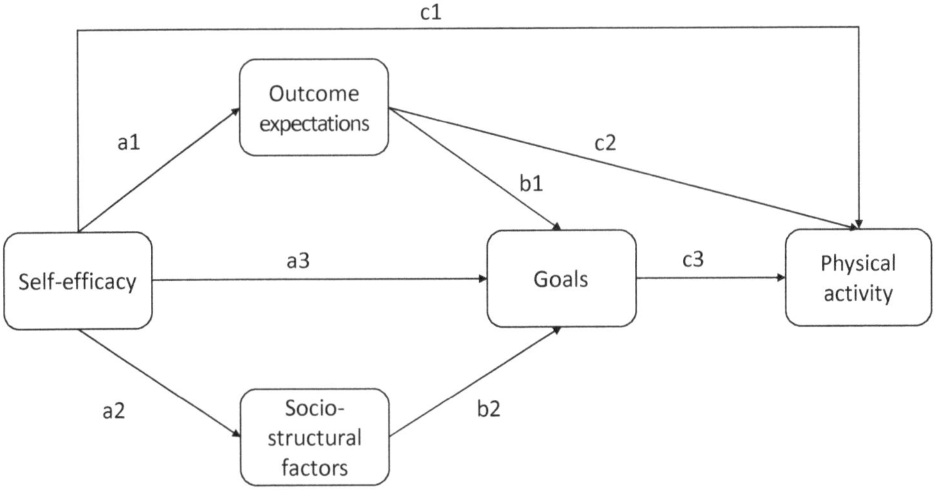

Figure 1. Schematic representation of the relationships between the constructs of social cognitive theory, as proposed by Bandura (2000).

Previous studies confirmed the central role of self-efficacy and pointed to its direct and indirect effects on physical activity behavior (see, for example, Young et al., 2014 meta-analysis). The role of outcome expectations as a mediator in the SCT model has also been confirmed (Tulloch et al., 2020; Wójcicki et al., 2009). Furthermore, it can be inferred from previous empirical findings that goal setting has a direct effect on physical activity behavior (Zechner & Gill, 2016), and there is evidence that social environmental factors, which operate from the outside, also influence physical activity (Gothe, 2018; Hamilton et al., 2017; Sweeney et al., 2017).

However, evidence for the predictive and explanatory power of SCT concerning physical activity was shown predominantly for specific samples, for example, populations with diseases such as multiple sclerosis (e.g., Baird et al., 2021; Silveira & Motl, 2019), type 2 diabetes (e.g., Sebastian et al., 2021), severe mental illness (e.g., Zechner & Gill, 2016), cancer (e.g., Auster-Gussman et al., 2022; Stacey et al., 2015), and obesity (e.g., Young et al., 2016). Relatively little research addresses healthy adult populations (Young et al., 2014).

Secondly, SCT has rarely been fully tested and modeled, as intended by Bandura. Bandura himself criticized this early on, as stated by Luszczynska and Schwarzer (2015, p. 229): "Some authors seem to believe that SCT is equivalent to self-efficacy theory (SET), provoking repeated statements by Bandura (1997) that SCT is not a 'one-factor theory'". Similarly, in their systematic review of studies concerning SCT in the context of physical activity, Young et al. (2014) criticize "the majority of SCT research has focused solely upon self-efficacy or examined self-efficacy in combination with only one or two other variables" (p. 985). Accordingly, the recommendations for research on SCT are as follows: "To generate more valid data regarding the utility of SCT to explain PA, it is crucial that future studies include measures for all constructs in appropriately specified structural equation models and report the direct, indirect, and total effects of all variables." (Young et al., 2016, p. N184).

Thirdly, there is a lack of evidence on the explanatory and predictive power of SCT concerning physical activity in Germany. To the best of our knowledge, there is exactly one study that has this focus. However, this study by Gellert et al. (2012) examined older adults aged 60–95 years and focused on affective and health-related outcome expectations. This, in turn, meets points 1 and 2 of the above-mentioned critique and confirms the need for a study on the explanatory power of SCT in the healthy general population in Germany that considers all the constructs and relationships between the elements envisaged by Bandura and verifies their tenability.

Therefore, the present study centers on three lines of inquiry:

We assume that the model fits the data and that it describes the theoretically stated relations between self-efficacy, outcome expectations, socio-structural factors, goal setting, and physical activity in its entity (RQ1).

Additionally, we examine the direct effect of self-efficacy on physical activity, as well as the direct effects of outcome expectations and goal setting on physical activity (RQ2).

Furthermore, we investigate the indirect effects of self-efficacy, outcome expectations, and socio-structural factors on physical activity (RQ3).

2. Materials and Methods

2.1. Sample and Procedure

Participants were recruited by posting notices on campus and in cultural centers in Saarland, Germany, in addition to placing online advertisements. The study was conducted on subjects between 18 and 64 years of age who had a command of the German language at the native speaker level and who did not have any health restrictions that would preclude participation in physical activity. Prior to analysis, data from subjects under the age of 18 ($n = 2$) or over the age of 64 ($n = 3$) were excluded. The survey was terminated for respondents indicating a lower language proficiency than the established requirement ($n = 1$) or reporting physical limitations ($n = 0$). Consequently, the data from these participants was not incorporated into the analyses.

The survey was fully conducted online with SosciSurvey (Leiner, 2024). Accordingly, a self-selected random sample was available for analysis in this study. Figure 2 depicts the course of the data collection. Data collection comprised two questionnaires. Prior to their participation in this study, all subjects provided written informed consent. In the initial questionnaire, subjects were instructed to provide answers regarding their demographic data, and their expressions on the SCT scale were assessed. The second point of measurement occurred seven days later to assess physical activity. The analyses were conducted on a dataset that exclusively comprised responses from subjects who had completed both questionnaires. Consequently, subjects who had only completed the first questionnaire ($n = 46$) or had discontinued the completion of the first ($n = 15$) or second ($n = 0$) questionnaire were excluded from the analyses.

The final sample consisted of 194 (109 male, 85 female) participants with a mean age of 26.03 years (SD = 10.33). The average amount of physical activity per week in the sample was 2478.30 MET minutes (SD = 2687.70). Although this is considerably more than 600 MET minutes of total physical activity per week, which is recommended by the WHO, it is not unusually high. For example, the national report for Germany shows that 85% of Germans report exercising for much more than 600 MET minutes (Der DKV-Report | DKV, 2023), and international studies also show that this level of activity is not unusual (Kyu et al., 2016).

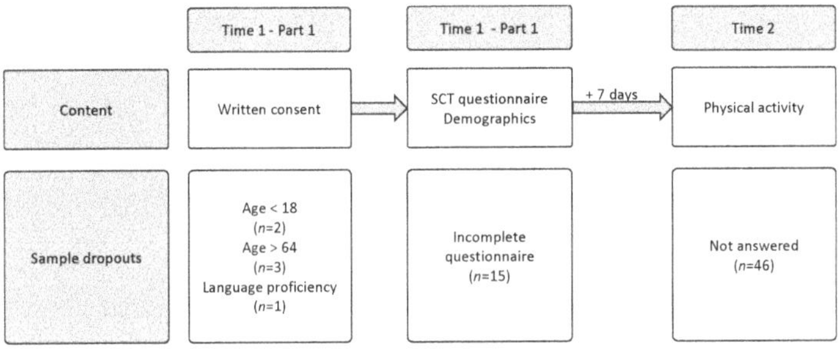

Figure 2. Course of the data collection.

2.2. Measures

Scales to measure the SCT components: A validated German scale to specifically assess the SCT components in the context of physical activity was applied (Egele & Stark, 2024). The scale consists of 18 items and has appropriate psychometric properties. We used an 11-point rating scale ranging from 0 (do not agree at all) to 10 (fully agree) for all items. Self-efficacy was measured by five items, its reliability was $\omega = 0.904$. Outcome expectations were also measured by five items, and their reliability was $\omega = 0.776$. The scale to measure goals comprised four items and its reliability was $\omega = 0.891$. Finally, social cognitive factors were measured by four items, with a reliability of $\omega = 0.741$.

Physical activity: Physical activity was assessed using the International Physical Activity Questionnaire—Short Form (Booth et al., 1996). The IPAQ-SF is a retrospective self-report questionnaire in which respondents rate their physical activity over the past seven days. The questions record the number of days with physical activity and the average time (measured in minutes) spent walking, performing moderate, and vigorous physical activity in an open-ended response format. All items for moderate and vigorous physical activity were presented with additional descriptions of example activities to foster a better understanding. We calculated the metabolic equivalent of task (MET) according to the formulas provided in the IPAQ manual. To achieve a total score of physical activity, the METs for walking, moderate, and vigorous physical activity were added. The resulting score was multiplied by the factor 1/1000 to avoid too large variances.

2.3. Statistical Analysis

All calculations were performed in R (R Core Team, 2020) using the packages lavaan (Rosseel, 2012) and psych (Revelle, 2023). To test our hypotheses, we set up the model shown in Figure 1 as a structural equation model (SEM) with latent variables. The SEM is composed of a measurement model part and a structural model part, the latter of which describes the theoretically stated relations between the individual constructs in SCT. Physical activity in terms of MET was included as a manifest variable. Because some of the latent variables' indicators and MET had skewed distributions, we used the MLM estimator with the Satorra–Bentler-scaled χ^2-test statistic and robust standard errors. Indirect and total effects were implemented through defined parameters.

To investigate the RQ1, we considered the model fit. Firstly, we investigated the measurement model of each latent variable separately with a one-factor confirmatory factor analysis (CFA). Afterwards, we also investigated a complete CFA model with all latent variables to investigate the model fit of the whole measurement model. The model fit was evaluated according to the criteria of Schermelleh-Engel et al. (2003). According to this classification, a model with a good fit should have a χ^2-test statistic with a p-value greater than 0.05, and the RMSEA should be smaller than 0.05 with a p-value for the test of close fit greater than 0.10. For CFI, a value greater than 0.97, and for the SRMR, a value smaller than 0.05 reflects a good model fit.

Secondly, we estimated the SEM. The model with evaluation was performed with the before-mentioned criteria. The SEM's fit measures are global measures that simultaneously assess the fit of the measurement and the structural part of the SEM and thus do not allow the separate assessment of the SEM's structural part that consists of the theoretically stated relations (Lance et al., 2016). To obtain an evaluation of the structural part, Lance et al. (2016) propose to consider the C9 and C10 indices. The C9 index reflects a model comparison in which the assumed theoretical model is compared to a model that specifies no directional relationships among the latent variables, i.e., a model that only contains the latent variables' variances. The C9 index is a goodness-of-fit index that ranges between 0 and 1, i.e., the closer its value to 1, the better the structural model's fit. The C10 index refers to the absence of direct causal effects between specified variables, and stems from a model comparison between the assumed theoretical model and a model that contains the paths that were omitted in the theoretical model, which in our case is a model that contains a path between social–structural factors and physical activity. The C10 index is a badness-of-fit index that ranges between 0 and 1, i.e., the closer its value to 0 the better the structural model's fit. To calculate the C9 and C10 indices, we used the formulas provided by Lance et al. (2016) that rely on the model's χ^2-test statistics. Additionally, to obtain some indications concerning the usual fit indices, we fitted a further CFA model that contained the latent variables' covariances with MET. We used this model's covariance matrix to estimate a structural model part only. Hereafter, this model is referred to as a partial structural model. For this estimation, we used the ML estimator to obtain the usual χ^2-test statistic and the usual fit indices.

To investigate RQ2, we refer to the unstandardized path coefficients between the constructs of SCT and physical activity. For RQ3, we calculated the indirect effects (products of the path coefficients) and total effects (sum of direct and indirect effects).

For all effects, we also reported the standardized coefficients. All significance tests referring to RQ2 and RQ3 were conducted with a nominal significance level of $\alpha = 0.05$. Data are available from the corresponding author upon reasonable request.

3. Results

Table 1 shows the correlational analyses of the latent variables with physical activity. A close examination reveals a robust correlation between self-efficacy and outcome expectations, both with respect to goals and physical activity behavior. Notably, goals and physical activity behavior exhibit a lack of significant correlation with each other, as well as with sociostructural factors.

Table 1. Correlations of the latent variables with physical activity.

	Physical Activity	Self-Efficacy	Goals	Outcome Expectations	Sociostructural Factors
Physical activity	-				
Self-efficacy	0.378 ***	-			
Goals	0.069	0.516 ***	-		
Outcome expectations	0.196 ***	0.608 ***	0.479 ***	-	
Sociostructural factors	−0.021	−0.091	0.041	−0.040	-

Note. *** $p < 0.001$.

3.1. Results Concerning Research Question 1

The results concerning RQ1 are presented in Table 2. The one-factorial measurement models and the complete CFA models indicate a good fit for each model. The SEM also indicates a good global model fit for the combined measurement and structural model parts. Concerning the separate assessment of the structural model part, the C9 index is 0.999, which hints at an exceptionally good fit for the structural model part. The C10 index, which is 0.0013, indicates the same conclusion. Thus, the structural part separated from the measurement model also indicates a good fit. To sum up, the investigation provides evidence for the relations as stated in the SCT.

Table 2. Fit measure of the measurement and structural equation models.

	χ^2	*df*	*p*	CFI	SRMR	RMSEA	p_{close}
Self-efficacy	4.262	5	0.512	1.000	0.018	0.000	0.822
Goals	0.487	2	0.784	1.000	0.007	0.000	0.918
Outcome expectations	3.801	5	0.578	1.000	0.027	0.000	0.846
Socio-structural factors	1.451	2	0.484	1.000	0.023	0.000	0.689
Complete CFA	148.477	129	0.116	0.986	0.079	0.028	0.986
SEM	159.284	145	0.197	0.990	0.077	0.023	0.997
Null model *	294.195	-	-	-	-	-	-
All paths SEM *	158.795	-	-	-	-	-	-
Partial structural model	0.264	2	0.876	1.000	0.008	0.000	0.922

Note. * The null model and the all-paths SEM are used for the calculation of the C9 and C10 indices. For these calculations, the χ^2-test statistic and the models as such are not judged concerning their model fit. Therefore, the table only reports the χ^2-test statistics.

3.2. Results Concerning Research Question 2

Table 3 (upper panel) presents the results concerning the direct effects; see also Figure 1 for the names of the path coefficients, and Figure 3 for a path model depicting the standardized coefficients and the explained variance. The results indicate that there are significant direct effects between self-efficacy and outcome expectations (path a1), self-efficacy and goals (path a3), outcome expectations and goals (path b1), as well as self-efficacy and physical activity (path c1).

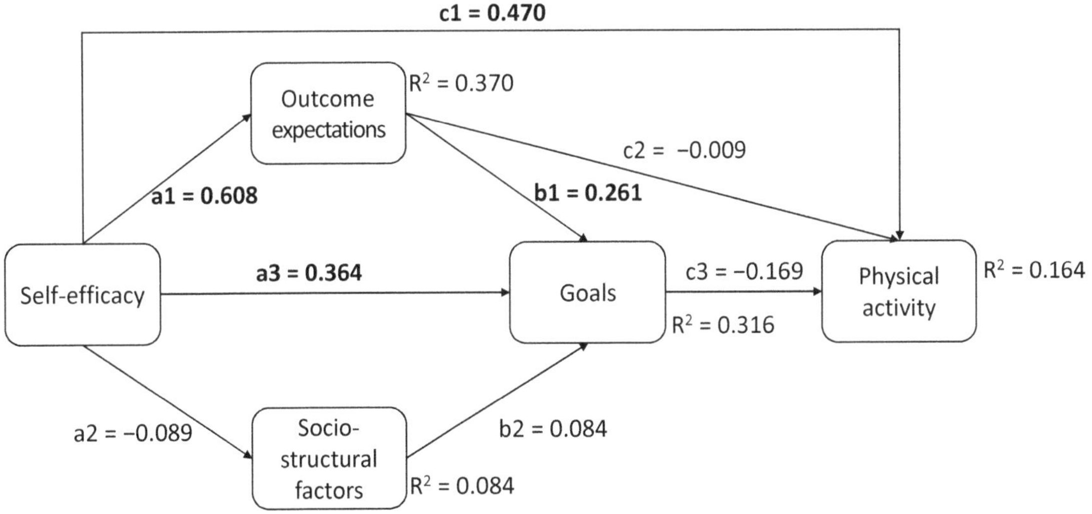

Figure 3. Path coefficients. Note: significant paths are marked in bold.

Table 3. Direct, indirect, and total effects for the standardized regression coefficients.

Paths	Estimate	*SE*	*z*	*p*
Total effect				
Total effect	**0.377**	0.057	6.661	<0.001
Direct effects (RQ2)				
a1	**0.608**	0.060	10.175	<0.001
a2	−0.089	0.083	−1.073	0.283
a3	**0.364**	0.095	3.824	<0.001
b1	**0.261**	0.107	2.441	0.015
b2	0.084	0.071	1.180	0.238
c1	**0.470**	0.107	4.391	<0.001
c2	−0.009	0.093	−0.095	0.924
c3	−0.169	0.095	−1.774	0.076
Indirect effects (RQ3)				
a1*c2	−0.005	0.057	−0.095	0.924
a1*b1	**0.159**	0.067	2.383	0.017
a1*b1*c3	−0.027	0.020	−1.324	0.186
a3*c3	−0.061	0.035	−1.747	0.081
a2*b2	−0.007	0.010	−0.717	0.474
a2*b2*c3	0.001	0.002	0.639	0.523
b1*c3	−0.044	0.033	−1.330	0.184
b2*c3	−0.014	0.015	−0.936	0.349
a1*c2+ a1*b1+c3+a2*b2*c3+a3*c3	−0.092	0.075	−1.237	0.216

Note. See Figure 1 for the designation of the path coefficients. All significance tests referring to RQ2 and RQ3 were conducted with a nominal significance level of $\alpha = 0.05$. Significant paths are marked in bold.

From an interpretative perspective, the results indicate, in combination with the good model fit of the structural part, that relations described by SCT are valid. However, some insignificant direct paths indicate that not all theoretically described relations are important, for example, the direct effect of self-efficacy on socio-structural factors, of socio-structural factors on goals, and of outcome expectations on physical activity.

3.3. Results Concerning Research Question 3

Concerning the indirect and total effects, the results are shown in Table 3 (lower panel). Only one indirect effect is statistically significant, namely the path from self-efficacy via outcome expectations to goals (path a1*b1). This result is in line with the results concerning the direct effects. The results indicate that the theoretically assumed relations seem valid but unimportant.

4. Discussion

4.1. Interpretation of Findings

This study aimed to examine the predictive power of SCT concerning physical activity behavior in a non-clinical sample. Therefore, all of Bandura's (2004) assumed relationships between the elements were taken into consideration, which has rarely been performed in the past. The present study makes a significant contribution to the field, as it employs an innovative analytical approach by considering the structural model independently from the measurement model. This enabled us to provide substantiated insights into the theoretical fit of Banduras assumptions concerning the relations of the constructs of SCT. The differentiation between the structural model and the measurement model is pivotal in facilitating the acquisition of substantiated insights into the validity of Bandura's assumptions concerning the relations of the constructs of SCT. The prevailing standard of the SEM procedure is characterized by its inability to differentiate between these models (Lance et al., 2016). As a consequence, the procedure fails to enable the independent evaluation of theoretical assumptions vis à vis the measurement assumptions, thus impeding a comprehensive and systematic examination of the theoretical underpinnings. Results showed the very good fit of the structural model, indicating that the theoretically stated relations between the constructs in SCT seem corroborated. However, it seems that some of the theoretically assumed relations are less important than others despite being valid, which will be discussed in the following.

Taking a closer look at the results, the significant direct effect of self-efficacy on physical activity in the present study joins many similar findings in the literature. This finding also corresponds to the fact that many interventions that promote physical activity behavior focus on self-efficacy (Tang et al., 2019).

The indirect effect of self-efficacy on physical activity is rarely reported, and in the cases where it is reported, evidence for significance is often absent, as in the present study. Perhaps the complexity of the indirect effect plays a role here, as it includes several paths. Given the analysis of the individual pathways that follow later, which together result in the indirect effect of self-efficacy on physical activity, the question arises whether some of these pathways are more relevant than others. Subsequently, it could be considered if the assumed indirect effect could be slimmed down, i.e., whether it is possible to distance oneself from the assumption of an all-encompassing indirect effect. A second consideration, however, is the relevance of the indirect effect of self-efficacy on physical activity against the background of the direct effect of self-efficacy on physical activity being so well documented. The question arises to what extent a potential indirect effect is of importance if a direct effect on physical activity behavior can be achieved in interventions by promoting self-efficacy.

As suggested by previous findings, outcome expectations would have a significant direct effect on physical activity behavior in our study. However, in the Young et al. (2014) meta-analysis, a positive and significant effect of outcome expectations on physical activity behavior was reported in about 30% of studies that examined the effect of outcome expectancies on physical activity. Our findings may contribute to the body of studies that investigated the effect but have been unable to prove it. It is similarly conceivable that this finding can be attributed to the measurement of outcome expectations, given that only positive outcome expectations were queried on the scale employed. Perhaps the impact of negative action outcome expectations on exercise behavior is more pronounced than that of positive experiences, explaining the non-significant relation. Alternatively, it would also be plausible that outcome expectations are of greater importance for individuals with lower levels of physical activity than for those who are more active. As the present sample was already active, it is possible that outcome expectations were not the deciding factor for physical activity. Therefore, it seems relevant to examine which factors influence the occurrence and the direction of the effect.

A significant indirect effect of outcome expectations on physical activity is rarely reported (c.f. Young et al., 2014). No evidence for this indirect effect was found in the present study either. However, the fact that goals had no significant effect on physical activity behavior in the present study (see the next section)—in contrast to previous findings in the literature—may also have had an influence. Studies that report an indirect effect of outcome expectations on physical activity like Gellert et al. (2012) demonstrate an indirect pathway mediated by "intention". Goals may be conceptualized more broadly than intentions, which might explain why the effect was not significant in our study.

Goals are usually consistently associated with physical activity behavior in the literature. In this study, the effect was not significant, hinting at a possible intention–behavior gap. The absence of a discernible correlation is further substantiated by the bivariate correlation analysis of goals and exercise behavior. The absence of a substantial correlation could be ascribed, at least in part, to the item formulation. Nevertheless, the observation that goals are closely associated with self-efficacy and outcome expectations provides a compelling counterargument to this assertion. Consequently, it can be deduced that a discordance exists between goals and physical activity behavior, as recorded in this study. Future studies should re-examine this relation, especially as more recent research results also show that it might be beneficial to assess goals more specifically tailored, i.e., adapted, to the type, quantity, and intensity of the respective physical activity (Conner & Norman, 2022).

Bandura does not include the direct effect of socio-structural factors on behavior. This restriction seems appropriate, as the structural model fit with this restriction was good. The fact that also no indirect effect of socio-structural factors on physical activity behavior was found is consistent with previous findings reporting that socio-structural factors do not seem to have a significant indirect effect on physical activity. Nevertheless, the question arises to what extent socio-structural factors play a role in physical activity behavior if neither a direct nor an indirect influence on physical activity behavior can be confirmed. Potentially, it would be beneficial to conduct moderator analyses to ascertain whether the effect is present under specific circumstances.

At this juncture, a discussion of the correlation matrix of the social–cognitive factors with each other, as well as with the criterion, is warranted, with a special focus on the socio-structural factors. While the majority of the bivariate correlations are consistent, it is evident that the socio-structural factors do not exhibit a significant correlation with any other construct. This may be attributable to the heterogeneity of the construct; alternatively, it is plausible that the sample utilized led to a restriction of variance in this domain. Notwithstanding, given the absence of a statistically significant correlation between the socio-structural factors and physical activity behavior, it is not unexpected that the model with a corresponding path restriction exhibits a satisfactory fit.

Overall, our findings are broadly consistent with previous findings, supporting the utility of SCT to explain physical activity. Yet, some differences between the present findings and common previous findings need to be discussed.

Despite a good model fit, the variance explained in physical activity behavior was smaller than in similar studies (e.g., meta-analysis by Young et al., 2016: R2 = 0.30). Multiple aspects can be mentioned. Firstly, meta-analyses show that the average age of the subjects is a moderator of the variance explained in the criterion. While more variance can be explained in older subjects (Young et al., 2014), the relatively young average age in the present sample could be one explanation for the smaller variance explained. Secondly, the homogeneity of our sample may have limited the extent to which the observed variance could be explained. Finally, the criterion of physical activity behavior was recorded employing IPAQ. The IPAQ is a common tool for recording physical activity, but is not free of criticism—for example, it is susceptible to bias based on self-reporting (Egele et al., 2021; Straßburg et al., 2019). The IPAQ captures a total physical activity score, which includes vigorous and moderate physical activity as well as walking. While several studies use a similar criterion, "a measure of total PA" (Young et al., 2014, p. 987), some have also captured physical activity more precisely and more objectively, such as via a number of steps. Therefore, the criterion capture per se may have an impact on the variance explained.

It also seems important to consider that behavior often proves less predictable than the goals or the intention to exhibit certain behaviors. This phenomenon, referred to as the "intention–behavior gap", is a well-documented occurrence, especially in the context of physical activity (Feil et al., 2023), and was also shown in the present study. While the variance explained in physical activity was rather small, a far larger share of the variance of goals could be explained. Meta-analyses show that while intentions or goals seem necessary for behavior, it seems like the probability of translating this intention into behavior is random at best (Feil et al., 2023; Rhodes & de Bruijn, 2013). Recent research shows that assessing not only goals but also the strength or stability of these goals could lead to a more accurate explanation of behavior (Conner & Norman, 2022). This was not explicitly included in Bandura's goal construct but might be worth adding in the future to reduce the intention–behavior gap.

If we consider the findings and their classification in the previous literature and research, we conclude that SCT seems to be suitable to explain physical activity behavior in a healthy sample. However, more research is needed to delve deeper into the indirect pathways and underlying mechanisms that influence physical activity behavior within the SCT framework.

In addition, potential moderators (e.g., age, sex, physical activity level, and other personal characteristics) should be investigated regarding their effect on the adequacy of the theoretical assumptions.

4.2. Limitations

It is important to note that the representativeness of the sample may be limited by the distorted gender ratio. Consequently, the results should be replicated in further studies to secure external validity. Further studies could illuminate the question of whether some paths are truly non-significant in a non-clinical sample, as found in the present study, or whether sample characteristics lead to non-significant paths. Furthermore, to generalize the results, it would be beneficial to replicate the study with a criterion that is more objectively recorded.

Another possible issue is the sample size. Typical recommendations for the MLM estimator are sample sizes of 250 or greater (e.g., Hu & Bentler, 1999). Our sample only amounts to 194 participants, so it undercuts the recommendation by about 22%. A possible problem with a smaller sample size than recommended is overcorrecting the standard errors. However, this issue does not likely affect our results, as we did not find as many significant paths as theoretically expected. In this respect, we want to point out that such sample size boundaries are only recommendations that should not be considered definitive. Nonetheless, the sample size may have constrained the capacity to discern potentially substantial pathways. This limitation could serve as a rationale for the observed insignificance of certain pathways.

Additionally, based on our findings, we cannot determine whether the good fit of the theoretical assumptions of SCT actually corresponds to the interaction of the constructs. Recently, for example, the directionality of the paths has been increasingly questioned (e.g., Beauchamp et al., 2019) and this matter cannot be clarified based on the data of this study.

4.3. Theoretical and Practical Implications

The present study confirms the tenability of the theoretical assumptions of social-cognitive theory as set out by Bandura. This conclusion seems particularly solid due to the distinction made between the structural model and the measurement model, which enabled the provision of substantiated insights into the theoretical fit of Bandura's assumptions concerning the relations of the constructs of SCT. The standard SEM procedure fails to differentiate between the structural and measurement models, thereby precluding the independent evaluation of theoretical assumptions against the measurement assumptions. In contrast, the approach adopted in this study to address the specified research question is commendable. The verification of the theoretical assumptions is of paramount importance, given the persistent utilization of social–cognitive theory as a foundational framework for behavioral explanation and modification studies (Luszczynska & Schwarzer, 2015). Consequently, it was imperative to ascertain the empirical validity of the theoretically postulated relations.

Despite the ostensible validity of the theoretical underpinnings of SCT, it has been demonstrated that certain pathways hold greater significance than others. At the forefront of this discourse lies the role of self-efficacy, which exerts a strong direct influence on behavior. The significant direct impact of self-efficacy on behavior, as compared to the seemingly lesser relevance of alternate pathways, prompts the examination of whether the implementation of SCT is warranted. Alternatively, the inquiry extends to whether the adoption of self-efficacy theory (Bandura, 1977) as a fundamental framework might yield equivalent outcomes.

The validation of the theoretical assumptions underlying SCT has significant ramifications for the field of practice. For instance, further studies grounded in SCT can be pursued to elucidate and modify behaviors. It can be contended that the present findings provide a robust basis for the initiation of additional studies, as a prevailing criticism of the theory—namely, the absence of a holistic model (Beyera et al., 2021)—has been addressed. In light of our findings, we would advocate for the prominent role of self-efficacy as a potential starting point for behavior change interventions and recommend targeting it due to its strong effect. Behavior change research offers numerous approaches for fostering self-efficacy concerning physical activity (e.g., Stojanovic et al., 2021; Warner & Schwarzer, 2020). The findings of this study can also be significant in everyday life, both for health practitioners and for individuals. For instance, the role of mastery experiences, which have been demonstrated to influence self-efficacy (Wiedenman et al., 2024), can be leveraged to enhance self-efficacy, which in turn can impact physical activity behavior. Analogous considerations can be drawn when examining outcome expectations; it may be feasible to deliberately focus on positive outcome expectations in order to manifest a desired behavior. Consequently, the present study provides important theoretical implications while also highlighting potential practical consequences.

5. Conclusions

The current study supports previous studies finding that SCT is useful in explaining physical activity behavior. Previous findings were extended by a holistic examination of the theory and a specific focus on the fit of the structural model assumed by Bandura. Nonetheless, previous studies that only investigated selected elements of the theory were also corroborated in that this study demonstrated the greater importance of certain model elements, including, in particular, self-efficacy and expected outcomes.

Author Contributions: Conceptualization, V.S.E., E.K. and R.S.; methodology, V.S.E. and E.K.; software, V.S.E. and E.K.; validation, V.S.E. and E.K.; formal analysis, E.K.; investigation, V.S.E.; resources, R.S.; data curation, V.S.E.; writing—original draft preparation, V.S.E.; writing—review and editing, V.S.E., E.K. and R.S.; visualization, V.S.E. and E.K.; supervision, R.S.; project administration, R.S. All authors have read and agreed to the published version of the manuscript.

Funding: This research received no external funding.

Institutional Review Board Statement: Ethical approval was not required for the studies involving humans because of local legislation and institutional requirements. The studies were conducted in accordance with the local legislation and institutional requirements. The ethical committee confirmed that ethics approval is not required for this type of study.

Informed Consent Statement: Informed consent was obtained from all subjects involved in the study.

Data Availability Statement: Data are available from the authors upon request.

Conflicts of Interest: The authors declare no conflicts of interest.

References

Auster-Gussman, L. A., Gavin, K. L., Siddique, J., Welch, W. A., Solk, P., Whitaker, M., Cullather, E., Fanning, J., Maria, C. S., Gradishar, W., Khan, S., Kulkarni, S., & Phillips, S. M. (2022). Social cognitive variables and physical activity during chemotherapy for breast cancer: An intensive longitudinal examination. *Psycho-Oncology, 31*(3), 425–435. [CrossRef] [PubMed]

Baird, J. F., Silveira, S. L., & Motl, R. W. (2021). Social cognitive theory and physical activity in older adults with multiple sclerosis. *International Journal of MS Care, 23*(1), 21–25. [CrossRef] [PubMed]

Bandura, A. (1977). Self-efficacy: Toward a unifying theory of behavioral change. *Psychological Review, 84*, 191–215. [CrossRef] [PubMed]

Bandura, A. (1986). *Social foundations of thought and action: A social cognitive theory* (pp. xiii, 617). Prentice-Hall, Inc.

Bandura, A. (1997). *Self-efficacy: The exercise of control.* Freeman.

Bandura, A. (2000). Health promotion from the perspective of social cognitive theory. In C. Abraham, P. Norman, & M. Conner (Eds.), *Understanding and changing health behaviour: From health beliefs to self-regulation* (1st ed., pp. 299–339). Psychology Press.

Bandura, A. (2004). Health promotion by social cognitive means. *Health Education & Behavior, 31*(2), 143–164. [CrossRef]

Beauchamp, M. R., Crawford, K. L., & Jackson, B. (2019). Social cognitive theory and physical activity: Mechanisms of behavior change, critique, and legacy. *Psychology of Sport and Exercise, 42*, 110–117. [CrossRef]

Beyera, G. K., O'Brien, J., & Campbell, S. (2021). Choosing a health behaviour theory or model for related research projects: A narrative review. *Journal of Research in Nursing, 27*(5), 436—446. [CrossRef]

Booth, M. L., Owen, N., Bauman, A. E., & Gore, C. J. (1996). Retest reliability of recall measures of leisure-time physical activity in Australian adults. *International Journal of Epidemiology, 25*(1), 153–159. [CrossRef]

Conner, M., & Norman, P. (2022). Understanding the intention-behavior gap: The role of intention strength. *Frontiers in Psychology, 13*, 923464. [CrossRef]

Der DKV-Report | DKV. (2023). Available online: https://www.dkv.com/der-dkv-report.html (accessed on 5 December 2023).

Egele, V. S., & Stark, R. (2024). Operationalization of the social cognitive theory to explain and predict physical activity in Germany: A scale development. *Frontiers in Sports and Active Living, 6*, 1508602. [CrossRef]

Egele, V. S., Kiefer, L. H., & Stark, R. (2021). Faking self-reports of health behavior: A comparison between a within-and a between-subjects design. *Health Psychology and Behavioral Medicine, 9*(1), 895–916. [CrossRef]

Feil, K., Fritsch, J., & Rhodes, R. E. (2023). The intention-behaviour gap in physical activity: A systematic review and meta-analysis of the action control framework. *British Journal of Sports Medicine, 57*(19), 1265–1271. [CrossRef] [PubMed]

Gellert, P., Ziegelmann, J. P., & Schwarzer, R. (2012). Affective and health-related outcome expectancies for physical activity in older adults. *Psychology & Health, 27*(7), 816–828. [CrossRef]

Gothe, N. P. (2018). Correlates of physical activity in urban African American adults and older adults: Testing the social cognitive theory. *Annals of Behavioral Medicine, 52*(9), 743–751. [CrossRef] [PubMed]

Hamilton, K., Warner, L. M., & Schwarzer, R. (2017). The role of self-efficacy and friend support on adolescent vigorous physical activity. *Health Education & Behavior, 44*(1), 175–181. [CrossRef]

Heiss, V. J., & Petosa, R. L. (2016). Social cognitive theory correlates of moderate-intensity exercise among adults with type 2 diabetes. *Psychology, Health & Medicine, 21*(1), 92–101. [CrossRef]

Hu, L. T., & Bentler, P. M. (1999). Cutoff criteria for fit indexes in covariance structure analysis: Conventional criteria versus new alternatives. *Structural Equation Modeling: A Multidisciplinary Journal, 6*(1), 1–55. [CrossRef]

Kyu, H. H., Bachman, V. F., Alexander, L. T., Mumford, J. E., Afshin, A., Estep, K., Veerman, J. L., Delwiche, K., Iannarone, M. L., Moyer, M. L., Cercy, K., Vos, T., Murray, C. J. L., & Forouzanfar, M. H. (2016). Physical activity and risk of breast cancer, colon cancer, diabetes, ischemic heart disease, and ischemic stroke events: Systematic review and dose-response meta-analysis for the Global Burden of Disease Study 2013. *BMJ, 354*, i3857. [CrossRef]

Lance, C. E., Beck, S. S., Fan, Y., & Carter, N. T. (2016). A taxonomy of path-related goodness-of-fit indices and recommended criterion values. *Psychological Methods, 21*(3), 388. [CrossRef]

Leiner, D. J. (2024). *SoSci Survey* (Version 3.1.06) [Computer software]. Available online: https://www.soscisurvey.de (accessed on 12 December 2024).

Luszczynska, A., & Schwarzer, R. K. (2015). *Social cognitive theory.* McGraw Hill. Available online: https://acuresearchbank.acu.edu.au/item/87306/social-cognitive-theory (accessed on 12 December 2024).

Miko, H.-C., Zillmann, N., Ring-Dimitriou, S., Dorner, T. E., Titze, S., & Bauer, R. (2020). Auswirkungen von Bewegung auf die Gesundheit. *Das Gesundheitswesen, 82*(S 3), S184–S195. [CrossRef]

R Core Team. (2020). *European Environment Agency.* (n.d.). [Methodology Reference]. Available online: https://www.eea.europa.eu/data-and-maps/indicators/oxygen-consuming-substances-in-rivers/r-development-core-team-2006 (accessed on 12 December 2024).

Revelle, W. (2023). *psych: Procedures for psychological, psychometric, and personality research* (2.3.3) [Computer software]. Available online: https://cran.r-project.org/web/packages/psych/index.html (accessed on 12 December 2024).

Rhodes, R. E., & de Bruijn, G.-J. (2013). How big is the physical activity intention–behaviour gap? A meta-analysis using the action control framework. *British Journal of Health Psychology*, *18*(2), 296–309. [CrossRef]

Rosseel, Y. (2012). lavaan: An R package for structural equation modeling. *Journal of Statistical Software*, *48*, 1–36. [CrossRef]

Schermelleh-Engel, K., Moosbrugger, H., & Müller, H. (2003). Evaluating the fit of structural equation models: Tests of significance and descriptive goodness-of-fit measures. *Methods of Psychological Research*, *8*, 23–74.

Sebastian, A. T., Rajkumar, E., Tejaswini, P., Lakshmi, R., & Romate, J. (2021). Applying social cognitive theory to predict physical activity and dietary behavior among patients with type-2 diabetes. *Health Psychology Research*, *9*(1), 24510. [CrossRef] [PubMed]

Silveira, S. L., & Motl, R. W. (2019). Do Social Cognitive Theory constructs explain response heterogeneity with a physical activity behavioral intervention in multiple sclerosis? *Contemporary Clinical Trials Communications*, *15*, 100366. [CrossRef]

Stacey, F. G., James, E. L., Chapman, K., Courneya, K. S., & Lubans, D. R. (2015). A systematic review and meta-analysis of social cognitive theory-based physical activity and/or nutrition behavior change interventions for cancer survivors. *Journal of Cancer Survivorship: Research and Practice*, *9*(2), 305–338. [CrossRef] [PubMed]

Stojanovic, M., Fries, S., & Grund, A. (2021). Self-Efficacy in habit building: How general and habit-specific self-efficacy influence behavioral automatization and motivational interference. *Frontiers in Psychology*, *12*, 643753. [CrossRef]

Strain, T., Flaxman, S., Guthold, R., Semenova, E., Cowan, M., Riley, L. M., Bull, F. C., & Stevens, G. A. (2024). National, regional, and global trends in insufficient physical activity among adults from 2000 to 2022: A pooled analysis of 507 population-based surveys with 5· 7 million participants. *The Lancet Global Health*, *12*(8), e1232−e1243. [CrossRef]

Straßburg, A., Eisinger-Watzl, M., Krems, C., Roth, A., & Hoffmann, I. (2019). Comparison of food consumption and nutrient intake assessed with three dietary assessment methods: Results of the German National Nutrition Survey II. *European Journal of Nutrition*, *58*(1), 193–210. [CrossRef]

Sweeney, A. M., Wilson, D. K., Lee, & Van Horn, M. (2017). Longitudinal relationships between self-concept for physical activity and neighborhood social life as predictors of physical activity among older African American adults. *International Journal of Behavioral Nutrition and Physical Activity*, *14*(1), 67. [CrossRef]

Tang, M. Y., Smith, D. M., Mc Sharry, J., Hann, M., & French, D. P. (2019). Behavior change techniques associated with changes in postintervention and maintained changes in self-efficacy for physical activity: A systematic review with meta-analysis. *Annals of Behavioral Medicine*, *53*(9), 801–815. [CrossRef]

Taylor, L. M., Raine, K. D., Plotnikoff, R. C., Vallance, J. K., Sharma, A. M., & Spence, J. C. (2016). Understanding physical activity in individuals with prediabetes: An application of social cognitive theory. *Psychology, Health & Medicine*, *21*(2), 254–260. [CrossRef]

Tulloch, H., Heenan, A., Sweet, S., Goldfield, G. S., Kenny, G. P., Alberga, A. S., & Sigal, R. J. (2020). Depressive symptoms, perceived stress, self-efficacy, and outcome expectations: Predict fitness among adolescents with obesity. *Journal of Health Psychology*, *25*(6), 798–809. [CrossRef] [PubMed]

Warner, L. M., & Schwarzer, R. (2020). Self-efficacy and health. In K. Sweeny, M. L. Robbins, & L. M. Cohen (Eds.), *The wiley encyclopedia of health psychology: Volume II, the social bases of health behavior* (pp. 605–613). Wiley-Blackwell. [CrossRef]

Wiedenman, E. M., Kruse-Diehr, A. J., Bice, M. R., McDaniel, J., Wallace, J. P., & Partridge, J. A. (2024). The role of sport participation on exercise self-efficacy, psychological need satisfaction, and resilience among college freshmen. *Journal of American College Health*, *72*(9), 3507–3514. [CrossRef] [PubMed]

World Health Organization. (2018). *Global action plan on physical activity 2018–2030: More active people for a healthier world*. World Health Organization. Available online: https://apps.who.int/iris/handle/10665/272722 (accessed on 12 December 2024).

Wójcicki, T. R., White, S. M., & McAuley, E. (2009). Assessing outcome expectations in older adults: The multidimensional outcome expectations for exercise scale. *The Journals of Gerontology: Series B*, *64B*(1), 33–40. [CrossRef] [PubMed]

Young, M. D., Plotnikoff, R. C., Collins, C. E., Callister, R., & Morgan, P. J. (2014). Social cognitive theory and physical activity: A systematic review and meta-analysis. *Obesity Reviews*, *15*(12), 983–995. [CrossRef] [PubMed]

Young, M. D., Plotnikoff, R. C., Collins, C. E., Callister, R., & Morgan, P. J. (2016). A test of social cognitive theory to explain men's physical activity during a gender-tailored weight loss program. *American Journal of Men's Health*, *10*(6), NP176–NP187. [CrossRef]

Zechner, M. R., & Gill, K. J. (2016). Predictors of physical activity in persons with mental illness: Testing a social cognitive model. *Psychiatric Rehabilitation Journal*, *39*, 321–327. [CrossRef] *healthcare* MDPI

Article

Exploring Telemedicine Usage Intention Using Technology Acceptance Model and Social Capital Theory

Liang-Hsi Kung [1,2], Yu-Hua Yan [2,*] and Chih-Ming Kung [3]

1 Department of Nursing, College of Medicine, National Cheng Kung University, No. 1, University Road, Tainan City 701, Taiwan; 2u0635@mail.tmh.org.tw
2 Tainan Municipal Hospital (Managed by Show Chwan Medical Care Corporation), No. 670, Chongde Road, East District, Tainan City 701, Taiwan
3 Department of Information Technology and Communication, Shih Chien University Kaohsiung, No. 200, Daxue Road, Neimen District, Kaohsiung City 84550, Taiwan; alex@cvig.org
* Correspondence: 2d0003@mail.tmh.org.tw; Tel.: +886-6-260-9926; Fax: +886-6-260-6351

Abstract: Telemedicine technology has emerged as a pivotal solution to enhance the accessibility and efficiency of healthcare services. This study investigates the factors influencing the acceptance of telemedicine technology among healthcare professionals in Taiwan. Employing a quantitative research approach, we utilized a survey instrument adapted from the Unified Theory of Acceptance and Use of Technology (UTAUT) model. Data were collected from 325 healthcare professionals across diverse medical fields. The results indicate that perceived usefulness, ease of use, social influence, and convenience significantly influence intention to use telemedicine. Moreover, age moderates the relationship between perceived usefulness and usage intention. These findings underscore the importance of addressing both technological and social factors in promoting the adoption of telemedicine among healthcare professionals. Policy implications and recommendations for enhancing telemedicine implementation are discussed based on the study findings. Specifically, our findings highlight that perceived usefulness, ease of use, social influence, and convenience significantly impact the intention to use telemedicine technology. Age significantly moderates the relationship between perceived usefulness and usage intention. These results not only theoretically support the UTAUT model but also provide practical strategies to advance the application of telemedicine technology.

Keywords: telemedicine; technology acceptance model; urban; rural; healthcare consumers; Taiwan

1. Introduction

The global outbreak of Coronavirus Disease 2019 (COVID-19) has had profound impacts worldwide, presenting significant challenges to physical health and imposing substantial burdens on public mental health [1–3]. In response to the pandemic's strain on healthcare systems, telemedicine has emerged as a critical tool, transcending temporal and spatial barriers between healthcare providers and patients, thereby preventing system collapse and substituting traditional face-to-face consultations [4]. This paradigm shift has garnered unprecedented attention and is increasingly recognized as a pivotal direction in many advanced countries [5].

In Taiwan, the rapid adoption of telemedicine during the COVID-19 pandemic has highlighted challenges related to regulatory frameworks, system flexibility, and cost-effectiveness [6,7]. Overcoming these hurdles requires strategic planning to integrate telemedicine into existing medical processes while ensuring the delivery of high-quality care and fostering patient trust [8]. The severity of the COVID-19 epidemic in Taiwan prompted proactive measures, including the issuance of operational guidelines by the National Health Insurance Special Medical Institutions, expanding telemedicine services to encompass a broader segment of the population beyond their initial scope [9]. This initiative marks a significant milestone towards the widespread adoption of telemedicine in Taiwan.

The successful establishment of telemedicine services hinges on several critical factors, including institutional norms, technological advancements, healthcare providers' readiness, and patient acceptance [10]. These factors are widely acknowledged as crucial in promoting telemedicine adoption across diverse healthcare settings [11,12]. Specifically, reference #11 emphasizes that perceived usefulness, perceived ease of use, and user attitudes significantly influence acceptance levels. Our study extends this foundational research by validating and expanding upon these findings within the specific context of telemedicine adoption in Taiwan. By doing so, we contribute novel empirical insights that enhance the theoretical foundations essential for informed policy-making and implementation strategies.

Telemedicine necessitates transformative shifts in patient–provider communication and engagement [13,14], reshaping user behavior through various applications [15]. Davis, Bagozzi, and Warshaw's Technology Acceptance Model (TAM) provides a robust framework for understanding user behaviors towards information technology systems, emphasizing internal factors such as perceived usefulness, ease of use, attitude, and intention to use [16]. TAM is instrumental in elucidating user attitudes towards new technologies and analyzing the factors that influence their acceptance.

Social Capital Theory (SCT), proposed by Bourdieu [17] and Coleman [18], underscores the role of social networks in cultivating trust and achieving individual goals [19]. Trust, a fundamental element of social capital, facilitates cooperation and enhances organizational efficiency [20,21]. Social influence within networks significantly impacts technology adoption [22–24], illustrating how established trust and influence contribute to resource accumulation [25]. A comprehensive understanding of these factors is imperative for advancing telemedicine adoption and guiding future governmental policies.

This study aims to explore behavioral intentions towards telemedicine adoption using TAM and SCT as theoretical frameworks, thereby providing insights crucial for policy-making. The empirical validation of our research model further enhances our understanding of these dynamics.

2. Materials and Methods

2.1. Theoretical Frameworks and Hypotheses

In this study, the TAM and SCT were employed as theoretical frameworks to investigate factors influencing patients' adoption of telemedicine. TAM components include perceived ease of use, perceived usefulness, and attitude, while SCT encompasses social influence and trust. By concurrently applying and integrating these theories, the study examines their combined impact on usage intention. The research hypotheses formulated are as follows (See Figure 1):

Hypothesis 1 (H1). *Perceived ease of use positively affects patients' perceived usefulness of participating in telemedicine.*

Hypothesis 2 (H2). *Perceived usefulness has a positive effect on patients' attitude toward telemedicine participation.*

Hypothesis 3 (H3). *Perceived ease of use has a positive effect on patients' attitude toward using telemedicine participation.*

Hypothesis 4 (H4). *Trust has a positive effect on patients' attitude toward participating in telemedicine.*

Hypothesis 5 (H5). *Social influence has a positive effect on patients' attitude toward participating in telemedicine.*

Hypothesis 6 (H6). *Patients' participation in telemedicine has a positive impact on usage intention.*

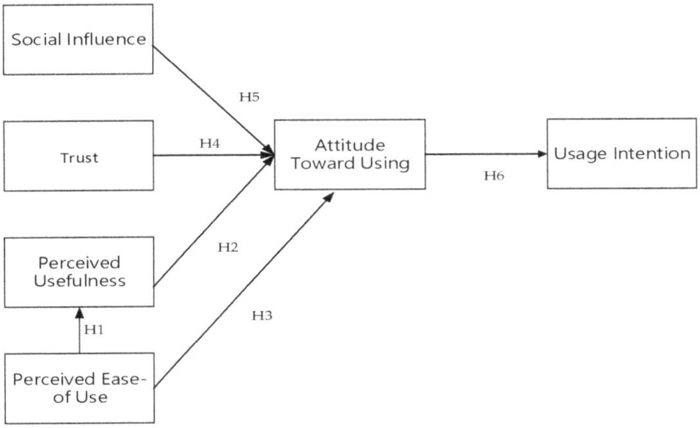

Figure 1. Research model.

2.2. *Sample Size Determination and Sampling*

Sample size determination followed the principles recommended for structural equation modeling (SEM) studies, aiming for a minimum ratio of 10 participants per estimated parameter. Considering the study's inclusion of 21 observed variables and a hypothesized structural model, a targeted minimum sample size of 210 participants was established.

The study population comprised patients who had previously utilized telemedicine services within [specific healthcare settings or geographic region]. A convenience sampling method was employed to recruit participants based on accessibility and willingness to participate in the study. Demographic factors such as age, gender, educational background, and marital status were considered to ensure a diverse representation.

2.3. *Questionnaire Development and Validation*

The questionnaire development process involved a comprehensive review of established scales from both the domestic and international literature to construct the research scale and measurement items. Previous studies have identified key factors influencing telemedicine adoption, including demographic characteristics and technical attributes such as perceived ease of use and usefulness [26,27], as well as the role of trust and social influence [23,28–31].

2.4. *The Questionnaire Encompassed the following Components*

Demographic Variables: This included personal attributes such as gender, age, education level, and marital status, reflecting the findings from studies by Mensah and Mi [26], Granić and Marangunić [27], and Parra et al. [32] highlighting the correlations between demographic variables and technology adoption.

Questionnaire Variables: The scale comprised six factors: perceived ease of use, perceived usefulness, trust, social influence, attitude toward using telemedicine, and usage intention. Each factor was assessed using a five-point Likert scale ranging from "strongly agree" to "strongly disagree", ensuring a comprehensive measurement of participant perceptions and intentions [23,33–39].

Measurement of Outcome Variables: Outcome variables such as intention for continued usage, perceived ease of use, and others were assessed using a five-point Likert scale. These variables were treated as continuous parametric variables in our analysis. Prior to statistical analysis, we conducted normality tests and assessments of skewness and kurtosis to confirm the appropriateness of assuming a parametric distribution.

2.5. Handling Missing Data

Approximately 14% of collected surveys were excluded due to missing data. We considered employing missing data imputation techniques to assess the potential biases introduced by excluding incomplete responses. Our analysis indicated that missingness did not correlate systematically with key demographic variables, including educational attainment. Sensitivity analyses further confirmed that the exclusion of incomplete responses did not significantly impact the robustness of our findings.

2.6. Consistency in Telemedicine Platforms

All participants in our study utilized the same standardized telemedicine platform to ensure uniformity in technological interactions and minimize potential variability in association results stemming from platform differences.

2.7. Ethical Considerations and Data Analysis

Ethical approval for the study was obtained from the Institutional Review Board of Show Chwann Memorial Hospital (Approval No. 1101001). Data analysis commenced with descriptive statistics and reliability analysis using SPSS 21.0 to assess data quality and internal consistency. Structural Equation Modeling (SEM) was subsequently conducted using AMOS 21.0 to validate the study's hypotheses and explore relationships among variables.

2.8. Software Licensing

All software used in data analysis, including SPSS 21.0 and AMOS 21.0, were licensed versions obtained through institutional agreements. The licensing details for these software applications are available upon request from the respective vendors.

3. Results

For the survey of 646 telemedicine patients in this institute, the gender distribution of participants was 234 (36.2%) males and 412 (63.8%) females. The majority age group was between the ages of 41 and 50 years, representing 29.7%. In terms of education, university degree holders representing 61.9% were the majority, and the minimum qualification was elementary school holders representing 0.8%. Table 1 shows the complete descriptions of the respondents.

Table 1. Descriptions of respondents.

Measure	Item	Frequency N = 646	Percentage (%)
Gender	Male	234	36.2
	Female	412	63.8
Age group	<30	157	24.3
	31–40	131	20.3
	41–50	192	29.7
	51–60	127	19.7
	>61	39	6.0
Education level	Elementary school	5	0.8
	Junior high school	14	2.2
	Senior high school	133	20.6
	Bachelor's degree	400	61.9
	Postgraduate (Master's/Doctoral)	94	14.6
Marital status	Married	323	42.6
	Single	275	50.0
	Widowed (divorced)	48	7.4

This study used a self-response method to collect information from a single subject, which might lead to the problem of CMV. Harman's single factor test was used [40]. The results showed that perceived usefulness, perceived ease of use, attitude, social influence, trust, and behavioral intention were six factors whose eigenvalues were >1. The explained variance of the first factor was 19.35%. It did not exceed 50% of the total explained variance (73.28%), indicating that CMV did not cause serious problems [41].

When conducting SEM analysis, it needs to include two stages: measurement and structural model analyses. First, for the measurement mode analysis stage, Bagozzi and Yi [42] proposed to adopt the following: (1) individual item reliability, (2) composite reliability (CR) of latent variables, and (3) average variance extracted (AVE) of latent variables. In the reliability part, the factor loadings (factor loading) of all variable measurement items in this research model ranged from 0.552 to 0.822, which were all >0.5 and reached statistical significance ($p < 0.05$). In the reliability analysis (reliability analysis), the Cronbach's alpha value of each variable in this study ranged from 0.766 to 0.918, which was in line with the criteria suggested by Hair et al. [43] to an acceptable level.

In the CR part, the CR values of the variables ranged from 0.634 to 0.869, which met the criteria suggested by Fornell and Larcker [44] that CR values should be >0.6. Finally, in the mean variation extraction (AVE) part, the AVE value of each variable ranged from 0.369 to 0.624, which met the standard of AVE values suggested by Fornell and Larcker [44] that should be at least >0.3. The above results showed that the internal consistency of the questionnaire in this study is"quit' good, with a high degree of credibility. The questionnaire dimensions are also acceptable. In the discriminant validity test, the correlation coefficient values among all aspects are significantly <1.0, which is in line with the basic assumption of discriminant validity [45] (Table 2).

Table 2. Reliability and validity and correlation analysis.

Measure	PU	PEOU	ATU	SI	Trust	UI
Perceived Usefulness (PU)						
Perceived Ease of Use (PEOU)	0.507					
Attitude Toward Using (ATU)	0.658	0.640				
Social Influence (SI)	0.568	0.508	0.556			
Trust	0.597	0.616	0.675	0.642		
Usage Intention (UI)	0.710	0.590	0.747	0.706	0.750	
Cronbach's α	0.766	0.867	0.780	0.918	0.879	0.927
CR	0.705	0.847	0.634	0.869	0.716	0.850
AVE	0.445	0.582	0.369	0.624	0.457	0.416
Mean	3.647	3.837	4.018	3.356	4.005	3.741
Standard Deviation	0.649	0.682	0.624	0.725	0.639	0.639

Note: CR (Composite Reliability) indicates internal consistency; values > 0.6 are acceptable. AVE (Average Variance Extracted) indicates convergent validity; values > 0.3 are acceptable.

Structural pattern analysis mainly verified the proposed research framework and illustrated the explanatory power of the overall pattern. In this study, AMOS 21.0 software was used for analysis, and its path coefficients were standardized to verify the four hypotheses of the research model. The results indicated that perceived ease of use has a significant positive impact on perceived usefulness ($\beta = 0.51$, $p < 0.001$); perceived usefulness has a significant positive impact on attitude toward using ($\beta = 0.51$, $p < 0.001$) = 0.37, $p < 0.001$); permitted ease of use has a significant positive effect on attitude toward using ($\beta = 0.32$, $p < 0.001$); trust has a significant positive effect on attitude toward using ($\beta = 0.32$, $p < 0.001$); social influence has no significant effect on attitude toward using ($\beta = 0.06$, $p > 0.001$); and attitude toward using has a significant positive effect on usage intention ($\beta = 0.70$, $p < 0.001$). Figure 2 illustrates the related research model path pattern.

H1–H4 and H6 were supported, but not H5. Figure 2 displays the explanatory power of each endogenous latent variable of the research model to the overall model. The path values between each dimension adopted standardized coefficients. The variation explanatory power (R^2) of each endogenous latent variable in the research model to the overall model is as follows: the R^2 of perceived ease of use to perceived usefulness was 26% (0.26); the R^2

of perceived usefulness, social influence, trust, and attitude toward using was 47% (0.47); and the R^2 of attitude toward using and usage intention was 48% (0.48).

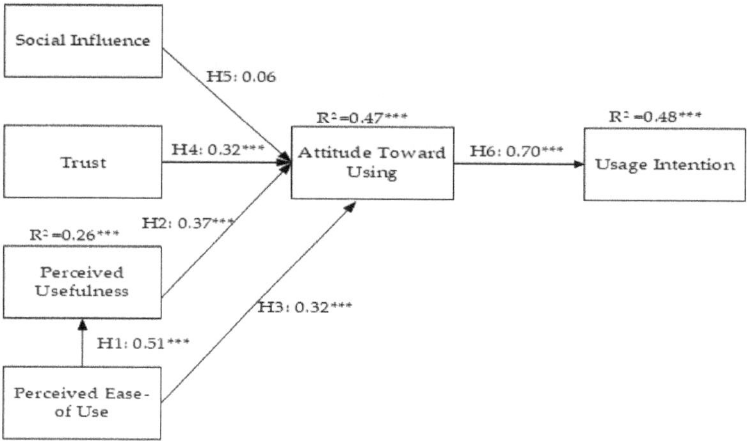

Figure 2. Structural model with path coefficient and R^2 values. Note: *** indicates significance at $p < 0.001$.

4. Discussion and Implication

This study integrates the SCT and the TAM to investigate the determinants of telemedicine adoption among patients. Our results confirm that SCT and TAM effectively evaluate the variables influencing the intention to use telemedicine, with most hypotheses being substantiated. Specifically, we found significant relationships between perceived ease of use, perceived usefulness, and usage intention. However, contrary to our initial hypothesis (Hypothesis 5), social influence did not significantly impact telemedicine usage intention.

The finding that social influence was not a significant predictor contrasts with previous studies [46,47]. This discrepancy may be due to the specific context of the COVID-19 pandemic, where social interactions were limited, reducing the potential impact of social influence on telemedicine adoption.

Perceived ease of use and perceived usefulness showed a strong positive correlation, consistent with the findings of Morton et al. and Melas et al. [12,48,49]. This supports the established view that perceived ease of use indirectly affects usage intention through perceived usefulness [16,24,48,50]. Furthermore, attitude towards using telemedicine significantly influences usage intention, aligning with the results obtained by Almojaibel et al. [51], Doma et al. [52], and Shadangi et al. [53]. The more positive the attitude towards telemedicine, the higher the intention to adopt such services.

Trust emerged as a critical factor, significantly correlating with usage intention and mediating the relationship between perceived usefulness and intention. This finding aligns with van Velsen et al. [46] and Park et al. [47], highlighting trust's role in patient acceptance of telemedicine.

5. Conclusions

The COVID-19 pandemic has underscored the necessity of telemedicine as a vital tool in healthcare delivery. Our study's findings emphasize the importance of perceived ease of use, perceived usefulness, and trust in telemedicine adoption. These insights provide a comprehensive understanding of the factors influencing telemedicine acceptance and offer valuable guidance for future research and practical applications.

6. Recommendations

Governments and healthcare providers should collaborate to develop standardized telemedicine platforms integrated with existing medical information systems to streamline user experience and improve accessibility. Policies should be adapted to allow the broader use of telemedicine, especially for chronic disease management, reducing the need for in-person hospital visits and increasing patient satisfaction. Educating patients about the functionalities and operation of telemedicine systems is crucial. Developing user-friendly interfaces and comprehensive training materials will improve patient attitudes and increase usage intention. Initiatives to build and maintain trust in telemedicine, such as ensuring the security and efficacy of these services, are essential for enhancing patient acceptance and usage.

7. Limitations and Future Research Directions

While this study provides valuable insights, several limitations must be acknowledged. The self-reported nature of the questionnaire may introduce response bias, and the cross-sectional design limits causal interpretations. Future studies should adopt longitudinal designs and incorporate qualitative methods to address these limitations.

Conducting longitudinal studies will provide deeper insights into the sustained effects of telemedicine on patient outcomes and engagement. Field interviews and case studies can uncover underlying reasons for the observed lack of significant social influence, providing a richer understanding of patient attitudes. Including healthcare providers' viewpoints can reveal additional barriers and facilitators to telemedicine adoption, offering a more comprehensive perspective. Exploring advanced technologies such as AI, machine learning, and blockchain in telemedicine can lead to innovative solutions for personalized care and enhanced data security. Comparative studies across different cultural contexts can identify unique challenges and opportunities in telemedicine adoption, informing more tailored implementation strategies.

In conclusion, this study advances our understanding of the factors influencing telemedicine adoption, providing both theoretical and practical contributions. By addressing the identified limitations and exploring future research directions, we can further enhance the efficacy and acceptance of telemedicine, ultimately improving healthcare delivery and patient outcomes.

Author Contributions: Data curation, L.-H.K., Y.-H.Y. and C.-M.K.; Methodology, L.-H.K. and Y.-H.Y.; Project administration, Y.-H.Y.; Supervision, C.-M.K.; Writing—original draft, Writing—review and editing, Y.-H.Y.; L.-H.K., C.-M.K. and Y.-H.Y. revised and approved the final version. All authors have read and agreed to the published version of the manuscript.

Funding: This study was supported by grant funds (MOST 111-2410-H-217-001-MY2) from the Taiwan National Science and Technology Council. The funding period was from August 2022 to July 2024, with a total grant amount of NT$1,169,000.

Institutional Review Board Statement: The study protocol was reviewed and approved by the institutional review board of the Tainan Municipal Hospital (managed by Show Chwan Medical Care Corporation), Taiwan (SCMH_IRB No: 1101001, 10 December 2021).

Informed Consent Statement: Informed consent was obtained online from all respondents before answering and returning an online questionnaire. The names of participants and their organizations were anonymous.

Data Availability Statement: Data cannot be made publicly available owing to the fact that the privacy of individual participants cannot be compromised. However, the dataset is available from the corresponding author on reasonable request.

Conflicts of Interest: The authors declare no conflicts of interest.

References

1. Gao, J.; Zheng, P.; Jia, Y.; Chen, H.; Mao, Y.; Chen, S.; Wang, Y.; Fu, H.; Dai, J. Mental health problems and social media exposure during COVID-19 outbreak. *PLoS ONE* **2020**, *15*, e0231924.
2. Huang, Y.; Zhao, N. Generalized anxiety disorder, depressive symptoms and sleep quality during COVID-19 outbreak in China: A web-based cross-sectional survey. *Psychiatry Res.* **2020**, *288*, 112954. [CrossRef] [PubMed]
3. Wang, C.; Pan, R.; Wan, X.; Tan, Y.; Xu, L.; Ho, C.S.; Ho, R.C. Immediate psychological responses and associated factors during the initial stage of the 2019 coronavirus disease (COVID-19) epidemic among the general population in China. *Int. J. Environ. Res. Public Health* **2020**, *17*, 1729. [CrossRef] [PubMed]
4. Shachar, C.; Engel, J.; Elwyn, G. Implications for telehealth in a postpandemic future: Regulatory and privacy issues. *JAMA* **2020**, *323*, 2375–2376. [CrossRef] [PubMed]
5. Hollander, J.E.; Carr, B.G. Virtually perfect? Telemedicine for COVID-19. *N. Engl. J. Med.* **2020**, *382*, 1679–1681. [CrossRef] [PubMed]
6. Chuang, M.M.; Lin, C.Y.; Sung, K.T.; Tsai, J.P.; Kuo, J.Y.; Huang, W.H.; Chen, Y.C.; Tsai, C.T.; Su, C.H.; Hou, J.Y.C.; et al. Contemporary Practice in Telemedicine through Telecommunication Technology during COVID-19 Pandemic in Taiwan-A Single Center Experience. *Int. J. Gerontol.* **2022**, *16*, 196–201.
7. Wu, T.C.; Ho, C.T.B. Barriers to telemedicine adoption during the COVID-19 pandemic in Taiwan: Comparison of perceived risks by socioeconomic status correlates. *Int. J. Environ. Res. Public Health* **2023**, *20*, 3504. [CrossRef] [PubMed]
8. Ho, P.H.; Huang, C.C.; Liu, Y.S. Exploring the Key Factors that Affect Patient Willingness to Use Telemedicine. *Cheng Ching Med. J.* **2021**, *17*, 27–36. (In Taiwanese)
9. National Health Insurance Administration. Telemedicine in Response to COVID-19. Available online: https://www.nhi.gov.tw/Content_List.aspx?n=1482911120B73697&topn=787128DAD5F71B1A (accessed on 30 June 2023).
10. Tseng, H.M.; Chung, P.J.; Wang, H.H.; Chuang, Y.J. Examining Factors Related to Acceptance of Telemedicine among Taiwan's Expatriate Workers Living in Shang Hai of China. *J. Taiwan Assoc. Med. Inform.* **2020**, *18*, 13–28. (In Taiwanese)
11. Harst, L.; Lantzsch, H.; Scheibe, M. Theories predicting end-user acceptance of telemedicine use: Systematic review. *J. Med. Internet Res.* **2019**, *21*, e13117. [CrossRef] [PubMed]
12. Holtz, B.; Mitchell, K.; Hirko, K.; Ford, S. Using the Technology Acceptance Model to Characterize Barriers and Opportunities of Telemedicine in Rural Populations: Survey and Interview Study. *JMIR. Form. Res.* **2022**, *6*, e35130. [CrossRef] [PubMed]
13. Aguilar, K.M.; Campbell, R.S.; Fiester, A.; Simpson, R.L.; Hertel, C. Bringing care home: How telemonitoring can expand population health management beyond the hospital. *Nurs. Adm. Q.* **2014**, *38*, 166–172. [CrossRef] [PubMed]
14. Esser, P.E.; Goossens, R.H. A framework for the design of user-centred teleconsulting systems. *J. Telemed. Telecare* **2009**, *15*, 32–39. [CrossRef] [PubMed]
15. Riley, W.T.; Rivera, D.E.; Atienza, A.A.; Nilsen, W.; Allison, S.M.; Mermelstein, R. Health behavior models in the age of mobile interventions: Are our theories up to the task? *Transl. Behav. Med.* **2011**, *1*, 53–71. [CrossRef] [PubMed]
16. Davis, F.D. Perceived usefulness, perceived ease of use, and user acceptance of information technology. *MIS Q.* **1989**, *13*, 319–340. [CrossRef]
17. Bourdieu, P. The forms of capttal. In *Handbook of Theory and Research for the Sociology of Education*; Richardson, J., Ed.; Greenwood: New York, NY, USA, 1986; pp. 241–258.
18. Coleman, J.S. Social capital in the creation of human capital. *Am. J. Sociol.* **1988**, *94*, S95–S120. [CrossRef]
19. Dika, S.L.; Singh, K. Applications of social capital in educational literature: A critical synthesis. *Rev. Educ. Res.* **2002**, *72*, 31–60. [CrossRef]
20. Lin, K.Y.; Lu, H.P. Intention to continue using Facebook fan pages from the perspective of social capital theory. *Cyberpsychol. Behav. Soc. Netw.* **2011**, *14*, 565–570. [CrossRef] [PubMed]
21. Putnam, R. The prosperous community: Social capital and public life. *Am. Prospect* **1993**, *13*, 35–42.
22. Schneider, G.E.; Griffith, W.H.; Knoedler, J.T. *The Great Disruption: Human Nature and the Reconstitution of Social Order*; The Free Press: New York, NY, USA, 2000.
23. Baptista, G.; Oliveira, T. Understanding mobile banking: The unified theory of acceptance and use of technology combined with cultural moderators. *Comput. Hum. Behav.* **2015**, *50*, 418–430. [CrossRef]
24. Kissi, J.; Dai, B.; Dogbe, C.S.; Banahene, J.; Ernest, O. Predictive factors of physicians' satisfaction with telemedicine services acceptance. *Health Inform. J.* **2020**, *26*, 1866–1880. [CrossRef] [PubMed]
25. Naqvi, M.H.A.; Jiang, Y.; Miao, M.; Naqvi, M.H. The effect of social influence, trust, and entertainment value on social media use: Evidence from Pakistan. *Cogent. Bus. Manag.* **2020**, *7*, 1723825. [CrossRef]
26. Mensah, I.K.; Mi, J. Computer self-efficacy and e-government service adoption: The moderating role of age as a demographic factor. *Int. J. Public Adm.* **2019**, *42*, 158–167. [CrossRef]
27. Granić, A.; Marangunić, N. Technology acceptance model in educational context: A systematic literature review. *Br. J. Educ. Technol.* **2019**, *50*, 2572–2593. [CrossRef]
28. Kamal, S.A.; Shafiq, M.; Kakria, P. Investigating acceptance of telemedicine services through an extended technology acceptance model (TAM). *Technol. Soc.* **2020**, *60*, 101212. [CrossRef]
29. Venkatesh, V.; Morris, M.G.; Davis, G.B.; Davis, F.D. User acceptance of information technology: Toward a unified view. *MIS Q.* **2003**, *27*, 425–478. [CrossRef]

30. Lu, J.; Yao, J.E.; Yu, C.S. Personal innovativeness, social influences and adoption of wireless Internet services via mobile technology. *J. Strate Inform. Syst.* **2005**, *14*, 245–268. [CrossRef]
31. Zhou, L.; Bao, J.; Watzlaf, V.; Parmanto, B. Barriers to and facilitators of the use of mobile health apps from a security perspective: Mixed-methods study. *JMIR mHealth uHealth* **2019**, *7*, e11223. [CrossRef] [PubMed]
32. Parra, C.; Jódar-Sánchez, F.; Jiménez-Hernández, M.D.; Vigil, E.; Palomino-García, A.; Moniche-Álvarez, F.; De la Torre Laviana, F.J.; Bonachela, P.; Fernández, F.J.; Cayuela-Domínguez, A.; et al. Development, implementation, and evaluation of a telemedicine service for the treatment of acute stroke patients: Tele Stroke. *Interact. J. Med. Res.* **2012**, *1*, e2163. [CrossRef] [PubMed]
33. Kao, M.Y.; Wu, C.I. Self-rated health and social capital: Cross-national analysis of international social survey data. *Taiwan J. Public Health* **2020**, *39*, 509–521. (In Taiwanese)
34. Davis, F.D.; Bagozzi, R.P.; Warshaw, P.R. User acceptance of computer technology: A comparison of two theoretical models. *Manag. Sci.* **1989**, *35*, 982–1003. [CrossRef]
35. Chakraborty, R.; Lee, J.; Bagchi-Sen, S.; Upadhyaya, S.; Rao, H.R. Online shopping intention in the context of data breach in online retail stores: An examination of older and younger adults. *Decis. Support Syst.* **2016**, *83*, 47–56. [CrossRef]
36. Kim, H.W.; Chan, H.C.; Gupta, S. Value-based adoption of mobile internet: An empirical investigation. *Decis. Support Syst.* **2007**, *43*, 111–126. [CrossRef]
37. Martins, C.; Oliveira, T.; Popovi, A. Understanding the Internet banking adoption: A unified theory of acceptance and use of technology and perceived risk application. *Int. J. Inf. Manag.* **2014**, *34*, 1–13. [CrossRef]
38. Smith, R.; Deitz, G.; Royne, M.B.; Hansen, J.D.; Grünhagen, M.; Witte, C. Cross-cultural examination of online shopping behavior: A comparison of Norway, Germany, and the United States. *J. Bus. Res.* **2013**, *66*, 328–335. [CrossRef]
39. Scherer, R.; Siddiq, F.; Tondeur, J. The technology acceptance model (TAM): A meta-analytic structural equation modeling approach to explaining teachers' adoption of digital technology in education. *Comput. Edu.* **2019**, *128*, 13–35. [CrossRef]
40. Harman, H.H. *Modern Factor Analysis*, 3rd ed.; The University of Chicago Press: Chicago, IL, USA, 1976.
41. Podsakoff, P.M.; MacKenzie, S.B.; Lee, J.Y.; Podsakoff, N.P. Common method biases in behavioral research: A critical review of the literature and recommended remedies. *J. Appl. Psychol.* **2003**, *88*, 879–903. [CrossRef] [PubMed]
42. Bagozzi, R.P.; Yi, Y. Specification, evaluation, and interpretation of structural equation models. *J. Acad. Mark. Sci.* **2012**, *40*, 8–34. [CrossRef]
43. Hair, J.F.; Black, W.C.; Babin, B.J.; Anderson, R.E. *Multivariate Data Analysis: A Global Perspective*, 7th ed.; MacMillan: New York, NY, USA, 2010.
44. Fornell, C.; Larcker, D.F. Evaluating structural equation models with unobservable variables and measurement error. *J. Mark. Res.* **1981**, *18*, 39–50. [CrossRef]
45. Bagozzi, R.P.; Yi, Y.; Phillips, L.W. Assessing construct validity in organizational research. *Adm. Sci. Q.* **1991**, *36*, 421–458. [CrossRef]
46. van Velsen, L.; van der Geest, T.; van de Wijngaert, L.; van den Berg, S.; Steehouder, M. Personalization has a Price, Controllability is the Currency: Predictors for the Intention to use Personalized eGovernment Websites. *J. Organ. Comput. Electron. Commer.* **2015**, *25*, 76–97. [CrossRef]
47. Park, H.; Chon, Y.; Lee, J.; Choi, I.J.; Yoon, K.H. Service design attributes affecting diabetic patient preferences of telemedicine in South Korea. *Telemed. J. eHealth* **2011**, *17*, 442–451. [CrossRef] [PubMed]
48. Morton, M.E.; Wiedenbeck, S. EHR acceptance factors in ambulatory care: A survey of physician perceptions. *Perspect. Health Inf. Manag.* **2010**, *7*, 1c. [PubMed]
49. Melas, C.D.; Zampetakis, L.A.; Dimopoulou, A.; Moustakis, V. Modeling the acceptance of clinical information systems among hospital medical staff: An extended TAM model. *J. Biomed. Inform.* **2011**, *44*, 553–564. [CrossRef] [PubMed]
50. Aggelidis, V.P.; Chatzoglou, P.D. Using a modified technology acceptance model in hospitals. *Int. J. Med. Inform.* **2009**, *78*, 115–126. [CrossRef] [PubMed]
51. Almojaibel, A.A.; Munk, N.; Goodfellow, L.T.; Fisher, T.F.; Miller, K.K.; Comer, A.R.; Bakas, T.; Justiss, M.D. Development and validation of the tele-pulmonary rehabilitation acceptance scale. *Respir. Care.* **2019**, *64*, 1057–1064. [CrossRef] [PubMed]
52. Doma, S.S.; Elaref, N.A.; Abo Elnaga, M.A. Factors affecting electronic word-of-mouth on social networking websites in Egypt: An application of the technology acceptance model. *Int. J. Netw. Virtual. Organ.* **2015**, *2015*, 1–31. [CrossRef]
53. Shadangi, P.Y.; Kar, S.; Mohanty, A.K.; Dash, M. Physician's attitude towards acceptance of telemedicine technology for delivering health care services. *Int. J. Mech. Eng. Technol.* **2018**, *9*, 715–722.

European Journal of
Investigation in Health, Psychology and Education

MDPI

Article

Segmenting Preventive Health Behavior: Gender Disparities and Psychosocial Predictors in a Culturally Diverse Italian Region

Dietmar Ausserhofer [1,2], Verena Barbieri [1], Stefano Lombardo [3], Timon Gärtner [3], Klaus Eisendle [4], Giuliano Piccoliori [1], Adolf Engl [1] and Christian J. Wiedermann [1,*]

[1] Institute of General Practice and Public Health, Claudiana—College of Health Professions, 39100 Bolzano, Italy
[2] Claudiana Research, Claudiana—College of Health Professions, 39100 Bolzano, Italy
[3] Provincial Institute for Statistics of the Autonomous Province of Bolzano—South Tyrol (ASTAT), 39100 Bolzano, Italy
[4] Directorate, Claudiana—College of Health Professions, 39100 Bolzano, Italy
* Correspondence: christian.wiedermann@am-mg.claudiana.bz.it

Abstract

Grounded in health behavior theory, this study examined patterns of preventive health behavior in a culturally diverse, multilingual region of northern Italy using data from a representative population survey (n = 2090). Preventive behaviors were assessed using the 16-item Good Health Practices (GHP-16) scale. Latent profile analysis (LPA) identified five behavioral profiles, ranging from 'Globally Low Engagers' to 'Comprehensive High Engagers'. Binary logistic regression compared 'Globally Low Engagers' to 'Broadly Moderate Preventers', examining predictors including gender, age, education, language, chronic disease status, health literacy (HLS-EU-Q16), patient activation (PAM-10), mistrust of health information, living situation, and healthcare employment. The results showed that men, younger adults, individuals with low patient activation, those living alone, and respondents with high mistrust of health information had higher odds of belonging to the low engagement group. Health literacy and language group membership were not significantly associated with the profile membership. Item-level comparisons revealed gender differences in information-seeking, oral hygiene, and dietary behaviors, with men reporting lower engagement. These findings support a segmentation-based understanding of preventive health behavior and highlight the need to address personal capacities and contextual barriers in interventions while challenging assumptions of uniformly higher female health vigilance.

Keywords: latent profile analysis; preventive health behavior; patient activation; health literacy; gender differences; mistrust; behavioral segmentation; population-based study; health promotion; social determinants of health

1. Introduction

Preventive health behaviors, including maintaining a healthy diet, engaging in regular physical activity, avoiding tobacco use, and participating in screening programs, are essential for reducing chronic diseases and improving population health outcomes. These behaviors address modifiable risk factors contributing to cardiovascular disease, cancer, diabetes, and other non-communicable conditions that impose substantial burdens on healthcare systems worldwide (Halpin et al., 2010; Corrêa et al., 2024; Gokhale, 2020; Martin Obianyo et al., 2024). Evidence from systematic reviews demonstrates that behavioral interventions, including framing techniques and incentives, can increase adherence to preventive care and improve health outcomes (Corrêa et al., 2024; Martin Obianyo et al., 2024). Additionally, promoting preventive behaviors through public policies and health promotion initiatives has been shown to reduce health disparities among disadvantaged groups (Higgins, 2015; Airhihenbuwa et al., 2021; Da Silva et al., 2024). The promotion of preventive health behaviors remains central to public health strategies for curbing chronic diseases and enhancing health equity.

Health behavior is often explained using theoretical models that describe how individuals make decisions regarding prevention and self-care. Two of the most widely used frameworks are the Health Belief Model (HBM) and Theory of Planned Behavior (TPB).

The HBM focuses on how people weigh the perceived benefits and barriers to taking action, as well as how vulnerable they feel to a given health risk. For example, someone may choose to get a flu shot because they believe it will protect them (benefit), even if they dislike injections (barrier), especially if they feel at high risk due to a chronic condition. Meta-analyses have shown that perceived benefits and barriers are consistently strong predictors of behavior in this model, while perceptions of severity (how serious the illness would be) are less influential (Carpenter, 2010; Sulat et al., 2018).

In contrast, the TPB adds a stronger emphasis on social influences and personal confidence. It explains behavior through three key drivers: behavioral intentions, subjective norms (e.g., what important others think one should do), and perceived control or self-efficacy. For instance, a person may intend to start exercising because they believe it is beneficial, their friends support the idea, and they feel confident that they can do it. The TPB often outperforms the HBM in predicting actual behavior, particularly when intentions and self-efficacy are strong (Gerend & Shepherd, 2012; Montanaro & Bryan, 2014).

Studies that combine elements of the HBM and the TPB often show greater explanatory power than either model alone. This is particularly true when both individual perceptions (such as perceived susceptibility, expected benefits, and perceived control) and social influences (like subjective norms and social support) are taken into account (Huang et al., 2020). While latent profile analysis (LPA) applications are limited here, structural equation modeling using these frameworks identifies subgroups with distinct behavioral profiles, aligning with LPA's goal of uncovering hidden typologies within populations (Huang et al., 2020). These integrated models provide an improved understanding of behavioral variability and a solid foundation for segmentation approaches targeting interventions.

Health literacy and patient activation are key enablers of preventive health behaviors; however, empirical findings are mixed.

- Higher health literacy is consistently linked to improved preventive practices in chronic disease contexts, including cardiovascular care, COVID-19 adherence, and cancer screening (Gautam et al., 2021; Aaby et al., 2017; Lee et al., 2021). However, its predictive power varies by population and behavior type, with some studies finding no association after controlling for confounders (Mohan et al., 2017).
- Patient activation, which reflects confidence and motivation to manage health, showed weaker associations. While it may enhance health-seeking behavior in some contexts (Erişen, 2024), it is not a reliable predictor of self-care adherence, particularly in chronic disease populations (Meraz et al., 2023).

Studies using behavioral clustering approaches suggest that preventive behaviors polarize into high- and low-adherence groups, and these clusters are better explained by clinical or structural variables than by literacy or activation alone (Zhao et al., 2023). These findings underscore the importance of typology-based analyses that extend beyond linear predictors.

Preventive health behaviors are shaped by individual-level factors and broader cultural and linguistic contexts. In multilingual regions of Italy, these factors strongly influence how individuals engage with preventive care and health information. Studies in Northern Italy have highlighted intercultural mediators in bilingual healthcare settings, showing that cultural assumptions shape health-related communication and behavior (Anderson & Cirillo, 2020). A multicenter trial demonstrated that co-designed, culturally tailored interventions improved lifestyle behaviors and therapy adherence among immigrant patients with type 2 diabetes (Bonvicini et al., 2025). Digital and community-based health promotion initiatives targeting disadvantaged youth have shown promise in improving health literacy and preventive knowledge (Franceschi et al., 2021). In South Tyrol, linguistic group membership has been linked to patterns of health information use, with German speakers favoring traditional medical sources and Italian speakers engaging more with digital platforms (Ausserhofer et al., 2022; Wiedermann et al., 2025). These findings support the relevance of culturally sensitive, segmentation-based approaches to behavioral health research. While the importance of preventive health behaviors has been established, current research often relies on linear models that overlook the complexity of behavioral patterns across populations. In culturally diverse contexts like South Tyrol, segmentation approaches like LPA can uncover distinct behavioral profiles hidden by aggregate methods (Figure 1). Research suggests that health literacy and patient activation may not uniformly predict preventive engagement, and that sociocultural context shapes how individuals access, interpret, and act on health information (Smith et al., 2013; Couture et al., 2018; Palumbo, 2021).

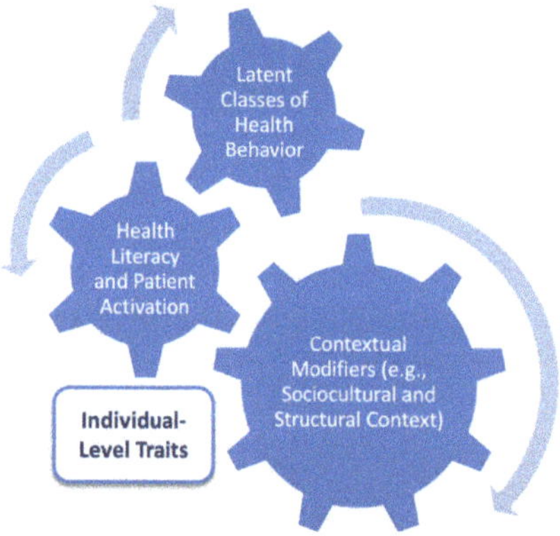

Figure 1. Analytic model guiding the identification of latent profiles of preventive health behavior. This model shows how health literacy and patient activation contribute to distinct latent profiles of preventive health behaviors. These behavioral profiles are shaped by personal capacities and contextual modifiers, including sociocultural and structural factors. The arrows indicate the interactions between the constructs.

Guided by the HBM, which emphasizes perceptions of susceptibility, benefits, and barriers, this study applied LPA to identify subgroups within a representative adult population based on preventive behaviors. The aim was to characterize these behavioral profiles and explore their associations with sociodemographic factors, health literacy, and patient activation, laying the groundwork for tailored interventions in multilingual and culturally heterogeneous settings.

2. Methods

2.1. Study Design and Sampling

This analysis was part of a population-based cross-sectional survey conducted in the Autonomous Province of Bolzano (South Tyrol), Italy, between March and May 2024. The province is characterized by cultural and linguistic heterogeneity, with German, Italian, and Ladin-speaking communities and a decentralized health system. The Provincial Institute of Statistics (ASTAT) designed the survey in collaboration with the Institute of General Practice and Public Health. Earlier studies using this dataset investigated the associations between mistrust and sleep quality (Wiedermann et al., 2025) and health information behavior (Ausserhofer et al., 2025). The current study focuses on behavioral typologies related to preventive health behaviors.

A total of 4000 individuals ($\geq$18 years) were randomly selected from the provincial population registry to provide robust estimates across strata and enable post-stratification weighting using ReGenesees software (version 2.3, ISTAT, Rome, Italy). The stratification criteria included age group (18–34, 35–54, and 55+ years), sex, citizenship, and municipality of residence. Participants received paper-based or online survey invitations in German and Italian. Of the 4000 individuals invited, 2120 responded, yielding a response rate of 53%. After data cleaning, 2090 cases were included in the analysis, corresponding to a completion rate of 98.6%. All respondents provided informed consent, and participation was voluntary and anonymous. The present analysis was based on 2090 completed responses.

2.2. Sociodemographic and Health Measures

Participants reported their biological sex, age (in years), and language group, with response options for German, Italian, Ladin, or others. For analytical purposes, the Ladin and "Other" groups were combined. Educational attainment was recorded in four categories: primary school, vocational/technical education, high school diploma, and university degrees.

Living situation was captured using a binary item indicating whether the respondent lived alone or with others (e.g., family or partner). Chronic illness status was assessed using a self-reported checklist. Respondents were asked whether they had ever been diagnosed with a range of common chronic conditions (e.g., cardiovascular disease, hypertension, diabetes, and mental health disorders). For the present analysis, a dichotomous variable (presence or absence of any condition) was constructed. Additional variables included employment in the health or social care sector (yes/no). For operational definitions of these and other background variables, readers are referred to prior methodological reports from this study series (Ausserhofer et al., 2025; Wiedermann et al., 2025).

2.3. Preventive Health Behavior (GHP-16)

Preventive behavior was assessed using the Good Health Practices scale (GHP-16) (Hampson et al., 2019), a validated short-form inventory derived from the original Health Behavior Checklist (HBC) (Vickers et al., 1990). The GHP-16 measures engagement in 16 diverse health-promoting practices across the lifestyle, medical, and hygiene domains. Items include:

- "I exercise regularly",
- "I follow a balanced diet",
- "I get routine medical check-ups",
- "I floss my teeth regularly", and
- "I avoid smoking" (phrased as "I don't smoke").

Each behavior was rated on a 4-point Likert scale ranging from 1 ("does not apply at all") to 4 ("fully applies"). To facilitate comparison with international studies using a 5-point format, responses were linearly rescaled using the following formula: rescaled score = 1 + (original score − 1) × (4/3). This preserved the ordinal structure while aligning the scale values with previously published work on the GHP-16. Higher scores indicate more consistent engagement in the preventive practices. No reverse coding was required because all items were positively phrased. The total score was computed as the arithmetic mean of non-missing items, resulting in a scale ranging from 1.0 (minimal engagement) to 5.0 (maximum engagement). The original GHP-16 validation study reported an internal consistency of $\alpha = 0.83$ (Hampson et al., 2019). In our analytic sample, the internal consistency of the GHP-16 was acceptable (Cronbach's $\alpha = 0.77$). Participants missing more than two items were excluded from the score-based analyses.

The GHP-16 items were translated into German and Italian by the ASTAT team using standard translation procedures, including pretesting and back-translation. However, a formal psychometric validation of the translated versions was not conducted. Therefore, observed differences between language groups may, in part, reflect language- or culture-specific interpretation effects. The GHP-16 served two purposes in this study: (1) as the input for latent profile analysis, modeling patterns of behavior across the 16 items, and (2) as the basis for item-level gender comparisons in descriptive analyses.

2.4. Health Literacy (HLS-EU-Q16)

Health literacy was measured using the 16-item European Health Literacy Survey Questionnaire (HLS-EU-Q16). The instrument captures the perceived difficulty in accessing, understanding, appraising, and applying health-related information. Items include:

- "How easy is it for you to understand what your doctor says to you?"
- "How easy is it for you to judge which everyday behaviors are related to your health?"
- "How easy is it for you to find information about treatments of illnesses that concern you?"

Validated Italian and German versions of the HLS-EU-Q16 were used in this study, as developed and published by (Lorini et al., 2019) and (Pelikan et al., 2014), respectively. Each question was rated on a four-point Likert scale (1 = very difficult to 4 = very easy). In accordance with the scoring guidelines (Lorini et al., 2019; Pelikan et al., 2019; Sørensen et al., 2015), each response of "very easy" or "easy" was scored as 1, while "difficult" and "very difficult" were scored as 0. The total score was computed as the sum of the valid items, resulting in a summary index ranging from 0 (low health literacy) to 16 (high health literacy). Respondents were required to answer at least 14 items to obtain valid scores. Those with fewer valid responses were categorized as "missing" for health literacy and retained in all models as separate categories. Based on standard cutoffs, valid scores were categorized as follows: 0–8, inadequate; 9–12, problematic; and 13–16, sufficient. These categories were used for all group-wise and regression analyses. The internal consistency of the HLS-EU-Q16 has been previously reported as $\alpha = 0.82$ for the German version (Pelikan et al., 2014) and $\alpha = 0.84$ for the Italian version (Lorini et al., 2019). In our analytic sample, Cronbach's alpha for the HLS-EU-Q16 was 0.89, indicating high internal consistency.

2.5. Patient Activation (PAM-10)

Patient activation was assessed using the PAM-10, a validated 10-item short form of the Patient Activation Measure. The instrument captures an individual's confidence, motivation, and self-management skills in relation to healthcare and daily routines. Sample items include:

- "I know how to prevent further problems with my health"
- "I can stick to positive health routines even during stress"
- "I am confident that I can tell my doctor concerns I have even when he or she does not ask."

Items were answered on a 4-point Likert scale, with higher scores indicating greater agreement. The raw scores were converted to a 0–100 scale using the standard conversion table provided by Insignia Health (Brenk-Franz et al., 2013; Graffigna et al., 2017; Lin et al., 2023). We used the validated German (PAM13-D) and Italian (PAM13-I) versions of the instrument, which have demonstrated robust psychometric properties in previous studies and were adapted for 10-item scoring. Participants were then categorized into four levels of activation: Level, disengaged and overwhelmed; Level 2, becoming aware but struggling; Level 3, taking action; and Level 4, maintaining behaviors and pushing further. These ordinal categories were used to examine the differences in health behavior profiles and predictors of profile membership. Cronbach's alpha for the PAM–10 was 0.86 (Lin et al., 2023). In our sample, Cronbach's alpha for the PAM-10 was 0.81, supporting its reliability.

2.6. *Mistrust of Professional Health Information*

Perceived mistrust in formal health information was assessed using a previously described 4-item Mistrust Index (Wiedermann et al., 2025). Participants rated their trust in general practitioners, outpatient specialists, pharmacists, and nurses on a 4-point Likert scale ranging from 1 ("very trustworthy") to 4 ("not at all trustworthy"). Item scores were summed to yield a composite index ranging from 4 to 16, with higher values indicating greater mistrust of professional health sources.

2.7. *Statistical Analysis*

Statistical analyses were conducted using a combination of IBM SPSS Statistics Version 29.0.2.0 (20) (IBM Corp., Armonk, NY, USA) and RStudio Version 2025.05.1+513 (Posit, PBC, Boston, MA, USA). General descriptive, comparative, and regression analyses were implemented in SPSS, while latent profile analysis was performed in R.

2.7.1. Latent Profile Analysis

Latent profile analysis (LPA) was used to identify behavioral subgroups based on the 16 rescaled items from the GHP-16. The items were treated as continuous indicators. Models with 1 to 6 latent profiles were estimated using Gaussian finite mixture models assuming profile-invariant variances and zero covariances, implemented via the R package (tidyLPA v1.1.0) (R Foundation for Statistical Computing, Vienna, Austria). Model estimation relied on the Expectation-Maximization (EM) algorithm with default convergence settings.

Model selection followed current best practice guidelines (Van Lissa et al., 2023), considering Bayesian Information Criterion (BIC), Integrated Completed Likelihood (ICL), and classification precision. The final model was selected based on a balance of statistical fit and substantive interpretability. To assess measurement quality, average posterior probabilities (AvePP) for profile membership were examined, with values ≥ 0.70 indicating adequate assignment quality. The tidyLPA package used for latent profile analysis, based on the mclust framework, does not provide LMR or BLRT tests for determining the number of classes. Consequently, model selection was based on BIC, ICL, and AvePP, as recommended (Van Lissa et al., 2023).

2.7.2. Descriptive and Comparative Statistics

Descriptive statistics were computed for all the variables included in the analysis. Means and standard deviations (SD) were reported for continuous variables, such as GHP-16 item scores, while proportions and absolute counts were reported for categorical variables.

To compare behavioral patterns across groups, gender-stratified analyses of GHP-16 item responses were conducted using Mann–Whitney U tests, as the item-level data showed non-normal distribution. The corresponding effect sizes were calculated using Cliff's delta.

To assess the potential impact of common method variance (CMV) due to the use of self-reported measures in a cross-sectional design, we conducted Harman's single-factor test. An unrotated exploratory factor analysis was performed, including all items from the GHP-16, PAM-10, and HLS-EU-Q16 instruments. The first factor accounted for 16.13% of the total variance, and ten factors had eigenvalues greater than 1. These results suggest that CMV is not a serious concern in this dataset.

2.7.3. Binary Logistic Regression Analysis

To examine predictors of minimal engagement in preventive health behaviors, a binary logistic regression analysis was conducted comparing individuals assigned to Profile 5 ('Globally Low Engagers') versus Profile 2 ('Broadly Moderate Preventers') of the five-profile latent profile solution. This contrast was chosen due to its public health relevance: Profile 5 members reported the lowest overall engagement across the GHP-16 behavioral domains, whereas Profile 2 represented a moderately engaged and demographically broad reference group.

The binary outcome variable was coded as 1 for 'Globally Low Engagers' and 0 for 'Broadly Moderate Preventers'. All other cases were excluded from the analysis.

The following predictors were included based on theoretical and empirical relevance: Gender, age, education level, language group, living arrangement (living alone vs. with others), presence of chronic disease, health literacy score, patient activation score, and mistrust of health information. All categorical variables were dummy coded using the lowest engagement or most neutral category as the reference level. Continuous variables were treated as linear predictors unless assumptions were violated. The final model included only participants with complete data on all covariates.

The regression model was estimated using the Binary Logistic Regression procedure in SPSS with the enter method. Results are reported as odds ratios (Exp(B)) with 95% confidence intervals and *p*-values. Model fit was assessed using the Hosmer–Lemeshow goodness-of-fit test. To ensure the validity of model assumptions, a series of diagnostic checks were conducted: Linearity of the logit was tested for continuous predictors (age, health literacy, patient activation, mistrust) using the Box–Tidwell transformation. Non-significant interaction terms ($p > 0.05$) confirmed the assumption of linearity. Independence of residuals was approximated using a Durbin–Watson statistic from a linear regression with the same covariates. The value was within the acceptable range (1.5–2.5). Multicollinearity was evaluated through Variance Inflation Factors (VIFs), which were all below 2.5. Outlier and influence diagnostics were performed using standardized residuals (flagged if $> |3.0|$) and Cook's distance (flagged if >1.0). No influential cases were found that warranted exclusion.

3. Results

3.1. Latent Profile Analysis of Preventive Health Behavior

To identify subgroups based on patterns of preventive health behavior, LPA was conducted using the 16 rescaled items of the GHP-16 as continuous indicators. Models with one to six latent profiles were estimated using

Model selection was guided by the BIC, interpretability, and parsimony. Although the 6-profile solution yielded the lowest BIC (−97,250), the 5-profile solution (BIC = −97,344) was selected as the optimal model due to its clearer conceptual distinction between profiles and better distribution of participants. All profiles contained more than 10% of the sample, and entropy-based classification quality was high, with average posterior AvePP ranging from 0.835 to 1.000, indicating strong assignment certainty. Although the 6-profile model had a marginally lower BIC, its substantive interpretability and profile distinctiveness were inferior to the 5-profile solution.

The five behavioral profiles were labeled as follows:

- Profile 1—'Medically Compliant, Lifestyle Passive' (29.2%): The largest profile, characterized by high scores for vaccinations and medical check-ups but lower engagement in exercise, supplementation, and information-seeking.
- Profile 2—'Broadly Moderate Preventers' (22.9%): Showed moderate engagement across most domains, with strengths in oral hygiene and sleep.
- Profile 3—'Comprehensive High Engagers' (20.6%): Exhibited uniformly high scores across lifestyle and medical prevention, reflecting a broadly health-conscious profile.
- Profile 4—'Peripherally Engaged' (16.7%): Displayed modest engagement across domains, with particularly low use of preventive dental and screening services.
- Profile 5—'Globally Low Engagers' (10.7%): Demonstrated the lowest scores on nearly all behaviors, including diet, supplementation, and preventive visits.

Profile assignment was based on the highest posterior probability for each individual. Table 1 presents the item-level means and SDs for each profile.

Table 1. GHP-16 scores per latent profile of preventive health behavior (n = 2090 participants).

Health Behavior (GHP-16 Item)	GHP-16 Scores, Mean (SD)				
	Medically Compliant, Lifestyle Passive	**Broadly Moderate Preventers**	**Comprehensive High Engagers**	**Peripherally Engaged**	**Globally Low Engagers**
n	610	478	431	348	223
1—Exercise regularly	2.82 (1.16)	2.93 (1.18)	3.67 (1.11)	2.57 (1.05)	3.64 (1.05)
2—Follow a balanced diet	3.35 (1.14)	3.35 (1.06)	4.16 (0.86)	3.04 (1.02)	4.12 (0.78)
3—Take vitamins or dietary supplements	2.26 (1.17)	2.00 (1.06)	3.89 (0.94)	2.09 (1.05)	2.14 (1.00)
4—Visit the dentist regularly	3.35 (1.36)	3.05 (1.29)	4.13 (1.12)	2.78 (1.16)	4.20 (1.02)
5—Watch weight or try to lose weight	2.92 (1.18)	2.58 (1.07)	3.73 (1.10)	2.70 (1.03)	3.56 (1.06)
6—Limit intake of high-fat or high-sugar foods	2.84 (1.06)	2.86 (0.97)	3.76 (0.91)	2.79 (1.00)	3.61 (0.86)
7—Gather health information before making decisions	2.92 (1.14)	2.45 (0.97)	3.91 (0.91)	2.66 (1.01)	3.39 (1.00)
8—Pay attention to physical symptoms or health changes	3.45 (1.12)	3.07 (1.05)	4.26 (0.87)	3.31 (0.97)	4.27 (0.82)
9—Take supplements to prevent illness	1.92 (1.17)	1.55 (0.85)	3.86 (0.89)	1.81 (0.97)	1.62 (0.72)
10—Get routine medical check-ups	2.78 (1.11)	2.45 (0.93)	3.60 (1.17)	2.72 (1.03)	3.50 (1.10)
11—Floss teeth regularly	2.59 (1.43)	2.07 (1.21)	3.32 (1.44)	1.86 (0.98)	3.13 (1.45)
12—Talk with others about health	2.93 (1.06)	2.57 (0.93)	3.56 (0.92)	2.75 (1.03)	3.27 (0.93)
13—Don't smoke	1.54 (0.66)	4.86 (0.41)	4.91 (0.33)	4.87 (0.39)	4.91 (0.33)
14—Brush teeth twice a day	4.64 (0.80)	5.00 (0.00)	4.91 (0.33)	3.36 (0.67)	4.93 (0.30)
15—Get vaccinated	3.40 (1.31)	3.19 (1.29)	3.62 (1.29)	3.29 (1.18)	3.83 (1.23)
16—Get enough sleep	3.58 (1.01)	3.64 (0.93)	3.88 (0.92)	3.58 (0.94)	3.95 (0.89)

Values represent means and SDs (in parentheses) for each of the 16 preventive health behavior items from the Good Health Practices scale (GHP-16), stratified by latent profile membership. Higher scores indicate more frequent or consistent engagement in the behavior. Profile membership was derived from a latent profile analysis using Gaussian mixture modeling. The profile labels are arbitrary and do not imply ordering.

3.2. Sociodemographic and Health Characteristics by Behavioral Profile

Using population-weighted data, Table 2 presents the distribution of key sociodemographic and health-related characteristics across the five latent profiles of preventive health behavior. Several characteristics varied significantly across profiles, but only a few reached effect sizes indicative of practical relevance.

Table 2. Population-based sociodemographic and health characteristics across latent profiles of preventive health behavior (n = 2090).

Variable	Medically Compliant, Lifestyle Passive [1]	Broadly Moderate Preventers [1]	Compre-hensive High Engagers [1]	Peripherally Engaged [1]	Globally Low Engagers [1]	p-Value [2]	Cramer's V [3]
Gender						<0.001	0.241
Male	256 (44.4)	292 (58.6)	121 (29.2)	209 (55.2)	149 (66.5)		
Female	320 (55.6)	206 (41.4)	294 (70.8)	169 (44.8)	75 (33.5)		
Age Group						<0.001	0.144
18–34	93 (16.1)	135 (27.1)	92 (22.3)	128 (33.9)	47 (21.2)		
35–54	159 (27.6)	182 (36.5)	128 (30.9)	136 (36.0)	78 (34.8)		
55–99	324 (56.3)	181 (36.4)	194 (46.8)	114 (30.1)	98 (44.0)		
Education						<0.001	0.085
Middle school	129 (22.5)	116 (23.3)	62 (14.9)	79 (20.8)	55 (24.4)		
Vocational school	156 (27.1)	175 (35.0)	118 (28.5)	130 (34.4)	88 (39.3)		
High school	149 (25.9)	124 (24.9)	125 (30.2)	101 (26.6)	46 (20.8)		
University	141 (24.5)	84 (16.8)	110 (26.4)	69 (18.2)	35 (15.5)		
Language						<0.001	0.114
German	394 (68.5)	341 (68.5)	223 (53.8)	226 (59.8)	145 (64.9)		
Italian	131 (22.7)	82 (16.5)	136 (32.8)	85 (22.4)	46 (20.8)		
Other	50 (8.7)	75 (15.0)	55 (13.3)	67 (17.8)	32 (14.3)		
HLS-EU-Q16 category						<0.001	0.122
Inadequate	67 (14.0)	63 (17.5)	38 (10.7)	57 (19.8)	40 (24.0)		
Problematic	157 (32.8)	148 (40.9)	108 (30.5)	88 (30.9)	58 (34.4)		
Sufficient	254 (53.1)	150 (41.6)	208 (58.8)	141 (49.2)	70 (41.6)		
HLS-EU-Q16 score [4]	12.2 (3.24)	11.4 (3.47)	12.6 (3.06)	11.7 (3.52)	11.0 (3.80)	<0.001	0.018
PAM-10						<0.001	0.127
Disengaged and overwhelmed	79 (13.8)	99 (19.9)	39 (9.5)	67 (17.7)	51 (22.6)		
Becoming aware but still struggling	235 (40.8)	219 (44.0)	168 (40.6)	158 (41.8)	107 (48.1)		
Taking action	139 (24.1)	122 (24.5)	80 (19.2)	99 (26.1)	50 (22.5)		
Maintaining behaviors and pushing further	123 (21.3)	58 (11.6)	127 (30.7)	54 (14.4)	15 (6.8)		
Chronic disease						0.008	0.085
No	350 (60.7)	351 (70.5)	270 (65.2)	254 (67.0)	132 (59.2)		
Yes	226 (39.3)	147 (29.5)	144 (34.8)	125 (33.0)	91 (40.8)		

[1] Percentage (absolute count); due to population weighting and variable-specific missing data, the effective sample sizes used in statistical testing may differ from the unweighted totals indicated in the table header. [2] p-values were based on chi-square tests. [3] Effect sizes are presented as Cramér's V; values are interpreted as follows: ≤0.10 = negligible, 0.10–0.19 = small, 0.20–0.29 = moderate, ≥0.30 = large effect. [4] Mean (SD), p-value of Kruskal–Wallis test; effect size estimated using eta squared; interpretation thresholds for η^2: <0.01 = negligible, 0.01–0.06 = small, 0.06–0.14 = moderate, ≥0.14 = large.

Gender emerged as the strongest profile-defining characteristic, with a moderate effect size (Cramér's V = 0.241). Age group and patient activation were also associated with profile membership, each with small-to-moderate effect sizes (Cramér's V = 0.144 and 0.127, respectively). In contrast, differences in language group, educational attainment, chronic disease status, and health literacy level, while statistically significant, showed only small or negligible effect sizes, suggesting limited contribution to profile differentiation.

3.2.1. Post Hoc Comparisons

Post hoc pairwise comparisons using adjusted standardized residuals (Bonferroni-corrected threshold: $|z| > 2.81$) revealed significant overrepresentation of men in the 'Broadly Moderate Preventers' and 'Globally Low Engagers' profiles, and of women in the 'Comprehensive High Engagers' profile. These contrasts confirm gender as a central driver of behavioral segmentation.

Age group differences further supported profile distinctions: the 'Medically Compliant, Lifestyle Passive' profile was dominated by older individuals (55+), while the 'Peripherally Engaged' and 'Broadly Moderate Preventers' profiles included disproportionately more young adults (18–34). These patterns suggest age-related gradients in engagement, particularly with younger individuals clustering in less medically anchored profiles.

With respect to patient activation, the 'Comprehensive High Engagers' had significantly more individuals at the highest PAM level (z = 7.5), whereas both the Broadly Moderate and 'Globally Low Engagers' were more likely to be found in the lowest activation category. This highlights a meaningful relationship between behavioral engagement and self-management capacity, albeit with a small overall effect size.

3.2.2. Health Literacy

Differences in health literacy scores across behavioral profiles were assessed using both the non-parametric Kruskal–Wallis test and one-way ANOVA, given the non-normality of the data. Given the robustness of ANOVA to moderate deviations from normality in large samples, and the similar results across both approaches (Table 2), post hoc comparisons were based on Bonferroni-adjusted ANOVA tests.

A one-way ANOVA revealed a significant effect of behavioral profile on health literacy scores, $F(4, 1644) = 11.06$, $p < 0.001$, with a small effect size ($\eta^2 = 0.026$). Bonferroni-corrected post hoc tests indicated that the 'Medically Compliant, Lifestyle Passive' group had significantly higher HLS scores than the Broadly Moderate, 'Comprehensive High Engagers', and Globally Low Engagers. The 'Peripherally Engaged' profile also scored significantly higher than both the Broadly Moderate and Globally Low groups. These findings suggest that while health literacy varies significantly across behavioral profiles, it only modestly contributes to distinguishing low engagement from medically oriented subgroups.

3.3. Gender Differences in Individual Preventive Health Behaviors

Table 3 presents a population-weighted comparison of preventive health behavior items between women and men. Although several behaviors showed statistically significant differences, most of the observed effects were small or negligible in practical terms.

The strongest gender differences, indicated by small-to-medium Cliff's delta values, were observed in behaviors associated with information engagement, supplementation, and communication. Men reported higher frequencies of gathering health information before making decisions, talking with others about health, and taking vitamins or supplements to prevent illness. These differences, although not large, suggest that male participants may engage more actively in informational and instrumental self-care strategies than commonly assumed.

Differences were also evident in the dietary and oral health practices of the participants. Men reported higher engagement in following a balanced diet, limiting the intake of high-fat or sugary foods, and visiting the dentist regularly. They also showed modestly higher adherence to routine checkups and oral hygiene behaviors, such as flossing and brushing. These patterns contribute to the broader preventive engagement profiles previously observed in profil-based analyses and challenge gender stereotypes that typically associate women with greater health vigilance than men.

In contrast, smoking abstinence, physical activity, and sleep quality showed minimal or negligible gender differences. Self-reported exercise and sleep patterns were nearly identical between the sexes, and the already high levels of non-smoking behavior in both groups showed only minor variation.

Taken together, these findings confirm that while men and women differ in specific preventive behaviors, particularly in health information use and dietary vigilance, the overall magnitude of gender differences at the item level was limited.

Table 3. Population-based comparison of preventive health behavior between women and men (n = 2090).

Item	PHG-16 Score Female Mean (SD) [1]	PHG-16 Score Male Mean (SD) [1]	Mean Difference	p-Value [2]	Cliff's Delta [3]
1—Exercise regularly	3.23 (1.25)	3.24 (1.15)	0.01	0.482	−0.02
2—Follow a balanced diet	3.46 (1.11)	3.84 (1.02)	0.38	<0.001	−0.21
3—Take vitamins or dietary supplements	2.19 (1.19)	2.72 (1.28)	0.53	<0.001	−0.25
4—Visit the dentist regularly	3.34 (1.30)	3.77 (1.28)	0.43	<0.001	−0.21
5—Watch weight or try to lose weight	3.10 (1.19)	3.20 (1.18)	0.10	0.004	−0.07
6—Limit intake of high-fat or high-sugar foods	3.03 (1.06)	3.40 (1.01)	0.37	<0.001	−0.20
7—Gather health information before making decisions	2.85 (1.13)	3.37 (1.09)	0.52	<0.001	−0.24
8—Pay attention to physical symptoms or health changes	3.55 (1.12)	3.86 (1.07)	0.32	<0.001	−0.16
9—Take supplements to prevent illness	1.86 (1.14)	2.39 (1.31)	0.53	<0.001	−0.23
10—Get routine medical check-ups	2.82 (1.14)	3.20 (1.17)	0.38	<0.001	−0.19
11—Floss teeth regularly	2.46 (1.38)	2.92 (1.46)	0.45	<0.001	−0.18
12—Talk with others about health	2.79 (1.02)	3.29 (0.99)	0.49	<0.001	−0.26
13—Don't smoke	4.20 (1.40)	4.36 (1.31)	0.17	0.002	−0.06
14—Brush teeth twice a day	4.61 (0.79)	4.83 (0.51)	0.21	<0.001	−0.12
15—Get vaccinated	3.40 (1.29)	3.54 (1.30)	0.14	0.012	−0.06
16—Get enough sleep	3.71 (0.94)	3.77 (0.95)	0.06	0.021	−0.05

[1] Weighted means and SD. [2] Mann–Whitney U tests. [3] Effect size interpretation of Cliff's delta: <0.147 = negligible effect, 0.147–0.33 = small effect, 0.33–0.474 = medium effect, ≥0.474 = large effect.

3.4. Predictors of Low Preventive Engagement: Profile 2 ('Broadly Moderate Preventers') vs. Profile 1 (Globally Low Engagers)

To identify characteristics associated with minimal engagement in preventive health behaviors, a binary logistic regression was conducted comparing Profile 5 ('Globally Low Engagers') with Profile 2 ('Broadly Moderate Preventers') based on the five-profile latent profile solution (Table 4). A total of n = 577 participants with complete data on all predictors were included ('Globally Low Engagers': n = 266, BMP: n = 311).

The model was statistically significant ($\chi^2(12) = 35.90$, $p < 0.001$) and explained 8.1% of the variance in profile membership (Nagelkerke $R^2 = 0.081$). The Hosmer–Lemeshow test indicated acceptable model fit ($\chi^2(8) = 12.25$, $p = 0.140$), and the Durbin–Watson statistic from an auxiliary linear regression was 1.90—suggesting independence of residuals.

Linearity of the logit was tested using the Box–Tidwell procedure; none of the interaction terms with log-transformed predictors were statistically significant, confirming the assumption of linearity. No standardized residuals exceeded $|3.0|$, and the maximum Cook's Distance was well below 1 (max = 0.12), indicating the absence of influential outliers.

Age was a significant predictor: with each additional year, the odds of being in the 'Globally Low Engagers' group decreased by 1.7% (OR = 0.983, p = 0.004). Living alone was associated with higher odds of 'Globally Low Engagers' membership (OR = 1.80, p = 0.011). Chronic disease was also predictive: individuals with chronic conditions had increased odds of being disengaged (OR = 1.79, p = 0.004).

Gender, language group, and patient activation showed trends but did not reach statistical significance in the multivariable model. Health literacy and mistrust were not significantly associated with profile membership.

These findings suggest that structural vulnerabilities, particularly living alone, chronic illness, and younger age, are stronger predictors of globally low preventive engagement than motivational constructs such as activation or trust.

Table 4. Binary logistic regression predicting membership in Profile 5 'Globally Low Engagers' versus Profile 2 'Broadly Moderate Preventers' (n = 577; Profile 5 = 266; Profile 2 = 311).

Predictor	B	SE	Wald χ^2	p	OR (Exp(B))	95% CI for OR
Intercept	0.508	0.684	0.550	0.458	1.662	[0.438, 6.300]
Gender (1 = Male)	0.416	0.251	2.748	0.097	1.516	[0.930, 2.469]
Age (continuous)	−0.017	0.006	8.303	0.004 **	0.983	[0.972, 0.994]
Education (ref = Middle school or lower)						
Vocational school	0.063	0.312	0.040	0.841	1.065	[0.577, 1.965]
High school	−0.296	0.337	0.774	0.379	0.744	[0.384, 1.443]
University	−0.016	0.406	0.002	0.968	0.984	[0.444, 2.181]
Language (ref = German)						
Italian	−0.453	0.325	1.942	0.163	0.636	[0.336, 1.202]
Other	−0.032	0.419	0.006	0.939	0.969	[0.426, 2.207]
Lives Alone (1 = Yes)	0.588	0.231	6.475	0.011 *	1.801	[1.144, 2.832]
Chronic Disease (1 = Yes)	0.582	0.201	8.391	0.004 **	1.789	[1.209, 2.647]
Health Literacy Score	−0.017	0.032	0.288	0.592	0.983	[0.923, 1.047]
Patient Activation Score	−0.010	0.008	1.522	0.217	0.990	[0.974, 1.006]
Mistrust Index	0.039	0.056	0.481	0.488	1.040	[0.932, 1.160]

Reference categories: Female (Gender), Middle school or lower (Education), German (Language), Not living alone (Lives Alone), No chronic disease (Chronic Disease). * $p < 0.05$, ** $p < 0.01$. Abbreviations: CI, Confidence Interval; SE, Standard Error; OR, Odds Ratio.

4. Discussion

This study identified five distinct latent profiles of preventive health behavior using 16 items from the GHP-16 scale in a representative sample of adults in South Tyrol. The profiles ranged from globally low engagement (Profile 5) to high engagement across all domains (Profile 3), with the largest share of participants falling into the medically compliant but lifestyle-passive group (Profile 1). Patient activation showed a clear gradient across profiles, whereas health literacy and language groups had limited explanatory power. Binary logistic regression confirmed that younger age, living alone, and chronic disease were significant predictors of globally low engagement. Among these, younger age showed the strongest associations. These findings underscore the need to examine not only direct predictors but also potential interactions between personal capacities and contextual barriers in preventive health research.

4.1. Interpretation Within a Health Behavior Framework

The five behavioral profiles align with the study's conceptual model (Figure 1). In this model, individual factors like motivation, confidence, and self-management interact with social and structural conditions to shape different patterns of preventive behavior (Hagger, 2025). Instead of viewing preventive behavior as a direct result of knowledge or demographics, the profile structure reveals meaningful subgroups with distinct patterns of behavior (Hill et al., 2022; L. K. Tong et al., 2024).

Beyond statistical fit indices, the five-profile solution was also supported by its substantive interpretability and external validity. Each profile exhibited a distinct and theoretically meaningful pattern of behavior, such as Profile 2's across-the-board disengagement or Profile 3's passivity in self-care but not in medical checkups. Additionally, the profiles correlated in expected directions with age, gender, mistrust, and patient activation, factors well-established in health behavior research. These patterns, and their practical value for designing public health interventions, support the external validity of the model.

The contrast between Profile 2 (Globally Low Engagers) and Profile 1 ('Broadly Moderate Preventers') offers insights into the determinants of poor preventive engagement. Individuals in Profile 2 were significantly more likely to be male, younger, less activated, and to report higher levels of mistrust in professional health information. In contrast, those in Profile 1 tended to be older, more often female, and reported higher patient activation. These patterns align with the analytic model's dual emphasis on personal capacities (such as activation and self-regulation) and contextual modifiers, including mistrust and social isolation (Hagger, 2025; L. K. Tong et al., 2024). Those living alone had significantly higher odds of belonging to Profile 2, although the effect size was moderate

Gender was the strongest predictor of profile membership. Men were overrepresented in the least engaged behavioral profile and underrepresented in the moderate- and high-engagement profiles. This finding challenges the common belief that women are always more health-conscious than men. Although health literacy is often conceptualized as a key predictor of health behavior, it was not significantly associated with profile membership in this study. This disconnect supports the notion that knowledge alone is insufficient to ensure safety. Motivation, trust, and social context play equally critical roles in shaping actions (Young-Silva et al., 2024; Bermeo et al., 2023).

The item-level analyses of GHP-16 behaviors support this interpretation in the following ways. Men reported lower engagement in health information-seeking, oral hygiene, and dietary control behaviors, which were aligned with the moderate- and high-engagement profiles. However, they reported higher frequencies of behaviors such as dietary supplement use or discussing health. These findings show the value of behavior-based segmentation and question common gender stereotypes in preventive health. Rather than assuming uniform needs across demographic groups, these results support the development of tailored interventions that align with empirically derived behavioral profiles (Burgermaster & Rodriguez, 2022).

Cultural-linguistic identity, captured by the language group, showed minimal association with the behavioral profiles. While language may influence communication preferences or trust in health information—as shown in previous analyses—it appears less relevant in shaping the structure of preventive behavior. This reinforces the idea that sociocultural variables act more as moderators of access and perception than as direct determinants of behavioral engagement (Short & Mollborn, 2015).

The observation that men reported both lower overall engagement and higher frequencies of specific behaviors like supplement use and health discussions warrants examination. Gendered reporting tendencies or social desirability bias may contribute to these patterns (Oksuzyan et al., 2019). Men might overreport proactive behaviors when asked directly, while underreporting routine activities like oral hygiene. Women, however, might provide more accurate self-assessments across behaviors. These response biases highlight the need to triangulate self-report data with objective measures and avoid overgeneralizing sex-based patterns without context.

4.2. Socio-Behavioral Drivers of Low Engagement

The regression analysis comparing Profile 2 (Globally Low Engagers) to Profile 1 ('Broadly Moderate Preventers') identified individual and psychosocial characteristics linked to low preventive health behaviors. Although several sociodemographic variables were statistically significant, few were meaningful predictors of disengagement. Gender differences were notable: men had higher odds of being 'Globally Low Engagers' than women, indicating that male participants were overrepresented in the least engaged profile

(Laska et al., 2009; Tabacchi et al., 2018). Age also influenced profile membership, with older individuals (especially those aged 55 and above) less likely to be in Profile 2, suggesting that preventive disengagement is more common among younger men, aligning with research on life-stage health behavior influences (Collins et al., 2023).

Among psychosocial variables, mistrust of professional health information was the main driver of disengagement. Individuals with higher Mistrust Index scores had increased odds of being Globally Low Engagers, reinforcing that low trust in health professionals can undermine engagement with recommended practices (Jaiswal & Halkitis, 2019; White et al., 2016). This finding suggests that rebuilding trust, especially among younger men, may be essential for improving adherence. Social isolation, as indicated by living alone, was linked to low engagement. Those living alone were nearly three times more likely to be in Profile 2 than those living with others. This supports including social context in behavior models and shows how living alone can affect habits like diet, hygiene, or medical visits (Dreyer et al., 2018; Hanna & Collins, 2015).

Patient activation findings confirm the role of motivation and self-efficacy in adopting preventive behaviors (Smith et al., 2013; Hibbard, 2017). In contrast, health literacy, both as a categorical and continuous measure, did not meaningfully predict profile membership. Sensitivity analysis confirmed only negligible differences in HLS scores across profiles, further suggesting that informational competence alone does not translate into behavioral engagement when trust or personal agency are lacking (Meraz et al., 2023). This shows that knowing what to do is insufficient without perceived control, motivation, and supportive environments.

These findings indicate that low preventive engagement reflects an interaction between distrust, isolation, and low agency, beyond sociodemographic disadvantages. Interventions addressing these barriers may be more effective than generic educational campaigns. Engaging community peer supporters or targeting health messages through trusted intermediaries could prove more successful in shifting behavior among low-engagement groups (Schwartz & Sendor, 1999).

4.3. Practical and Regional Implications

One unexpected finding was the minimal role of the language group in shaping preventive health behavior profiles. Despite South Tyrol's linguistic diversity, where German, Italian, and Ladin speakers coexist, language group membership did not meaningfully predict profile membership in the latent profile model or regression analysis. This contrasts with earlier analyses showing differences in health information-seeking by language group (Ausserhofer et al., 2022). The findings suggest that while cultural identity may influence how individuals access health information (Zanchetta & Poureslami, 2006), it plays a lesser role in preventive behaviors when controlling for individual and psychosocial factors (Solis et al., 1990; Unger, 2011).

This has implications for the generalizability of the findings. Although situated in a unique region, the identified behavioral profiles appear to transcend local language boundaries. This segmentation approach could also be useful in other multilingual regions, like Switzerland. This finding reinforces that preventive behaviors are shaped more by psychological and structural factors such as mistrust, isolation, and perceived self-efficacy than by cultural affiliation (Yap et al., 2023).

Latent profile segmentation helps public health planning by identifying behavioral subgroups that need tailored interventions. 'Globally Low Engagers' may need trust-building and social support (Drageset, 2021; Wilkins, 2018), while High Engagers may benefit from feedback and reinforcement (Krukowski et al., 2020; DiClemente et al., 2001).

Medically Passive individuals may require lifestyle coaching despite adequate preventive check-up behavior (Conn & Curtain, 2019).

This approach challenges the assumptions underlying health communication strategies. The finding that health literacy did not distinguish behavioral profiles, while mistrust and activation levels did, shows the need for context-sensitive messaging targeting psychological readiness (Smith et al., 2013). This may include peer-based outreach or programs that build health-related confidence rather than just transmitting knowledge (Brinsley et al., 2025).

Segmenting the population into behavioral subgroups can enhance equity in health promotion. By identifying groups with the greatest need, such as younger men with high mistrust and limited social connections, interventions can be better targeted, ensuring that resources are used efficiently and fairly to maximize their public health impact.

The identified profiles suggest distinct intervention needs. 'Globally Low Engagers' may require trust-building and social support through outreach by community intermediaries and messaging focused on small, achievable steps (Ward, 2017). Medically Passive individuals might benefit from personalized feedback and low-threshold digital tools to support lifestyle changes beyond routine check-ups (H. L. Tong et al., 2021). Aligning strategies with behavioral profiles may enhance the relevance and impact of preventive efforts.

4.4. Strengths and Limitations

This study had several methodological strengths that enhanced its validity. First, it used a large, population-based stratified sample of South Tyrolean adults, with a standardized bilingual survey design supporting representativeness. The stratification across sociodemographic variables and calibrated weights ensured that the results reflected the general adult population. Second, the LPA of the GHP-16 items identified empirically derived behavioral profiles beyond traditional scoring methods. Third, the study included comprehensive psychosocial and contextual variables, including mistrust, living situation, and patient activation, enabling an integrative analysis of behavioral engagement reflecting individual and social health determinants.

However, there are some limitations to this approach. The analysis relied on self-reported behaviors that were subject to recall bias and social desirability effects. While the GHP-16 shows validity, self-assessments may not align with objective behaviors. The use of rescaled Likert data for GMM could limit comparability with the categorical LPA techniques.

LPA and binary logistic regression used unweighted data. Although this enhances the LPA model stability, it limits the generalizability of profile proportions. Population weights were applied post hoc to improve the representativeness of descriptive profiling and comparisons. Additionally, the software framework used for LPA estimation (tidyLPA, based on mclust) does not provide Lo-Mendell-Rubin (LMR) or bootstrap likelihood ratio tests (BLRT) for determining the number of profiles. Therefore, model selection relied on BIC, Integrated Completed Likelihood, and AvPP, in line with current recommendations. Furthermore, we did not apply BCH-adjusted comparisons when analyzing differences across profiles, which would account for classification uncertainty. While our approach was based on direct class assignment using maximum posterior probabilities, future studies could enhance precision by implementing BCH methods now available in packages like tidySEM.

Furthermore, the regression model did not include certain key structural determinants such as household income, employment type, or healthcare access, as these were not assessed in the survey. The absence of these variables may limit the explanatory power of the predictive model and hinder deeper understanding of the economic or occupational drivers of low preventive engagement. Future research should aim to integrate these dimensions to better capture the full range of social determinants influencing preventive health behavior.

The cross-sectional design precludes causal inferences about behavioral changes. The relationship between mistrust, activation, and preventive behaviors is still hypothetical. Additionally, factors such as health service access and income were not fully explored, although they may affect behavioral segmentation.

Despite these limitations, this study provides an empirical framework for understanding preventive engagement patterns and supports segmentation models in research and public health planning.

5. Conclusions

This study identified five distinct behavioral profiles of preventive health engagement in a population-based sample from South Tyrol using latent profile analysis of the GHP-16. While most individuals exhibited moderate or high levels of engagement, a small but important subgroup—Globally Low Engagers—emerged with consistently low scores across preventive domains. This group was disproportionately composed of younger, less activated men and individuals with higher mistrust of health professionals or limited social ties.

The results highlight that preventive actions are influenced not only by personal knowledge or demographic factors but also by a combination of individual abilities (such as confidence and self-management) and contextual factors (such as social isolation and trust in personal health information). The lack of a strong link between health literacy and behavioral categories indicates that information alone is insufficient to effect behavior change. Motivation, perceived control, and trust are the essential drivers.

This study lays the groundwork for more focused and fair health promotion strategies by dividing the population into groups with distinct behaviors. Efforts to enhance preventive actions should consider not only people's knowledge, but also their beliefs, the level of control they perceive they have, and the environment they inhabit. Employing person-centered, data-driven segmentation models, such as LPA, could pave the way for crafting more adaptive and successful prevention initiatives in South Tyrol and other similar contexts.

Author Contributions: Conceptualization, C.J.W., D.A., G.P., K.E. and A.E.; methodology, D.A., S.L., T.G. and V.B.; formal analysis, V.B., D.A. and C.J.W.; investigation, S.L. and T.G.; data curation, D.A. and V.B.; writing—original draft preparation, C.J.W.; writing—review and editing, D.A., S.L., T.G., G.P., K.E. and A.E.; supervision, A.E., K.E. and T.G. All authors have read and agreed to the published version of the manuscript.

Funding: This research received no external funding.

Institutional Review Board Statement: The study was conducted in accordance with the Decla-ration of Helsinki, and approved by the Institutional Review Board of the Institute of General Practice and Public Health, Bolzano, Italy (protocol code 20/11/2023, approved on 20 November 2023).

Informed Consent Statement: Informed consent was obtained from all subjects involved in the study.

Data Availability Statement: Data are available from the corresponding author upon reasonable request.

Conflicts of Interest: The authors declare no conflicts of interest.

Abbreviations

The following abbreviations are used in this manuscript.

ASTAT	Provincial Institute of Statistics of South Tyrol
AvePP	Average Posterior Probabilities
BHC	Bolck-Croon-Hagenaars
BIC	Bayesian Information Criterion
BLRT	Bootstrap Likelihood Ratio Tests
CI	Confidence Interval
GHP-16	Good Health Practice 16 Items
HBC	Health Behavior Checklist
HBM	Health Belief Model
HLS-EU-Q16	Health Literacy Survey EU Questionnaire 16 Items
ISTAT	National Institute of Statistics of Italy
LMR	Lo-Mendell-Rubin
LPA	Latent Profile Analysis
PAM-10	Patient Activation Measure 10 Items
SD	Standard Deviation
TPB	Theory of Planned Behavior
VIF	Variance Inflation Factors

References

Aaby, A., Friis, K., Christensen, B., Rowlands, G., & Maindal, H. T. (2017). Health literacy is associated with health behaviour and self-reported health: A large population-based study in individuals with cardiovascular disease. *European Journal of Preventive Cardiology, 24*(17), 1880–1888. [CrossRef] [PubMed]

Airhihenbuwa, C. O., Tseng, T., Sutton, V. D., & Price, L. (2021). Global perspectives on improving chronic disease prevention and management in diverse settings. *Preventing Chronic Disease, 18*, E33. [CrossRef] [PubMed]

Anderson, L. J., & Cirillo, L. (2020). The emergence and relevance of cultural difference in mediated health interactions. *Health Communication, 36*(9), 1101–1114. [CrossRef]

Ausserhofer, D., Piccoliori, G., Engl, A., Marino, P., Barbieri, V., Lombardo, S., Gärtner, T., & Wiedermann, C. J. (2025). Sleep problems and sleep quality in the general adult population living in South Tyrol (Italy): A cross-sectional survey study. *Clocks & Sleep, 7*(2), 23. [CrossRef]

Ausserhofer, D., Wiedermann, W., Becker, U., Vögele, A., Piccoliori, G., Wiedermann, C. J., & Engl, A. (2022). Health information-seeking behavior associated with linguistic group membership: Latent class analysis of a population-based cross-sectional survey in Italy, August to September 2014. *Archives of Public Health, 80*(1), 87. [CrossRef]

Bermeo, R. N. Z., Gonzalez, C. E., & Guerra, E. d. P. H. (2023). Influence of personal factors on health-promoting behavior in college students: A structural equation modeling approach. *Journal of Multidisciplinary Healthcare, 16*, 1259–1270. [CrossRef] [PubMed]

Bonvicini, L., Venturelli, F., Bononi, F., Balestra, G. L., Iorio, G., Ghirotto, L., Petrelli, A., Pierconti, S., Laurendi, G., Perticone, M., Pellegrino, A., Boddi, M., Modesti, P. A., Rossi, P. G., DIABETHIC Working Group & Dadras, O. (2025). A randomized trial to evaluate a complex, co-created, culture-sensitive intervention to promote healthy lifestyles and compliance to therapy in immigrants with type 2 diabetes: A protocol of a multicenter Italian study. *PLoS ONE, 20*(2), e0317994. [CrossRef]

Brenk-Franz, K., Hibbard, J. H., Herrmann, W. J., Freund, T., Szecsenyi, J., Djalali, S., Steurer-Stey, C., Sönnichsen, A., Tiesler, F., Storch, M., Schneider, N., Gensichen, J., & Janda, M. (2013). Validation of the German version of the patient activation measure 13 (PAM13-D) in an international multicentre study of primary care patients. *PLoS ONE, 8*(9), e74786. [CrossRef]

Brinsley, J., Schmidt, M., Curtis, R., Simpson, C. E., Edwards, J., Eglitis, E. E., Gosse, G., Broad, M., Jardine, B., Taddeo, E., Banati, P., & Maher, C. (2025). Effectiveness of peer-led health behaviour interventions on adolescent's mental health and wellbeing: A systematic review and meta-analysis. *Scientific Reports, 15*(1), 16480. [CrossRef]

Burgermaster, M., & Rodriguez, V. A. (2022). Psychosocial-behavioral phenotyping: A novel precision health approach to modeling behavioral, psychological, and social determinants of health using machine learning. *Annals of Behavioral Medicine, 56*(12), 1258–1271. [CrossRef]

Carpenter, C. J. (2010). A meta-analysis of the effectiveness of health belief model variables in predicting behavior. *Health Communication, 25*(8), 661–669. [CrossRef]

Collins, S., Hoare, E., Allender, S., Olive, L., Leech, R. M., Winpenny, E. M., Jacka, F., & Lotfalian, M. (2023). A longitudinal study of lifestyle behaviours in emerging adulthood and risk for symptoms of depression, anxiety, and stress. *Journal of Affective Disorders, 327*, 244–253. [CrossRef] [PubMed]

Conn, S., & Curtain, S. (2019). Health coaching as a lifestyle medicine process in primary care. *Australian Journal of General Practice, 48*(10), 677–680. [CrossRef]

Corrêa, R., Froner, M. B., & Tabak, B. M. (2024). Assessing the impact of behavioral sciences interventions on chronic disease prevention and management: A systematic review of randomized controlled trials. *International Journal of Environmental Research and Public Health, 21*(7), 837. [CrossRef] [PubMed]

Couture, É. M., Chouinard, M., Fortin, M., & Hudon, C. (2018). The relationship between health literacy and patient activation among frequent users of healthcare services: A cross-sectional study. *BMC Family Practice, 19*(1), 38. [CrossRef]

Da Silva, A. C. R., Da Silva, K. G. S., Costa, T. T., Dutra, M. d. O., De Oliveira, A. B. S., Silva, R. M. d. S., Tunes, R. A. M., De Barros, S. C., Da Costa, M. G., & Araújo, W. M. R. (2024). The importance of preventive medicine in reducing chronic diseases. *Revista de Gestão Social e Ambiental, 18*(2), e04380. [CrossRef]

DiClemente, C. C., Marinilli, A. S., Singh, M., & Bellino, L. E. (2001). The role of feedback in the process of health behavior change. *American Journal of Health Behavior, 25*(3), 217–227. [CrossRef]

Drageset, J. (2021). Social Support. In G. Haugan, & M. Eriksson (Eds.), *Health promotion in health care—Vital theories and research*. Springer. Available online: https://library.oapen.org/bitstream/handle/20.500.12657/47291/1/9783030631352.pdf (accessed on 21 July 2025).

Dreyer, K., Steventon, A., Fisher, R., & Deeny, S. R. (2018). The association between living alone and health care utilisation in older adults: A retrospective cohort study of electronic health records from a London general practice. *BMC Geriatrics, 18*(1), 269. [CrossRef]

Erişen, M. A. (2024). Effect of health literacy and patient activation on health-seeking behaviour: A cross-sectional study in turkey. *Health Expectations, 27*(5), e70052. [CrossRef] [PubMed]

Franceschi, R., Fornari, E., Ghezzi, M., Buzzi, E., Toschi, M., Longhi, S., Maimone, R., Forti, S., Carneri, S., Pirous, F. M., Agostini, B., Iori, T., Gibin, M., Porchia, S., Soffiati, M., & Maffeis, C. (2021). Educational intervention of healthy life promotion for children with a migrant background or at socioeconomic disadvantage in the North of Italy: Efficacy of telematic tools in improving nutritional and physical activity knowledge. *Nutrients, 13*(10), 3634. [CrossRef]

Gautam, V., S, D., Rustagi, N., Mittal, A., Patel, M., Shafi, S., Thirunavukkarasu, P., & Raghav, P. (2021). Health literacy, preventive COVID 19 behaviour and adherence to chronic disease treatment during lockdown among patients registered at primary health facility in urban Jodhpur, Rajasthan. *Diabetes & Metabolic Syndrome: Clinical Research & Reviews, 15*(1), 205–211. [CrossRef]

Gerend, M. A., & Shepherd, J. E. (2012). Predicting human papillomavirus vaccine uptake in young adult women: Comparing the health belief model and theory of planned behavior. *Annals of Behavioral Medicine, 44*(2), 171–180. [CrossRef]

Gokhale, S. S. (2020, December 7–10). *Comparing the impact of unhealthy behaviors and preventive services on chronic health outcomes*. 2020 IEEE/ACM International Conference on Advances in Social Networks Analysis and Mining (ASONAM) (pp. 798–802), The Hague, The Netherlands. [CrossRef]

Graffigna, G., Barello, S., & Bonanomi, A. (2017). The role of patient health engagement model (PHE-model) in affecting patient activation and medication adherence: A structural equation model. *PLoS ONE, 12*(6), e0179865. [CrossRef] [PubMed]

Hagger, M. S. (2025). Psychological determinants of health behavior. *Annual Review of Psychology, 76*(1), 821–850. [CrossRef]

Halpin, H. A., Morales-Suárez-Varela, M. M., & Martin-Moreno, J. M. (2010). Chronic disease prevention and the new public health. *Public Health Reviews, 32*(1), 120–154. [CrossRef]

Hampson, S. E., Edmonds, G. W., & Goldberg, L. R. (2019). The health behavior checklist: Factor structure in community samples and validity of a revised good health practices scale. *Journal of Health Psychology, 24*(8), 1103–1109. [CrossRef]

Hanna, K. L., & Collins, P. F. (2015). Relationship between living alone and food and nutrient intake. *Nutrition Reviews, 73*(9), 594–611. [CrossRef] [PubMed]

Hibbard, J. (2017). Patient activation and health literacy: What's the difference? how do each contribute to health outcomes. In *Health literacy* (pp. 251–262). IOS Press. [CrossRef]

Higgins, S. T. (2015). Editorial: 2nd special issue on behavior change, health, and health disparities. *Preventive Medicine, 80*, 1–4. [CrossRef] [PubMed]

Hill, M. S., Barnes, T., Wu, L., Tkatch, R., Kraemer, S., Schaeffer, J., & Yeh, C. (2022). Profiles of personal determinants of health and associated health outcomes in older adults: A latent class analysis. *Innovation in Aging, 6*(Suppl. 1), 651. [CrossRef]

Huang, X., Dai, S., & Xu, H. (2020). Predicting tourists' health risk preventative behaviour and travelling satisfaction in Tibet: Combining the theory of planned behaviour and health belief model. *Tourism Management Perspectives, 33*(January), 100589. [CrossRef]

Jaiswal, J., & Halkitis, P. N. (2019). Towards a more inclusive and dynamic understanding of medical mistrust informed by science. *Behavioral Medicine, 45*(2), 79–85. [CrossRef]

Krukowski, R., Kim, H., Stansbury, M., Li, Q., Sen, S., Farage, G., & West, D. (2020). Importance of multiple reinforcing comments and areas for change in optimizing dietary and exercise self-monitoring feedback in behavioral weight loss programs: Factorial design. *Journal of Medical Internet Research, 22*(11), e18104. [CrossRef]

Laska, M. N., Pasch, K. E., Lust, K., Story, M., & Ehlinger, E. (2009). Latent class analysis of lifestyle characteristics and health risk behaviors among college youth. *Prevention Science, 10*(4), 376–386. [CrossRef] [PubMed]

Lee, P. C., Mao, A., Dong, P., Wang, K., & Qiu, W. (2021). 951Can cancer-related health literacy predict cancer preventive behaviours? *International Journal of Epidemiology, 50*(Suppl. 1). [CrossRef]

Lin, C.-Y., Chung, M. L., Schuman, D. L., Biddle, M. J., Mudd-Martin, G., Miller, J. L., Hammash, M., Schooler, M. P., Rayens, M. K., Feltner, F. J., & Moser, D. K. (2023). Psychometric properties of the patient activation measure in family caregivers of patients with chronic illnesses. *Nursing Research, 72*(4), 292–300. [CrossRef] [PubMed]

Lorini, C., Lastrucci, V., Mantwill, S., Vettori, V., Bonaccorsi, G., & Florence Health Literacy Research Group. (2019). Measuring health literacy in Italy: A validation study of the HLS-EU-Q16 and of the HLS-EU-Q6 in Italian language, conducted in florence and its surroundings. *Annali Dell'Istituto Superiore Di Sanita, 55*(1), 10–18. [CrossRef]

Martin Obianyo, C., Ezeamii, V. C., Idoko, B., Adeyinka, T., Ejembi, E. V., Idoko, J. E., Obioma, L. O., & Ugwu, O. J. (2024). The role of preventive medicine in reducing chronic disease Burden in the USA: A systematic review. *Magna Scientia Advanced Biology and Pharmacy, 13*(1), 095–126. [CrossRef]

Meraz, R., Caldwell, E. P., & McGee, J. S. (2023). The relationships among health literacy, patient activation, and self-care behaviors in adults with heart failure: A cross sectional study. *Sage Open, 13*(1), 21582440231163779. [CrossRef]

Mohan, Y., Sidell, M., Tillman, L., & Young, D. (2017). Abstract P241: Health literacy and patient activation are not predictors of positive health behaviors among young adult women. *Circulation, 135*(Suppl. 1), AP241. [CrossRef]

Montanaro, E. A., & Bryan, A. D. (2014). Comparing theory-based condom interventions: Health belief model versus theory of planned behavior. *Health Psychology, 33*(10), 1251–1260. [CrossRef]

Oksuzyan, A., Dańko, M. J., Caputo, J., Jasilionis, D., & Shkolnikov, V. M. (2019). Is the story about sensitive women and stoical men true? Gender differences in health after adjustment for reporting behavior. *Social Science & Medicine, 228*, 41–50. [CrossRef] [PubMed]

Palumbo, R. (2021). Leveraging organizational health literacy to enhance health promotion and risk prevention: A narrative and interpretive literature review. *The Yale Journal of Biology and Medicine, 94*(1), 115–128.

Pelikan, J. M., Ganahl, K., Van den Broucke, S., & Sørensen, K. (2019). Measuring health literacy in Europe: Introducing the european health literacy survey questionnaire (HLS-EU-Q). In *International handbook of health literacy* (pp. 115–138). Policy Press.

Pelikan, J. M., Röthlin, F., Ganahl, K., & The HLSEU Consortium. (2014). *Comparative report on health literacy in eight EU member states (second extended and revised version)*. Maastricht University.

Schwartz, C. E., & Sendor, R. M. (1999). Helping others helps oneself: Response shift effects in peer support. *Social Science & Medicine, 48*(11), 1563–1575. [CrossRef]

Short, S. E., & Mollborn, S. (2015). Social determinants and health behaviors: Conceptual frames and empirical advances. *Current Opinion in Psychology, 5*, 78–84. [CrossRef]

Smith, S. G., Curtis, L. M., Wardle, J., von Wagner, C., & Wolf, M. S. (2013). Skill set or mind set? associations between health literacy, patient activation and health. *PLoS ONE, 8*(9), e74373. [CrossRef]

Solis, J. M., Marks, G., Garcia, M., & Shelton, D. (1990). Acculturation, access to care, and use of preventive services by Hispanics: Findings from HHANES 1982–84. *American Journal of Public Health, 80*(Suppl), 11–19. [CrossRef]

Sørensen, K., Pelikan, J. M., Röthlin, F., Ganahl, K., Slonska, Z., Doyle, G., Fullam, J., Kondilis, B., Agrafiotis, D., Uiters, E., Falcon, M., Mensing, M., Tchamov, K., Broucke, S. v. D., & Brand, H. (2015). Health literacy in Europe: Comparative results of the European health literacy survey (HLS-EU). *European Journal of Public Health, 25*(6), 1053–1058. [CrossRef]

Sulat, J. S., Prabandari, Y. S., Sanusi, R., Hapsari, E. D., & Santoso, B. (2018). The validity of health belief model variables in predicting behavioral change. *Health Education, 118*(6), 499–512. [CrossRef]

Tabacchi, G., Faigenbaum, A., Jemni, M., Thomas, E., Capranica, L., Palma, A., Breda, J., & Bianco, A. (2018). Profiles of physical fitness risk behaviours in school adolescents from the ASSO project: A latent class analysis. *International Journal of Environmental Research and Public Health, 15*(9), 1933. [CrossRef] [PubMed]

Tong, H. L., Quiroz, J. C., Kocaballi, A. B., Fat, S. C. M., Dao, K. P., Gehringer, H., Chow, C. K., & Laranjo, L. (2021). Personalized mobile technologies for lifestyle behavior change: A systematic review, meta-analysis, and meta-regression. *Preventive Medicine, 148*, 106532. [CrossRef]

Tong, L. K., Li, Y. Y., Liu, Y. B., Zheng, M. R., Fu, G. L., & Au, M. L. (2024). Social determinants of health and their relation to suboptimal health status in the context of 3PM: A latent profile analysis. *EPMA Journal, 15*(2), 221–232. [CrossRef]

Unger, J. B. (2011). Cultural Identity and Public Health. In S. J. Schwartz, K. Luyckx, & V. L. Vignoles (Eds.), *Handbook of identity theory and research* (pp. 811–825). Springer. [CrossRef]

Van Lissa, C. J., Garnier-Villarreal, M., & Anadria, D. (2023). Recommended practices in latent class analysis using the open-source R-package tidySEM. *Structural Equation Modeling: A Multidisciplinary Journal, 31*(3), 526–534. [CrossRef]

Vickers, R. R., Conway, T. L., & Hervig, L. K. (1990). Demonstration of replicable dimensions of health behaviors. *Preventive Medicine, 19*(4), 377–401. [CrossRef]

Ward, P. R. (2017). Improving access to, use of, and outcomes from public health programs: The importance of building and maintaining trust with patients/clients. *Frontiers in Public Health, 5*, 22. [CrossRef]

White, R. O., Chakkalakal, R. J., Presley, C. A., Bian, A., Schildcrout, J. S., Wallston, K. A., Barto, S., Kripalani, S., & Rothman, R. (2016). Perceptions of provider communication among vulnerable patients with diabetes: Influences of medical mistrust and health literacy. *Journal of Health Communication, 21*(sup2), 127–134. [CrossRef]

Wiedermann, C. J., Barbieri, V., Lombardo, S., Gärtner, T., Rina, P., Eisendle, K., Piccoliori, G., Engl, A., & Ausserhofer, D. (2025). Health information use and trust: The role of health literacy and patient activation in a multilingual european region. *International Journal of Environmental Research and Public Health, 22*(4), 570. [CrossRef]

Wilkins, C. H. (2018). Effective engagement requires trust and being trustworthy. *Medical Care, 56*(Suppl. 1), S6–S8. [CrossRef] [PubMed]

Yap, S., Lim, W. M., Gaur, S. S., & Lim, P. Y. (2023). A framework for preventive health marketing. *Journal of Strategic Marketing, 31*(4), 894–917. [CrossRef]

Young-Silva, Y., Berenguera, A., Juvinyà-Canal, D., Martí-Lluch, R., Arroyo-Uriarte, P., Tamayo-Morales, O., Marcilla-Toribio, I., Elizondo-Alzola, U., Méndez-López, F., Chela-Àlvarez, X., & Motrico, E. (2024). Exploring personal aptitudes and personality traits that, together with social determinants, shape health behaviors and conduct: A thematic analysis based on the Capability, Opportunity, Motivation and Behavior (COM-B) change system. *Frontiers in Public Health, 12*, 1387528. [CrossRef]

Zanchetta, M. S., & Poureslami, I. M. (2006). Health literacy within the realiTABLEty of immigrants' culture and language. *Canadian Journal of Public Health = Revue Canadienne De Sante Publique, 97*(Suppl. 2), S26–S30. [PubMed]

Zhao, R., Zhao, N., Wang, S., Zhang, X., Ding, B., Li, Y., Miao, W., Pan, L., & Fan, H. (2023). Assessment of type 2 diabetes mellitus patients' behavioral characteristics associated with integrated treatment and prevention services in community health centers in China. *Frontiers in Public Health, 10*, 1084946. [CrossRef] [PubMed] healthcare

MDPI

Article

Factors Affecting Physical Activity Adherence in Male Office Workers Based on Self-Determination Theory: The Mediating Effects of Psychological Need Satisfaction and Autonomous Motivation

Sangmi Han [1] and Yeongmi Ha [2,*]

[1] Department of Nursing, Gyeongnam Geochang University, Geochang 50147, Gyeongnam, Republic of Korea; y2k2509@nate.com
[2] College of Nursing and Sustainable Health Research Institute, Gyeongsang National University, Jinju 52727, Gyeongnam, Republic of Korea
* Correspondence: yha@gnu.ac.kr

Abstract

Background/Objectives: Despite the health benefit of regular physical activity, many adults often discontinue it within 3–6 months due to various obstacles. The purpose of this study was to investigate factors affecting physical activity adherence of male office workers based on self-determination theory by constructing a structural equation model. **Methods:** In total, 257 full-time male office workers who engage in regular physical activity participated. The participants from 15 companies completed a survey asking about perceived physical activity barriers, autonomy support, psychological need satisfaction in physical activity, autonomous motivation, and physical activity adherence. Data analysis was performed using the SPSS 28.0 and the AMOS 26.0 programs to verify the fit of the hypothetical model and identify the direct and indirect effects of variables on physical activity adherence for male office workers. **Results:** As a result, the path significance test results for the hypothetical model showed that five of the nine paths were significant. The results show that psychological need satisfaction in physical activity and autonomous motivation were significant variables that had a direct effect on physical activity adherence, while autonomy support from significant others and perceived physical activity barriers had a significant indirect effect through psychological need satisfaction and autonomous motivation, explaining 62.0%. **Conclusions:** Based on these findings, it is recommended to implement customized workplace-specific physical activity interventions to enhance autonomous motivation and the autonomy, competence, and relatedness aspects of psychological need satisfaction in physical activity.

Keywords: office workers; physical activity adherence; psychological need satisfaction; motivation; self-determination theory

1. Introduction

1.1. Background

According to the 2018 Physical Activity Guidelines for Americans [1] and 2023 Physical Activity Guidelines for Koreans [2], adults aged 18 through 64 years should do at least 150–300 min a week of moderate-intensity, or 75–150 min a week of vigorous-intensity aerobic physical activity, or an equivalent combination of moderate- and vigorous-intensity aerobic activity. Office workers are known to be at risk of insufficient physical activity due to their work characteristics, which require them to spend at least seven hours a day sitting [3]. The lack of physical activity caused by their job characteristics contributes to many adverse health outcomes, including all-cause mortality and the risk of developing chronic diseases such as stroke, coronary heart diseases, diabetes, and metabolic syndrome [1,4]. Despite the risks of physical inactivity, many adults often find it difficult to begin moderate–vigorous physical activity (MVPA) or tend to discontinue it within 3–6 months due to various barriers [5,6]. In particular, regarding its health benefits, physical activity adherence is recommended on three or more days a week, and adults should minimize prolonged sitting time throughout the day [1,2].

The definition of physical activity adherence varies among scholars, but it generally refers to the consistent practice of regular physical activity as an integral part of one's life, and it includes factors such as frequency, intensity, duration, and type of activity [4]. Most previous studies have focused on physical activity adherence among patients with various chronic diseases [7,8], while research examining the physical activity adherence of general adults is limited. According to a systematic review on physical activity adherence among patients prescribing exercise therapy, the factors that significantly affected physical activity adherence were support from family or health professionals, enjoyment of physical activity, and personal wellness goals [8]. Since long-term physical activity adherence clearly has positive effects on health, the factors affecting the physical activity adherence of office workers should be explored.

Self-determination theory, well known as explaining motivational processes for physical activity, has demonstrated how regular physical activity is initiated and maintained in the long-term through motivational processes [9,10]. Behavioral motivation is the most powerful driving force within an individual that impels them to pursue their positive behavioral changes [11]. A growing body of research and systematic reviews have been conducted on behavioral motivation toward physical activity—i.e., why some people show an enduring desire to pursue their activity, whereas others lose interest [12,13]. Behind the motivational process for physical activity, applying self-determination theory, is the premise that people are inherently active in their pursuit to satisfy three basic psychological needs: the need to feel a sense of engagement during physical activity (autonomy); a belief in one's ability to perform the physical activity well (competence); and feeling a meaningful connection with others participating in the same physical activity (relatedness) [10,12]. The fulfillment of these three basic needs for physical activity determines individuals' persistence toward engaging in intrinsically motivated activity behaviors, thereby leading to long-term physical activity adherence [13]. Pelletier et al. [14] developed a sports motivation scale based on self-determination theory, which allows for a precise assessment of an individual's intrinsic and extrinsic motivation to participate in sports and regular physical activity. Individuals with high intrinsic motivation for physical activity tend to find MVPA interesting and enjoyable, which drives them to continue engaging in it voluntarily over a long period [4,9,11].

Perceived barriers to physical activity can be an important factor that determines whether individuals continue or discontinue physical activity [15]. Adults generally discontinue regular physical activity for reasons such as 'time restriction,' 'lack of knowledge or exercise skills,' 'poor accessibility to physical activity facilities,' and 'burden of expenses for MVPA' [8,16]. According to previous research about barriers to reduce sedentary behaviors and increase physical activity of office workers, major barriers were personal factors such as lack of motivation, job characteristics such as lack of time, cost, distance, and job stress, or organizational factors such as poor accessibility [17,18]. These barriers are known to reduce confidence and decrease intrinsic motivation for physical activity, ultimately making physical activity adherence more difficult [8]. Several suggestions have emerged to decrease the sedentary behaviors and improve the physical activity of office workers such as that more support from companies, cultivating health supporting organizational culture, and high accessibility to exercise facilities in companies should be provided [18]. Therefore, this study aimed to identify predictors of physical activity adherence among office workers based on self-determination theory [19]. First, the purpose of this study is to build a hypothetical model for the physical activity adherence of male office workers based on self-determination theory and literature reviews. Second, it is verified whether the relationship between the hypothetical model and the actual data is suitable for the model of self-determination theory. Third, the study identifies the factors that affect the physical activity adherence of male office workers and identifies direct and indirect effects and total effects.

1.2. Conceptual Framework

The conceptual framework of this study was established based on self-determination theory [19] and literature reviews related to physical activity for adults. When three basic psychological needs for autonomy, competence, and relatedness in physical activity are fulfilled, people's intrinsic motivation is enhanced, leading them to actively engage in physical activity adherence. Self-determination theory and previous studies demonstrate autonomous motivation as a significant influencing factor for physical activity adherence [10,13]. In the hypothetical model of this study, exogenous variables such as perceived physical activity barriers and autonomy support from significant others affect the endogenous variables, such as psychological need satisfaction in physical activity and autonomous motivation; these factors, in turn, established both direct and indirect pathways toward physical activity adherence of office workers (Figure 1). The hypotheses in this study are as follows:

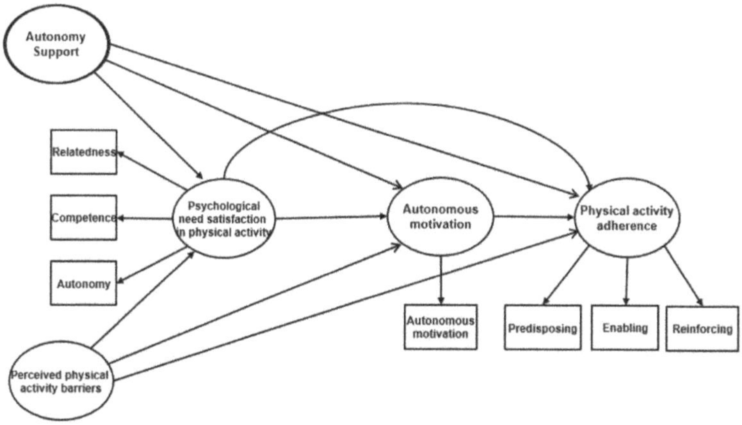

Figure 1. Hypothetical model.

1.2.1. Hypothesis with Psychological Need Satisfaction in Physical Activity as an Endogenous Variable

Autonomy support (Hypothesis 1, H1) and perceived physical activity barriers (Hypothesis 2, H2) are expected to be positively and significantly associated with psychological need satisfaction in physical activity.

1.2.2. Hypothesis with Autonomous Motivation as an Endogenous Variable

Hypothesis 3 (H3). *Autonomy support is expected to be positively and significantly associated with autonomous motivation.*

Hypothesis 4 (H4). *Perceived physical activity barriers are expected to be positively and significantly associated with autonomous motivation.*

Hypothesis 5 (H5). *Psychological need satisfaction in physical activity is expected to be positively and significantly associated with autonomous motivation (H5a), and psychological need satisfaction in physical activity is hypothesized to act as a mediator in the pathways between autonomy support, perceived physical activity barriers, and autonomous motivation (H5b).*

1.2.3. Hypothesis with Physical Activity Adherence as an Endogenous Variable

Hypothesis 6 (H6). *Autonomy support is expected to be positively and significantly associated with physical activity adherence.*

Hypothesis 7 (H7). *Perceived physical activity barriers are expected to be positively and significantly associated with physical activity adherence.*

Hypothesis 8 (H8). *Psychological need satisfaction in physical activity is expected to be positively and significantly associated with physical activity adherence.*

Hypothesis 9 (H9). *Autonomous motivation is expected to be positively and significantly associated with physical activity adherence (H9a); autonomous motivation is hypothesized to act as a mediator in the pathways between psychological need satisfaction in physical activity and physical activity adherence (H9b); and autonomous motivation is hypothesized to act as a mediator in the pathways between autonomy support, perceived physical activity barriers, and physical activity adherence (H9c).*

2. Methods

2.1. Participants

This study conveniently sampled male office workers working in the banking sector in a city in Korea. The inclusion criteria for the participants were as follows: (1) office workers aged between 19 and 60; (2) full-time workers working 40 h per week; and (3) individuals engaging in 150–300 min of moderate aerobic physical activity or 75–150 min of vigorous aerobic physical activity per week. The exclusion criteria were determined based on literature reviews that explore whether accessibility, preference for physical activity adherence, basic psychological needs, and activity barriers and facilitators have a moderating effect depending on gender [20–24]. First, previous studies demonstrated that men and women differ in their response to autonomy support, with men showing stronger associations between autonomy support and intrinsic motivation for physical activity [17,21–23]. Other research has shown that the relative importance of the three basic psychological needs (autonomy, competence, and relatedness) varies significantly between genders, with men typically showing higher sensitivity to competence-related factors while women place greater emphasis on relatedness aspects [18,21]. Second, workplace-based physical activity research has revealed distinct gender-specific barriers and facilitators [24]. Male office workers face unique challenges including workplace culture expectations around masculinity and physical performance, different social support structures, and varying responses to workplace interventions [24]. Hence, women were excluded from this study due to gender differences in physical activity adherence. Temporary or part-time workers were also excluded since their working hours and environments differ from those of full-time workers.

The sample size was determined according to current best practices for structural equation modeling [25–27]. Following recent recommendations [25–27], our sample of 257 participants meets current guidelines: (1) it exceeds the minimum 200 cases recommended for complex SEM models; (2) it satisfies the updated 10:1 participant-to-parameter ratio with 25 parameters estimated in our model; and (3) it provides adequate power (>0.80) for detecting medium effect sizes ($\beta = 0.30$) at $\alpha = 0.05$ based on Monte Carlo simulations. The final 257 cases in the dataset were used for analysis, after excluding 18 cases with missing data.

2.2. Measurements

The general characteristics of the participants included age, marital status, educational level, having a chronic disease, subjective health status, total working experience, daily amount of MVPA, weekly frequency of MVPA, years of MVPA, and physical activity adherence. The survey comprised a total of 66 items.

2.2.1. Physical Activity Adherence

Physical activity adherence was measured using the Physical Activity Adherence Questionnaire [4]. The English version of this instrument was translated into Korean using a double translation process, in which two bilingual individuals translated the English version into Korean and back-translated it into English, after which the finalized Korean version of the questionnaire was used for this study [28]. This instrument comprises three subdomains: predisposing, enabling, and reinforcing factors. Each subdomain has 4 items, for a total of 12 items. Examples of items include "I am very knowledgeable about physical activity (predisposing factor), I know how to plan my own physical activity (enabling factor), I have the support of my family for doing my regular physical activity (reinforcing factor)." Each item is rated on a 3-point Likert scale, with 1 point for "Not true," 2 points for "Somewhat true," and 3 points for "Very true," with higher scores indicating higher physical activity adherence. A score of 33–36 points indicates "Adherence likely," 27–32 points indicates "Adherence possible," and below 27 points indicates "Adherence unlikely." In this study, the overall Cronbach's α was 0.85, the Cronbach's α of the predisposing factor was 0.74, the enabling factor was 0.68, and the reinforcing factor was 0.70.

2.2.2. Autonomous Motivation

Autonomous motivation was measured using the Behavioral Regulation in Exercise Questionnaire-2 (BREQ-2) developed by Wilson and Rogers [29]. A previous study on physical activity by Ha and Han [30] translated the BREQ-2 into Korean and conducted tests for cultural appropriateness, with a Cronbach's α value of 0.89. The BREQ-2 consists of 19 items, but this study used 7 items measuring autonomous motivation including identified regulation and intrinsic regulation, which refers to actively participating in physical activity for enjoyment, satisfaction, and interest. Examples of items include "I take part in exercise because my friends/family/partner say I should, I enjoy my exercise sessions." The items are rated on a 5-point Likert scale, with 0 point for "Not true for me," and 4 points for "very true for me," with higher scores indicating higher autonomous motivation for physical activity. In this study, the overall Cronbach's α was 0.84.

2.2.3. Psychological Need Satisfaction in Physical Activity

Psychological need satisfaction in physical activity (autonomy, competence, and relatedness) was measured using the Psychological Need Satisfaction in Exercise (PNSE) questionnaire developed by Wilson et al. [31]. Previous study on physical activity by Ha and Han [30] translated the PNSE into Korean and conducted cultural appropriateness testing with a Cronbach's α value of 0.92~0.95. The PNSE comprises 18 items, with 6 items each for perceived autonomy, perceived competence, and perceived relatedness. Examples of items include "I feel free to exercise in my own way (perceived autonomy), I feel that I am able to complete exercises that are personally challenging (perceived competence), I feel connected to the people who I interact with while we exercise together (perceived relatedness)." The items are rated on a 6-point Likert scale, with higher scores indicating higher autonomy, competence, and relatedness. In this study, the overall Cronbach's α of psychological need satisfaction in physical activity was 0.94, the perceived autonomy was 0.87, the perceived competence was 0.95, and the perceived relatedness was 0.94.

2.2.4. Autonomy Support

Autonomy support was measured using the Important Other Climate Questionnaire (IOCQ) developed by Williams et al. [32]. A previous study using self-determination theory by Seo and Choi [33] translated the IOCQ into Korean and conducted cultural appropriateness testing with a Cronbach's α value of 0.87. Examples of items include "I feel that my important others have provided me with choices and options about physical activity, My important others encourage me to ask questions about physical activity." The IOCQ comprises 6 items rated on a 5-point Likert scale, with higher scores indicating higher autonomy support from significant others. The Cronbach's α in this study was 0.85.

2.2.5. Perceived Physical Activity Barriers

The Exercise Benefits/Barriers Scale [34] comprises 14 items on perceived exercise barriers and 14 items on perceived exercise benefits. A previous study on physical activity by Seo and Ha [35] translated the EBBS into Korean and conducted cultural appropriateness testing with a Cronbach's α value of 0.89. This study used only the perceived exercise barriers scale from the EBBS. Examples of items include "Physical activity takes too much of my time, Physical activity tires me" The instrument rated on a 4-point Likert scale, with higher scores indicating greater perceived barriers to physical activity. The Cronbach's α in this study was 0.86.

2.3. Data Collection

After obtaining Institutional Review Board (No: GIRB-A20-Y-0009) approval, data were collected from male office workers working at 15 banks in one city in Korea. The researcher contacted the human resources departments of each bank in advance by phone to explain the purpose and procedures of the study and to ask their permission. To recruit participants, the researcher visited the workplaces in person. Office workers were recruited to participate in the survey near the cafeterias or dining areas they use. The purpose and procedures of the study were explained to the male office workers and, after obtaining voluntary consent from those who voluntarily agreed to participate and met the inclusion and exclusion criteria of this study, written consent was obtained before distributing the paper-based questionnaires. The survey took 20 min to complete, and a small gift was given after completion.

2.4. Data Analysis

The data were analyzed as follows using SPSS 28.0 and AMOS 26.0 software. First, the general characteristics of the participants and measured variables were analyzed using descriptive statistics. Skewness and kurtosis were checked to verify the normality, and tolerance limits and variance inflation factors (VIFs) were calculated for multicollinearity. The general characteristics and physical activity-related characteristics were analyzed by frequency, percentage, mean, and standard deviation. The differences in physical activity adherence by the general characteristics and physical activity-related characteristics of participants were evaluated using *t*-tests, ANOVA, and the Scheffé post hoc test. Second, confirmatory factor analysis was conducted to examine the validity and reliability of the latent variables and test the fit of the measurement model. Third, absolute fit indices such as χ^2, χ^2/df, root mean square residual (RMR), root mean squared error of approximation (RMSEA), goodness-of-fit index (GFI), and adjusted goodness-of-fit index (AGFI) were calculated to verify the fit of the hypothetical model. The incremental fit indices used included the normed fit index (NFI), the Tucker–Lewis index (TLI), and the comparative fit index (CFI). Acceptable values as goodness of fit indicators are an RMR of less than 0.05, an RMSEA of less than 0.08, a GFI of 0.90 or higher, an AGFI of 0.90 or higher, an NFI of 0.90 or higher, a TLI of 0.90 or higher, and a CFI of 0.95 or higher [36]. Fourth, standardized regression weights, critical ratios, and *p*-values were utilized to analyze the significance of the path coefficients in the hypothetical model, and the explanatory power of the endogenous variables was measured using squared multiple correlations (SMCs). Moreover, the significance of the direct, indirect, and total effects was examined using Bootstrap Maximum Likelihood estimation with 5000 bootstrapping resamples (AMOS 26.0), and the effects were tested at a 95% confidence interval [37].

3. Results

3.1. Differences in Physical Activity Adherence by General Characteristics of Participants

The participants' age was 40.85 years. Of the participants, 68.5% were married, and 83.3% were at least college graduates. Over two-thirds of the participants (77.0%) reported no chronic diseases and perceived their health status as moderate or good. Total working experience was 12.39 years. The amount of daily MVPA was 85.21 min, the weekly MVPA frequency was 3.75 days, and average years of MVPA duration was 4.17 years. In terms of physical activity adherence, 44.7% of the participants were classified as "adherence unlikely" (below 27 points), 44.0% as "adherence possible" (27–32 points), and 11.3% as "adherence likely" (33–36 points).

Significant differences in physical activity adherence according to the general characteristics of the participants were found in education level ($F = 5.34$, $p = 0.005$), subjective health status ($F = 7.83$, $p = 0.001$), weekly frequency of MVPA ($t = -2.52$, $p = 0.012$), and years of MVPA duration ($F = 11.87$, $p < 0.001$). In terms of educational level, significant differences in physical activity adherence were found between those with associate's degree and those with bachelor's degree. For subjective health status, significant differences were observed between those who perceived their health as good and those who perceived their health as poor. In terms of MVPA, there were significant differences between more than 4 days of weekly MVPA and 3 days of weekly MVPA. In addition, significant differences in physical activity adherence were observed between more than 5 years of MVPA and less than 3 years of MVPA (Table 1).

Table 1. Differences in Physical Activity Adherence by General Characteristics and Physical Activity-Related Characteristics of Participants.

Characteristics	Categories	*n* (%)	Physical Activity Adherence	
			M ± SD	t/F (*p*)
Age (year)	<30	27 (10.5)	2.35 ± 0.37	0.88 (0.454)
	30~39	86 (33.5)	2.23 ± 0.39	
	40–49	91 (15.4)	2.26 ± 0.37	
	≥50	53 (20.6)	2.30 ± 0.30	
	M ± SD	40.85 ± 8.52		
Marital status	Unmarried	176 (68.5)	2.28 ± 0.37	−0.69 (0.493)
	Married	81 (31.5)	2.24 ± 0.36	
Educational level †	High school [a]	43 (16.7)	2.19 ± 0.58	5.34 (0.005)
	College [b]	56 (21.8)	2.16 ± 0.36	b < c
	University [c]	158 (61.5)	2.32 ± 0.35	
Having a chronic disease	Yes	59 (23.0)	2.26 ± 0.36	−0.14 (0.886)
	No	198 (77.0)	2.27 ± 0.37	
Subjective health status †	Poor [a]	17 (6.6)	2.01 ± 0.38	7.83 (0.001)
	Moderate [b]	80 (31.1)	2.20 ± 0.35	a < c
	Good [c]	160 (62.3)	2.33 ± 0.36	
Total working experience (years)	<10	110 (42.8)	2.27 ± 0.37	0.93 (0.395)
	10–19	80 (31.1)	2.23 ± 0.40	
	≥20	67 (26.1)	2.31 ± 0.31	
	M ± SD	12.39 ± 8.94		
Amount of MVPA (min/day)	30–59	28 (34.6)	2.21 ± 0.34	0.35 (0.705)
	60–89	104 (32.3)	2.27 ± 0.34	
	≥90	125 (33.1)	2.27 ± 0.39	
	M ± SD	85.21 ± 37.96		
Frequency of MVPA (days/week)	3	124 (48.2)	2.21 ± 0.39	−2.52 (0.012)
	4–7	133 (51.8)	2.32 ± 0.34	
	M ± SD	3.75 ± 1.23		
Years of MVPA duration †	<3 [a]	152 (59.2)	2.18 ± 0.36	11.87 (<0.001)
	3–5 [b]	36 (14.0)	2.29 ± 0.31	a < c
	>5 [c]	69 (26.8)	2.43 ± 0.36	
	M ± SD	4.17 ± 5.47		
Physical activity adherence †	Adherence unlikely [a]	115 (44.7)	-	-
	Adherence possible [b]	113 (44.0)	-	-
	Adherence likely [c]	29 (11.3)	-	-

Note: † Scheffé post hoc test.

3.2. Descriptive Statistics and Convergent Validity of Variables

The perceived physical activity barriers score was 1.69 ± 0.38 (range 1–4), autonomy support was 3.71 ± 0.62 (range 1–5), and psychological need satisfaction in physical activity was 4.64 ± 0.74 (range 1–6), with the subdomains of autonomy, competence, and relatedness obtaining scores of 4.88 ± 0.75, 4.40 ± 1.01, and 4.65 ± 0.87, respectively. The autonomous motivation score was 3.20 ± 0.56 (range 0–4), and physical activity adherence was 27.19 ± 4.39 (range 12–36).

Regarding the normality of the research variables, skewness ranged from −1.03 to 0.02 and kurtosis ranged from −0.75 to 2.08, meeting the assumption of normal distribution. Multicollinearity was not found among the measurement variables of the hypothetical model. Regarding convergent validity to test the validity of the latent variables, the average variance extracted (AVE) ranged from 0.63 to 0.87 and construct reliability ranged from 0.84 to 0.95; hence, the convergent validity of the variables was established (Table 2).

3.3. Direct, Indirect, and Total Effects of the Hypothetical Model

The goodness-of-fit test results of the hypothetical model showed that both absolute fit indices (RMR, RMSEA, GFI, and AGFI) and incremental fit indices (NFI, TLI, and CFI) met the recommended levels, indicating an acceptable model fit. The path significance test results for the hypothetical model showed that five out of nine paths were significant (Table 3, Figure 2). For psychological need satisfaction in physical activity, direct effects were observed from autonomy support ($\beta = 0.44$, $p < 0.001$) and perceived physical activity barriers ($\beta = -0.42$, $p < 0.001$). For autonomous motivation, direct effects from autonomy support (β = 0.01, p = 0.861) and perceived physical activity barriers (β = −0.09, p = 0.115) were not significant. Psychological need satisfaction in physical activity had a direct effect on autonomous motivation (β = 0.66, p < 0.001). For physical activity adherence, the direct effect (β = 0.03, p = 0.695) of autonomy support was not significant. The direct effect of perceived physical activity barriers (β = 0.02, p = 0.723) was not significant. The direct effect (β = 0.52, p < 0.001), indirect effect (β = 0.22, p = 0.004), and total effect (β = 0.74, p = 0.005) of psychological need satisfaction in physical activity were significant, while the direct effect of autonomous motivation (β = 0.33, p < 0.001) was significant.

Table 2. Descriptive Statistics and Convergent Validity of Variables.

Variables	Range	M ± SD	Skewness	Kurtosis	β	CR	AVE
Perceived physical activity barriers	1–4	1.69 ± 0.38	0.09	0.58	-	-	-
Autonomy support	1–5	3.71 ± 0.62	−0.45	0.12	-	-	-
Psychological need satisfaction in physical activity	1–6	4.64 ± 0.74	−0.74	0.92	-	0.84	0.63
Autonomy		4.88 ± 0.75	−0.98	1.86	0.63	-	-
Competence		4.40 ± 1.01	−0.62	0.17	0.81	-	-
Relatedness		4.65 ± 0.87	−1.03	2.08	0.81	-	-
Autonomous motivation	0–4	3.20 ± 0.56	−0.78	0.99	-	-	-
Physical activity adherence	12–36	27.19 ± 4.39	−0.19	−0.30	-	0.95	0.87
Predisposing		9.43 ± 1.84	−0.26	−0.58	0.84	-	-
Enabling		9.11 ± 1.77	−0.05	−0.75	0.79	-	-
Reinforcing		8.28 ± 1.82	−0.02	−0.30	0.66	-	-

Note: SD = standard deviation; CR = construct reliability; AVE = average variance extracted.

Table 3. Direct, Indirect, and Total Effects of the Hypothetical Model.

Endogenous Variables	Exogeneous Variables	Parameter Statistics		Direct Effect	Indirect Effect	Total Effect	SMC
		SE	C.R.	β (p)	β (p)	β (p)	
Psychological need satisfaction in physical activity	Autonomy support	0.44	6.67	0.44 (<0.001)	-	0.44 (<0.001)	0.46
	Perceived physical activity barriers	−0.42	−6.45	−0.42 (<0.001)	-	−0.42 (<0.001)	
Autonomous motivation	Autonomy support	0.01	0.18	0.01 (0.861)	0.29 (0.011)	0.30 (0.007)	0.51
	Perceived physical activity barriers	−0.09	−1.58	−0.09 (0.115)	−0.28 (0.005)	−0.37 (0.007)	
	Psychological need satisfaction in physical activity	0.66	7.02	0.66 (<0.001)		0.66 (<0.001)	
Physical activity adherence	Autonomy support	0.03	0.39	0.03 (0.695)	0.33 (0.005)	0.36 (0.011)	0.62
	Perceived physical activity barriers	0.02	−0.35	0.02 (0.723)	−0.34 (0.002)	−0.32 (0.014)	
	Psychological need satisfaction in physical activity	0.52	4.35	0.52 (<0.001)	0.22 (0.004)	0.74 (0.005)	
	Autonomous motivation	0.33	3.93	0.33 (<0.001)	-	0.33 (<0.001)	

Note: SE = standardized estimates; C.R. = construct reliability; SMC = squared multiple correlations.

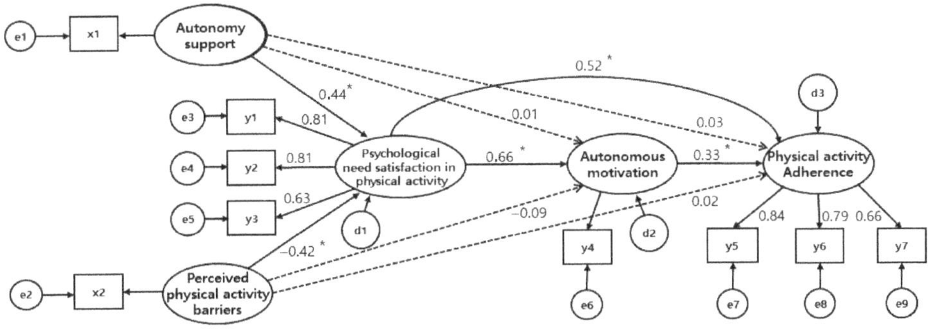

Figure 2. Path diagram for the final model. x1 = Autonomy support; x2 = Perceived physical activity barriers; y1 = Relatedness; y2 = Competence; y3 = Autonomy; y4 = Autonomous motivations; y5 = Predisposing; y6 = Enabling; y7 = Reinforcing (Goodness-of fit-indicators: $\chi^2 = 51.53$, $p < 0.001$, $\chi^2/df = 2.577$, RMR = 0.01, RMSEA = 0.07, GFI = 0.96, AGFI = 0.90, NFI = 0.95, TLI = 0.94, CFI = 0.97). * $p < 0.01$.

4. Discussion

The increase in office jobs due to the decline of labor-intensive jobs in South Korea, along with the inherent characteristics of office work, has raised the risk of chronic diseases among office workers. Hence, it is more important than ever to understand physical activity adherence in office workers. The participants in this study were male office workers with an average age of 40.85 years, and 44.7% of them fell into the category of "physical activity adherence unlikely." This raises the need for greater attention to improving physical activity adherence among office workers. It is crucial to create health promoting environments that support physical activity adherence among office workers working in sedentary jobs for 8 h a day, 5 days a week [3]. For instance, it may be helpful to create an environment that encourages office workers to use the stairs instead of elevators, develop a workplace physical activity program during lunch or break time, change the office environment to increase physical activity within the office, create an environment where workers can work standing up, and form walking paths to encourage workers to walk around the workplace [38]. Additionally, our findings specifically indicate that higher education levels, better subjective health status, higher weekly MVPA frequency, and longer MVPA duration are significantly associated with higher physical activity adherence. To ensure a more evidence-based discussion, it would be beneficial to focus on why these factors contribute to adherence to physical activity. For instance, individuals with higher education levels may have greater awareness of the benefits of physical activity, leading to stronger motivation for adherence. Similarly, those with better subjective health status may feel more capable of engaging in physical activity, reinforcing consistent participation [4]. Based on our findings, it is necessary to focus on the physical activity adherence of workers with lower education levels or poor subjective health status and to develop strategies to help them sustain their physical activity.

In this study, psychological need satisfaction in physical activity, a variable that directly affected physical activity adherence among office workers, was the factor that had the greatest direct impact. Moreover, it had a significant effect on physical activity adherence through the mediation of autonomous motivation. This finding is supported by previous studies, which reported that psychological need satisfaction in physical activity directly affected physical activity behaviors and significantly affected physical activity adherence through the mediation of autonomous motivation [21,39,40]. It is noted that psychological need satisfaction in physical activity involves autonomy (freely choosing the desired physical activity), competence (believing in one's ability to perform the physical activity successfully), and relatedness (forming close relationships with others participating in the same physical activity), through which physical activity is sustained [12,31]. Our study findings demonstrated that physical activity should be sustained by enhancing three factors of PNSE (psychological need satisfaction in exercise) which have the greatest impact on sustaining physical activity. This is why there is a need to develop strategies to increase autonomy, competence, and relatedness for physical activity adherence among male office workers. Strategies to enhance autonomy can include providing not only options for individuals to choose the physical activity they like and prefer but also the time and place for such activity [19]. Moreover, since individuals perform physical activities better when provided immediate feedback, personalized feedback must be provided after a physical activity to improve competence in workers [19]. Finally, strategies to improve relatedness should include warm support among people participating in the same activity. These strategies must be applied to the physical activity program, since individuals find greater enjoyment and satisfaction through physical activity carried out in close relationships with several others [41].

As expected, autonomous motivation was a significant factor directly affecting physical activity adherence. This finding is supported by the self-determination theory and numerous previous studies that demonstrate autonomous motivation as a significant influencing factor for sustaining physical activity [10,13,21,39,42]. Autonomous motivation refers to the enjoyment, satisfaction, and interest perceived by individuals in MVPA itself, which causes them to actively adopt physical activity and sustain long-term activity [10,12,29]. Considering both the direct and mediating effects of autonomous motivation on physical activity adherence in this study, a strategy that promotes autonomous motivation is needed. For instance, several studies have reported the effectiveness of physical activity programs applying motivational coaching to increase enjoyment and satisfaction with physical activity or mobile health programs using motivational interviewing [43]. Therefore, workplace physical activity programs that apply these strategies must be implemented to promote autonomous motivation.

Autonomy support from significant others was a significant factor that had a direct effect on psychological need satisfaction in physical activity and an indirect effect on physical activity adherence through the mediation of psychological need satisfaction in physical activity and autonomous motivation. According to the SDT, autonomy support from significant others has a direct effect on basic psychological needs and an indirect effect on health behaviors through basic psychological needs and motivation [19]. Autonomy support from significant others not only promotes sustained health behaviors but also enhances personal growth [19]. Therefore, a strategy that enhances autonomy support must be implemented for physical activity adherence among participants so that significant others such as family or colleagues of participants can actively support their MVPA.

Contrary to expectations, perceived physical activity barriers did not have a direct effect on the physical activity adherence, but it had an indirect effect on physical activity adherence through psychological needs and autonomous motivation. In general, obstacles for discontinuing physical activity are lack of time, the high costs associated with MVPA, and inconvenient locations, while intrinsic factors of physical activity obstacles are lack of motivation, negative emotions toward regular physical activity, and insufficient information and skills [8,16]. According to previous research, such obstacles reduce the autonomy and competence related to physical activity adherence, thereby lowering activity motivation and hindering the sustained performance of MVPA [16]. Although our findings show that physical activity barriers do not have a direct effect on physical activity adherence, considering that many previous studies have found significant effects of these barriers on adherence, it is necessary to re-examine the relationship between them in future studies.

This study is significant in that it developed a structural equation model of physical activity adherence based on the SDT and identified complex causal relationships including direct and indirect effects for the physical activity adherence of office workers. Despite this significance, however, this study has limitations. First, participants in this study were male office workers, which makes it difficult to generalize the results to all male office workers. Second, a study with limited participants such as workers in small and medium banks may not be representative of all office workers because our participants would show significant differences in terms of organizational support for physical activity compared to workers in large banks or companies. Third, self-report data could be susceptible to social desirability bias, memory distortions, and potential for exaggeration or omission of information which can affect the reliability of research findings.

5. Conclusions

This study aimed to test the hypothesized relationships based on self-determination theory to investigate factors affecting the physical activity adherence of male office workers, and to provide information for developing workplace physical activity programs. Our results show that psychological need satisfaction in physical activity and autonomous motivation were significant variables that had direct effects on physical activity adherence, while autonomy support from significant others and perceived physical activity barriers had significant indirect effects through psychological need satisfaction and autonomous motivation, explaining 62.0%. Psychological need satisfaction in physical activity directly affected physical activity adherence, and the total effect was significant as it indirectly affected physical activity adherence through autonomous motivation. Autonomous motivation directly affected physical activity adherence. Autonomy support and perceived physical activity barriers were not significant direct effects on physical activity adherence, but the total effect was significant by indirectly affecting psychological need satisfaction in physical activity and autonomous motivation.

Based on the results of this study, the following suggestions can be made for further research. First, this study targeted male workers from small to medium banks with around 50 workers. Since the financial and environmental support for the physical activity adherence of workers may vary by company size, further research is needed involving male workers from larger banks or companies. Considering the increasing employment rate of female workers in the job market, further research is needed to investigate the factors influencing physical activity adherence among female workers, to examine the predictors of physical activity adherence, including both male and female workers, and to validate the moderating effects of gender as well. Second, it is necessary to develop workplace activity programs to improve the autonomy, competence, and relatedness aspects of psychological need satisfaction in physical activity. In addition, office workers could continue their physical activity if they recognize the social support from significant others and customized workplace-specific physical activity programs to promote autonomous motivation should be implemented.

Author Contributions: Conceptualization, S.H., and Y.H.; methodology, Y.H.; formal analysis, S.H., and Y.H.; investigation, S.H., and Y.H.; data curation, S.H.; writing—original draft preparation, S.H., and Y.H.; writing—review and editing, S.H., and Y.H.; supervision, Y.H.; project administration, S.H., and Y.H. All authors have read and agreed to the published version of the manuscript.

Funding: This research received no external funding.

Institutional Review Board Statement: The study was conducted in accordance with the Declaration of Helsinki and approved by the Institutional Review Board of Gyeongsang National University in South Korea (IRB No.: GIRB-A20-Y-0009/date of approval: 24 February 2020).

Informed Consent Statement: Informed consent was obtained from all subjects involved in the study.

Data Availability Statement: The datasets generated and analyzed during the current study are not publicly available due to concerns regarding participant privacy. The data presented in the study can be available from the corresponding author upon reasonable request.

Conflicts of Interest: The authors declare no conflicts of interest.

References

1. Piercy, K.L.; Troiano, R.P.; Ballard, R.M.; Carlson, S.A.; Fulton, J.E.; Galuska, D.A.; George, S.M.; Olson, R.D. The Physical Activity Guidelines for Americans. *JAMA* **2018**, *320*, 2020–2028. [CrossRef] [PubMed]
2. Ministry of Health and Welfare. *The Physical Activity Guidelines for Koreans 2023*; Ministry of Health and Welfare: Sejong, Republic of Korean, 2023.
3. Michalchuk, V.F.; Lee, S.J.; Waters, C.M.; Hong, O.S.; Fukuoka, Y. Systematic review of the influence of physical work environment on office workers' physical activity behavior. *Workplace Health Saf.* **2022**, *70*, 97–119. [CrossRef] [PubMed]
4. Welk, G.J.; Corbin, C.B.; Corbin, W.R.; Welk, K.A. *Corbin's Concepts of Fitness and Wellness: A Comprehensive Lifestyle Approach*, 13th ed.; McGraw-Hill Companies: New York, NY, USA, 2023; p. 522.
5. Bannell, D.J.; France-Ratcliffe, M.; Buckley, B.J.R.; Crozier, A.; Davies, A.P.; Hesketh, K.L.; Jones, H.; Cocks, M.; Sprung, V.S.; MOTIVATE Team. Adherence to unsupervised exercise in sedentary individuals: A randomised feasibility trial of two mobile health interventions. *Digit Health* **2023**, *9*, 20552076231183552. [CrossRef]
6. Linke, S.E.; Gallo, L.C.; Norman, G.J. Attrition and adherence rates of sustained vs. intermittent exercise interventions. *Ann. Behav. Med.* **2011**, *42*, 197–209. [CrossRef]
7. Shaw, J.F.; Pilon, S.; Vierula, M.; McIsaac, D.I. Predictors of adherence to prescribed exercise programs for older adults with medical or surgical indications for exercise: A systematic review. *Syst. Rev.* **2022**, *11*, 80. [CrossRef]
8. Morgan, F.; Battersby, A.; Weightman, A.L.; Searchfield, L.; Turley, R.; Morgan, H.; Jagroo, J.; Ellis, S. Adherence to exercise referral schemes by participants—What do providers and commissioners need to know? A systematic review of barriers and facilitators. *BMC Public Health* **2016**, *16*, 27. [CrossRef]
9. Ryan, R.M.; Frederick, C.M.; Lepes, D.; Rubio, N.; Sheldon, K.M. Intrinsic motivation and exercise adherence. *Int. J. Sport Psychol.* **1997**, *28*, 335–354.
10. Ryan, R.M.; Deci, E.L. Active human nature: Self-Determination theory and the promotion and maintenance of sport, exercise, and health. In *Intrinsic Motivation and Self-Determination in Exercise and Sport*; Mshnld, C., Ed.; Human Kinetics: Champaign, IL, USA, 2007.
11. Bandhu, D.; Mohan, M.M.; Nittala, N.A.P.; Jadhav, P.; Bhadauria, A.; Saxena, K.K. Theories of motivation: A comprehensive analysis of human behavior drivers. *Acta Psychol.* **2024**, *244*, 104177. [CrossRef]
12. Wilson, P.M.; Mack, D.E.; Grattan, K.P. Understanding motivation for exercise: A Self-Determination Theory perspective. *Can. Psychol.* **2008**, *49*, 250–256. [CrossRef]
13. Teixeira, P.J.; Carraça, E.V.; Markland, D.; Silva, M.N.; Ryan, R.M. Exercise, physical activity, and Self-Determination Theory: A systematic review. *Int. J. Behav. Nutr. Phys. Act.* **2012**, *9*, 78. [CrossRef] [PubMed]
14. Pelletier, L.G.; Rocchi, M.A.; Vallerand, R.J.; Deci, E.L.; Ryan, R.M. Validation of revised sport motivation scale (SMS-II). *Psychol. Sport Exerc.* **2013**, *14*, 329–341. [CrossRef]
15. Pender, N.J. *Health Promotion in Nursing Practice*, 3rd ed.; Appleton & Lange: Stanford, CT, USA, 1996; p. 320.
16. Kennedy, A.; Narendran, P.; Andrews, R.C.; Daley, A.; Greenfield, S.M.; EXTOD Group. Attitudes and barriers to exercise in adults with a recent diagnosis of type 1 diabetes: A qualitative study of participants in the Exercise for Type 1 Diabetes (EXTOD) study. *BMJ Open* **2018**, *8*, e017813. [CrossRef]
17. Waters, C.N.; Ling, E.P.; Chu, A.H.; Ng, S.H.; Chia, A.; Lim, Y.W.; Müller-Riemenschneider, F. Assessing and understanding sedentary behaviour in office-based working adults: A mixed-method approach. *BMC Public Health* **2016**, *16*, 360. [CrossRef] [PubMed]
18. Hill-Mey, P.E.; Merrill, R.M.; Kumpfer, K.L.; Reel, J.; Hyatt-Neville, B. A focus group assessment to determine motivations, barriers and effectiveness of a university-based worksite wellness program. *Health Promot. Perspect.* **2013**, *3*, 154. [CrossRef] [PubMed]
19. Deci, E.L.; Ryan, R.M. *Handbook of Self-Determination Research*; University of Rochester Press: Rochester, NY, USA, 2002; p. 480.

20. Jun, H.J.; Park, S. The effect of cross-level interaction between community factors and social capital among individuals on physical activity: Considering gender difference. *Int. J. Environ. Res. Public Health* **2019**, *16*, 495. [CrossRef]
21. Weman-Josefsson, K.; Lindwall, M.; Ivarsson, A. Need satisfaction, motivational regulations and exercise: Moderation and mediation effects. *Int. J. Behav. Nutr. Phys. Act.* **2015**, *12*, 67. [CrossRef] [PubMed]
22. Zhang, S.; Huang, J.; Wang, H. Influencing factors of women's sports participation based on Self-Determination Theory: A systematic review and meta-analysis. *Psychol. Res. Behav. Manag.* **2024**, *17*, 2953–2969. [CrossRef]
23. Standage, M.; Sebire, S.J.; Loney, T. Does exercise motivation predict engagement in objectively assessed bouts of moderate intensity exercise?: A self-determination theory perspective. *J. Sport Exerc. Psychol.* **2008**, *30*, 337–352. [CrossRef]
24. Mailey, E.L.; Huberty, J.; Dinkel, D.; McAuley, E. Physical activity barriers and facilitators among working mothers and fathers. *BMC Public Health* **2014**, *14*, 657. [CrossRef]
25. Mitchell, R.J. Path analysis: Pollination. In *Design and Analysis of Ecological Experiments*, 2nd ed.; Scheiner, S.M., Gurevitch, J., Eds.; Oxford University Press: Oxford, UK, 2001; pp. 217–234.
26. Kyriazos, T.A. Applied psychometrics: Sample size and sample power considerations in factor analysis (EFA, CFA) and SEM in general. *Psychology* **2018**, *9*, 2207–2230. [CrossRef]
27. Wolf, E.J.; Harrington, K.M.; Clark, S.L.; Miller, M.W. Sample size requirements for structural equation models: An evaluation of power, bias, and solution propriety. *Educ. Psychol. Meas.* **2013**, *76*, 913–934. [CrossRef]
28. Waltz, C.F.; Strickland, O.L.; Lenz, E.R. *Measurement in Nursing and Health Research*, 5th ed.; Springer Publishing Company: New York, NY, USA, 2016; p. 632.
29. Wilson, P.M.; Rogers, W.M. The relationship between perceived autonomy support, exercise regulations and behavioral intentions in women. *Psychol. Sport Exerc.* **2004**, *5*, 229–242. [CrossRef]
30. Ha, Y.; Han, S. Relationships between psychological need satisfaction in exercise, motivation for exercise, and physical activity of female workers in retail and health service sectors. *Korean J. Occup. Health Nurs.* **2020**, *29*, 97–105. [CrossRef]
31. Wilson, P.M.; Rogers, W.T.; Rodgers, W.M.; Wild, T.C. The psychological need satisfaction in exercise scale. *J. Sport Exerc. Psychol.* **2006**, *28*, 231–251. [CrossRef]
32. Williams, G.C.; Lynch, M.F.; McGregor, H.A.; Sharp, D.; Deci, E.L. Validation of the "Important Other" climate questionnaire: Assessing autotomy support for health-related change. *Fam. Syst. Health* **2006**, *24*, 179–194. [CrossRef]
33. Seo, Y.M.; Choi, W.H. A predictive model on self-care behavior for patients with type 2 diabetes: Based on self-determination theory. *J. Korean Acad. Nurs.* **2011**, *41*, 491–499. [CrossRef]
34. Sechrist, K.R.; Walker, S.N.; Pender, N.J. Development and psychometric evaluation of the Exercise Benefits/Barriers scale. *Res. Nurs. Health* **1987**, *10*, 357–365. [CrossRef]
35. Seo, Y.; Ha, Y. Gender differences in predictors of physical activity among Korean college students based on the Health Promotion Model. *Asian Pac. Isl. Nurs. J.* **2019**, *4*, 1–10. [CrossRef]
36. Brown, T.A. *Confirmatory Factor Analysis for Applied Research*, 2nd ed.; The Guilford Press: New York, NY, USA, 2015; p. 462.
37. Schumacker, R.E.; Lomax, R.G. *A Beginner's Guide to Structural Equation Modeling*, 4th ed.; Routledge: London, UK, 2015; p. 372.
38. Zhou, L.; Deng, X.; Guo, K.; Hou, L.; Hui, X.; Wu, Y.; Xu, M.; Wang, Y.; Liang, S.; Yang, K.; et al. Effectiveness of multicomponent interventions in office-based workers to mitigate occupational sedentary behavior: Systematic review and meta-analysis. *JMIR Public Health Surveill.* **2023**, *9*, e44745. [CrossRef]
39. Hagger, M.S.; Chatzisarantis, N.L.D. Self-determination theory and the psychology of exercise. *Int. Rev. Sport Exerc. Psychol.* **2008**, *1*, 79–103. [CrossRef]
40. Williams, G.C.; McGregor, H.A.; Zeldman, A.; Freedman, Z.R.; Deci, E.L. Testing a Self-Determination Theory process model for promoting glycemic control through diabetes self-management. *Health Psychol.* **2004**, *23*, 58–66. [CrossRef] [PubMed]
41. Bartholomew, L.K.; Markham, C.M.; Ruiter, R.A.; Fernandez, M.E.; Kok, G.; Parcel, G.S. *Planning Health Promotion Programs: An Intervention Mapping Approach*, 4th ed.; Jossey-Bass Public Health: Hoboken, NJ, USA, 2016; p. 704.
42. Ng, J.Y.; Ntoumanis, N.; Thogersen-Ntoumai, G.; Deci, E.L.; Ran, R.M.; Duda, J.L.; Williams, G.C. Self-Determination Theory applied to health contexts: A meta-analysis. *Perspect. Psychol. Sci.* **2012**, *7*, 325–340. [CrossRef] [PubMed]
43. Gaesser, V.J.; Maakestad, W.M.; Hayes, E.S.; Snyder, S.J. Motivational coaching improves intrinsic motivation in adult fitness program participants. *Int. J. Exerc. Sci.* **2020**, *13*, 1167–1178. [CrossRef] [PubMed]

European Journal of
Investigation in Health, Psychology and Education

MDPI

Article

How to Promote Walking in Women with Fibromyalgia: A Look at Catastrophizing, Goal Conflict, and Avoidance from a Self-Emotional Regulatory Perspective

Carmen Ecija, Lorena Gutiérrez, Patricia Catalá and Cecilia Peñacoba *

Department of Psychology, Rey Juan Carlos University, Avda. de Atenas s/n, 28922 Alcorcón, Spain; carmen.ecija@urjc.es (C.E.); lorena.gutierrezh@urjc.es (L.G.); patricia.catala@urjc.es (P.C.)
* Correspondence: cecilia.penacoba@urjc.es; Tel.: 91-488-8864

Abstract: The aim of this study was twofold: to explore the concordance between two measures of physical activity (accelerometer and IPAQ) among female fibromyalgia (FM) patients, as well as to examine the impact of psychosocial variables (catastrophism, activity avoidance) on walking among these patients. Helplessness, activity avoidance, and commitment to physical activity were evaluated in 132 FM women. After the first assessment, an accelerometer was placed by a psychologist on each participant for seven consecutive days. Eight days later, accelerometers were collected, and participants were evaluated again using the IPAQ. Two models were tested to analyze mediation and a moderated mediation effect. The mediating role of activity avoidance between helplessness and minutes walked was corroborated regarding the objective measure of walking. The effect of helplessness on minutes walked during a week was mediated by activity avoidance and assessed by accelerometers. Cognitive variables played a contextual role when trying to promote exercise. Activity avoidance must be understood as a key variable in physical activity promotion, specifically in the promotion of walking with the aim to do exercise in individuals with FM.

Keywords: fibromyalgia; catastrophism; activity avoidance

1. Introduction

Fibromyalgia (FM) is a complex multidimensional disorder characterized by chronic diffuse musculoskeletal pain, low physical activity (PA), and a reduced quality of life [1–3] that usually leads to changes in the individual's ability to function physically [4–6]. An active lifestyle has been postulated as a resilience factor in FM [7,8], and exercise is one of the more commonly recommended non-pharmacological therapies for this population [2,7,9,10]. Specifically, walking as a type of exercise is easy and accessible, and it has a low musculoskeletal impact [11,12]. Moreover, its effect on pain relief, fatigue, anxiety, depression, number of falls, disability, balance, mobility, and quality of life has been widely demonstrated [11,13–16].

However, as studies have shown, FM patients rarely meet the guidelines for PA, including walking [17]. According to the fear-avoidance model [18], this could be due to the fact that FM patients frequently avoid walking as a way of minimizing the pain they feel [19]. In this sense, an activity avoidance pattern (AA) is a significant predictor of worse psychological and physical function as well as of greater pain interference in FM patients [20]. However, pain is not the only factor that explains low adherence to walking. The previous literature has shown that although AA implies fewer minutes spent walking, other factors also come into play, such as the conflict between PA and patients' perceptions of it, influencing well-being and quality of life in individuals with FM [21]. This has been observed specifically in the case of walking as a form of physical exercise [21–23].

Within the fear-avoidance model [18] regarding the chronification of pain, the motivational perspectives of goal conflict and catastrophizing play a key role. Catastrophizing has been proposed as one of the most important psychosocial predictors of pain, distress, and disability in individuals with FM [24–29]; it has a specific predictive power within the interpersonal context in which pain occurs [30]. In general terms, it entails processing pain through heightened (rumination) or exaggerated thoughts (magnification), which involve fixating excessively on the painful sensation, amplifying its severity and perceiving it as beyond control (helplessness), making it a pivotal factor influencing symptom severity. From a motivational perspective, catastrophizing could be defined as the result of the interference between attaining pain-controlling goals and other relevant goals [31,32]. Patients with chronic pain usually anticipate negative consequences from physical activity (as a possible relevant goal), which leads to avoiding activities that could prevent pain [33]. Along with this, the preference for completing goals has also emerged as a relevant factor in undertaking and maintaining function in patients with FM and has become a recent focus of research from contextual models [34] in which goals have been underscored as a way to explain different profiles of women with FM [35–40].

On the one hand, taking into consideration that psychological factors influence the relationship between chronic pain and disability—with behavioral (activity avoidance) and cognitive (catastrophizing and goals) factors being the most explored [41]—and, on the other hand, the relevant role of the clash between how people with chronic pain feel about their abilities and how they behave [42], there is a need to delve into the assessment and implementation of multicomponent interventions including both objective and subjective measures, specifically those related to maintaining patients' functioning despite ongoing pain [43]. Walking cannot be reduced solely to the patient's capacity or to mere observable motor behavior; it is necessary to analyze this behavior in the context in which it takes place, considering the effect of cognitive variables such as catastrophizing (and specifically hopelessness) and goal preference on PA while taking into account the influence of activity avoidance [27,38,44–47].

Biopsychosocial models posit that how individuals think and behave in relation to their pain plays a critical role in their pain experience, highlighting people's abilities to effectively (or not) manage pain. In this context, hopelessness and activity avoidance have been classified as inherently maladaptive variables related to escaping from activities that are anticipated to be unpleasant or pain-eliciting [48], establishing activity avoidance as a highly relevant predictor of disability [49]. This is in agreement with the framework of the behavioral activation (BA) approach, which suggests that if the individual's environment provides contact with reinforcement for unhealthy behaviors and lacks reinforcement for healthy behaviors, unhealthy behaviors will increase and healthy behaviors will decrease [50]. Based on this, we can hypothesize that catastrophizing, and specifically helplessness, may influence FM through the contextual role of activity avoidance. This could be in accordance with contextual–functional approaches [34] that put an adapted behavior to the service of a set personal goal [51]. Within this more integrative perspective, the effects of helplessness and avoidance on physical activity, specifically on walking, could be related to underlying personal goals and other contextual factors that need to be explored [52].

Therefore, the current study had two main objectives. The first was to analyze the concurrence between two measures of physical activity (accelerometer and IPAQ), focusing on the tendency to avoid walking among female FM patients. The second was to explore the role of the psychosocial variables discussed above (helplessness and activity avoidance), taking into account the contextual role of the tendency to avoid walking when pain appears. Meanwhile, walking was measured from the perspective of the emerging goal conflict (both from the patient's perception and actual behavior). We believe that the results from this study may be useful in healthcare contexts related to the implementation of effective treatments of physical activity in patients with FM, including both measures of actual performance and patient perception.

2. Materials and Methods

2.1. Participants

A sample of 132 women with FM were recruited from different FM mutual aid associations in the Communities of Madrid and Castilla-La Mancha (Spain), all having been diagnosed according to the American College of Rheumatology (ACR) criteria [1,53,54]. The occurrence of FM shows a variation based on gender, with it being more common in females. However, the prevalence in males can vary depending on the study methods used. A 2017 study by Marques and others [27] indicated that FM's prevalence in the general population across various countries spanned between 0.2% and 8.8%, with the rates for women lying between 2.4% and 6.8%. In accordance with these percentages, only women were included in our study, while the following additional criteria were included: being above 18 years old, providing written consent to participate, having a medical prescription to walk, and not presenting any physical impairments to carry out physical activity.

2.2. Procedure

The University Committee on Ethics approved this study. Based on the prospective nature of our study, two different assessments were conducted, with a one-week separation between each. The participants first gave their informed consent to take part in the project and were then given a booklet of questionnaires (this booklet contained questions from the measures noted below), which took 20–30 min to complete in their associations in the presence of a psychologist. Firstly, participants self-reported their sociodemographic and clinical data using an ad hoc questionnaire (pain). Then, using validated questionnaires, participants were evaluated regarding helplessness (pain catastrophizing), activity avoidance (AA), and commitment to physical activity (PA). Finally, after finishing the first assessment, levels of physical activity were evaluated and an accelerometer was placed by a psychologist on the wrist of each participant for 7 consecutive days, starting on the same day that they received the accelerometer. Participants were instructed to always wear the accelerometer, except during water-based activities such as showering or swimming. After 8 days, the accelerometers were collected in a second evaluation time, and participants were given a second booklet that included the IPAQ to be answered individually by each participant. The data from the accelerometers was finally downloaded onto a computer and processed using the manufacturer software.

2.3. Measures

2.3.1. First Assessment

Helplessness (H). The Spanish adaptation of the Pain Catastrophizing Scale (PCS) evaluates three components of pain catastrophizing. The Pain Catastrophizing Scale (PCS) stands out as the most widely utilized tool for assessing pain catastrophizing [30]. Its development was based on a multidimensional understanding of catastrophizing, encompassing aspects of magnification (e.g., pondering whether something serious might happen), rumination (e.g., unable to stop thinking about it), and helplessness (e.g., feeling powerless to alleviate pain intensity). It contains 13 items in a 4-point Likert response format [55,56]. In this study, the helplessness subscale was used. Specifically, we measured when women were feeling powerless to alleviate pain intensity. This subscale contains 6 responses, such as "there is nothing I can do to reduce the intensity of the pain". Higher scores on this scale represent higher helplessness. In the present study, the internal consistency of the helplessness subscale was 0.89.

Activity avoidance (AA). This activity pattern was measured through the Spanish version of the Activity Patterns Scale (POAM-P) [57]. The POAM-P (24 items on a 5-point Likert scale divided into 8 dimensions) allows assessment of three widely accepted general activity patterns (avoidance, persistence, and pacing). Avoidance patterns include pain avoidance (avoidance of a behavior in the presence or anticipation of changes in pain) and activity avoidance (avoidance refers to the patients' condition of being in pain rather than the fluctuating pain experience). In this study, the activity avoidance subscale was used. Studies so far support the validity of the Activity Patterns Scale to measure different activity patterns in chronic pain settings [57,58]. In the present study, the Cronbach alpha for the activity avoidance subscale was 0.82.

Avoidance goal (AG). Walking with the goal of avoiding physical exercise. The preference for pain-avoidance goals in relation to activities was assessed using the Spanish adaptation [39] of the Goal Pursuit Questionnaire for Pain (GPQ-P) [59]. The GPQ measures the goal pursuit of people with pain, considering achievement goals (performing activity) and hedonic goals (avoiding activities because of pain), which can be activated simultaneously or be in conflict. The adaptation of the GPQ to physical exercise was used specifically in relation to 5 specific situations: (1) walking while doing other activities, (2) walking with the goal of physical exercise, (3) mild physical activity, (4) moderate physical activity, and (5) intense physical activity. Higher mean scores in each factor indicate stronger preferences for a hedonic goal in comparison to an achievement goal, that is, to avoid pain (Factor I) or to maintain a positive mood (Factor II). For this study, the "Pain avoidance goals" factor was selected. Cronbach's alpha in this study was 0.81.

Pain severity (covariate). Pain severity was assessed by the mean score of the four pain severity items (maximum, minimum, overall pain intensity during the last 7 days, and pain intensity at the current time) from the Brief Pain Inventory (BPI) [60]. Each rating was evaluated using an 11-point numerical scale from 0 = "no pain" to 10 = "the worst pain you can imagine". This procedure has been widely used in the pain-focused literature [61]. Researchers have shown an excellent internal consistency in previous studies of the Spanish population with chronic pain ($\alpha = 0.93$) [62]. In this study, the internal consistency of this scale was 0.86.

2.3.2. Second Assessment: Physical Activity Measures

Regular walking behavior (IPAQ-walking). During the second evaluation, the Spanish version of the International Physical Activity Questionnaire (IPAQ) was used to assess the physical activity levels of patients. This questionnaire catalogs various activities undertaken in the past week, noting their intensity, duration, and frequency. From this, each participant's physical activity level was determined based on the IPAQ's data processing and analysis guidelines. High activity levels were defined as at least three days of vigorous activity totaling 1500 or more MET (metabolic equivalent of task) minutes weekly, or seven days of any combination of walking, moderate, or vigorous activities totaling at least 3000 MET minutes. Moderate activity levels were achieved by engaging in vigorous activities and/or walking for at least 30 min per day for three days, or moderate activities and/or walking for the same duration over five days, accumulating 600 or more MET minutes. Participants who did not meet the criteria for high or moderate levels were considered to have low activity levels. The IPAQ version used in this study was validated within the Spanish population, showing strong reliability in measuring total physical activity, vigorous and moderate activities, and walking time [63].The internal consistency for our sample was also robust, with Cronbach's alpha values reflecting the reliability of the vigorous, moderate, and walking activity measures (0.871 in vigorous activity, 0.721 in moderate activity, and 0.753 in walking activity). For the present study, MET-mins related to walking behavior were used. Additionally, to analyze sedentary behavior, the questionnaire included questions about the amount of time spent sitting down on a working day.

Physical activity (St; steps). ActiGraph wGT3X-BT (Pensacola, FL, USA) was used to quantify physical activity objectively by measuring accelerations in physical activity from three dimensions (anteroposterior, mediolateral, and longitudinal axis) (CE., 2005). It is measured in counts per minute, which is then translated to METs. Measurements can range from 1 to 18 METs, depending on the intensity of physical activity [22]. A total of 7 continuous days with a minimum of 10 valid hours per day was required for being included in the study analysis. Participants were instructed to wear an Actical accelerometer on their hip for up to 8 days, and to always wear it, except when performing water-based activities. Episodes of 20 continuous minutes with intensity 0 were excluded from the analysis. The Actical accelerometer has been validated to measure physical activity in adults (DP, 2006). We calculated mean counts per minute by dividing the sum of total counts per epoch for a valid day by the number of minutes of wear time on that day across all valid days. Time spent walking was consequently defined as minutes accumulated between 100 and 759 counts min^{-1}. We used the manufacturer software (ActilifeTM v.6.11.7 desktop) for data download, reduction, cleaning, and analysis purposes. Further details are available elsewhere [64]. The average minutes per day as a walking variable was used in the analyses.

2.4. Data Analysis

Data were analyzed using SPSS 27 (Windows). The characteristics of the sample were described using frequency distributions, percentages, and mean and standard deviations. Following the first aim of this study, differences between walking-IPAQ and accelerometers scores were assessed using the Bland and Altman method [65]. Second, bivariate Pearson correlation analyses were performed to assess the relationships between both measures of physical activity (walking) and hopelessness, avoidance goals regarding walking, activity avoidance, and pain. Statistical significance was established at a p value of less than 0.05. Third, two models were tested by the SPSS macro-PROCESS macro 3.5 to analyze mediation (Figure 1), and a moderated mediation model (Figure 2) (model 7) between variables. First, two mediation analyses were run to examine the mediation role of activity avoidance among hopelessness and both physical activity measures (accelerometer and IPAQ) (model 4, Figure 1). To test these two models, regression (to calculate statistics for specific paths) and bootstrapping (to generate a confidence interval [CI] for the mediation effects) analyses were used. Variables were centered before the analyses by subtracting the mean from the predictors to rescale them. It revealed the effect when the remaining predictors had a value of '0' [66] and created 'artificial' scores by rescaling the predictors. However, centering had no effect on model fit, significance tests, and standardized slope values. Trying to analyze effects described altogether, a moderated mediation model (model 7, Figure 2) was run. This model tested if the indirect effect of helplessness on physical activity (accelerometer), by way of activity avoidance, depended on avoidance goals regarding walking. Product terms of helplessness (centered) × avoidance goals regarding walking (centered) were added to the regression models predicting physical activity. Simple slope analyses were performed to illustrate significant interaction effects [67]. The index of moderated mediation was estimated as a measure of the association between an indirect effect and a moderator, together with a 95% confidence interval, from bootstrapping 10,000 samples [68]. Pain was specifically considered as a significant covariate in each model, controlling also for sociodemographic covariates that were related to the variables of interest.

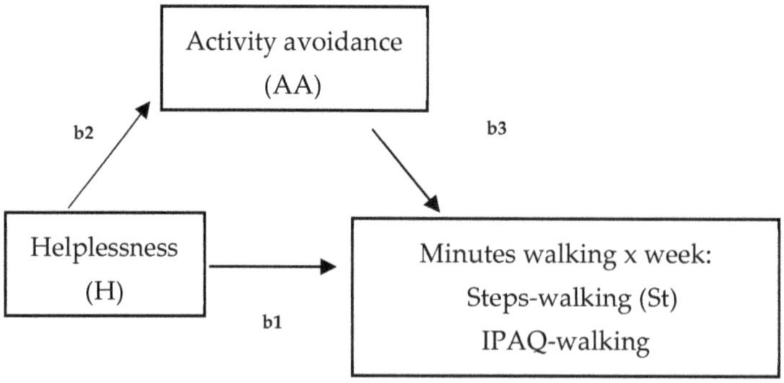

Figure 1. Hypothesized model of the mediated effect of helplessness on minutes walking (per week), measured by steps-walking (St, accelerometer) and IPAQ-walking by activity avoidance (b1 = total effect; b2 = direct effect; b3 = indirect effect).

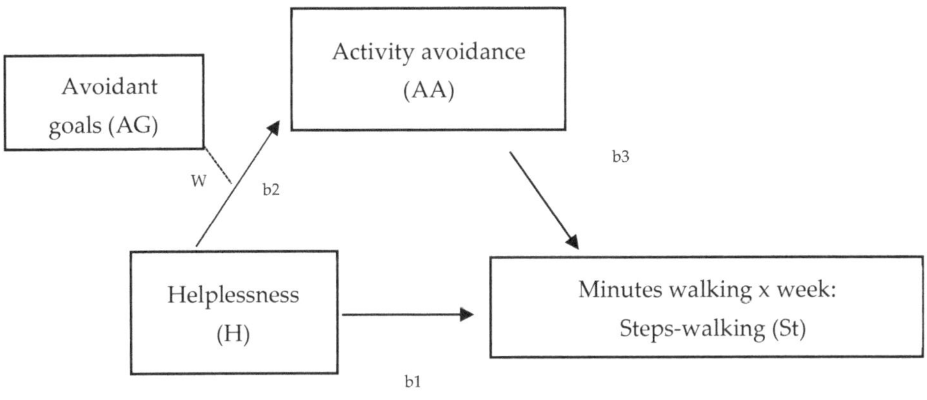

Figure 2. Hypothesized model of the moderated mediation effect of hopelessness on minutes walking (per week), measured by steps-walking (St, accelerometer) at different levels of avoidant goals (W) (W = moderation effect; b1 = total effect; b2 = direct effect; b3 = indirect effect).

3. Results

3.1. Participant Characteristics

The sample had a mean age of 56.91 years (SD = 8.9) (ranging between 30 and 78 years old). Related to employment status, 12% were employed (all of them part-time; mean of working hours = 5.49; SD = 2.92), 33.8% were homemakers, 32% were retired (18.8% reported chronic pain as a reason for retirement), 12.1% were unemployed, and 10% were employed but on sick leave. Half of the women were married (53%) or in a stable relationship. Regarding education level, 52.6% of women had completed elementary school as their highest level of education (according to the International Standard Classification of Education (ISCED, 2011). The average time since their fibromyalgia diagnosis was 12.14 years (SD = 8.45), ranging between 1 and 46 years. Finally, the pain mean BPI score was 7.15 (SD = 1.52).

3.2. Descriptive Data and Correlations

Table 1 shows Pearson correlations between the variables included in the analysis. Hopelessness was positively correlated with activity avoidance (r = 0.25; $p = 0.007$), and activity avoidance was negatively correlated with steps assessed by accelerometer (r = −0.32; $p = 0.02$). Regarding pain, positive correlations were found with hopelessness (r = 0.30; $p = 0.001$) and negative correlations with activity avoidance (r = −0.32; $p = 0.02$). No significant correlations were found related to exercise goals and regular walking with hopelessness, steps, activity avoidance, and pain.

Table 1. Pearson correlations between study variables.

	2	3	4	5	6
1. Helplessness	0.25 **	−0.16	−0.01	−0.07	0.30 **
2. Activity avoidance		−0.32 *	−0.05	−0.01	−0.32 *
3. Minutes walked (week) by steps			0.11	0.08	0.21
4. Minutes walked (week) by regular walking				0.002	−0.61
5. Avoidance goal					0.15
6. Pain					1

* $p < 0.05$; ** $p < 0.01$.

3.3. Differences between Physical Activity Measures: Accelerometer and Regular Walking

Following the first aim of this study, the results from differences estimated by the Bland and Altman method show significant variations in measurements between the IPAQ and the accelerometer in all physical activity intensities, including walking behavior [65].

Specifically related to their regular walking behavior (Table 2), steps measured by the accelerometer show higher minutes registered compared to the IPAQ. Moreover, although correlations with physical exercise intensities were significant, the most significant correlation was related to walking intensity (p = 0.008).

Table 2. Descriptive physical activity according to intensity of IPAQ and ActiGraph wGT3X-BT in a week.

	Sedentary Behavior		Walking		Moderate		Vigorous	
	IPAQ MET min Day^{-1}	Accelerometer Counts·min^{-1}	IPAQ MET min·Day^{-1}	Accelerometer Counts·min^{-1}	IPAQ MET min·Day^{-1}	Accelerometer Counts·min^{-1}	IPAQ MET min·Day^{-1}	Accelerometer Counts·min^{-1}
	496	18,567	636	1019	225	547	63	22
p	0.017		0.008		0.027		0.047	

3.4. Test of the Models

First, the mediating role of activity avoidance (AA) between helplessness (H) and physical activity measured by steps (St) (accelerometer) and IPAQ-walking was examined with pain as the covariate (Figure 1). For both mediating models, no significant total effects of the predictor (hopelessness) on steps (B = −7.95, SE = 5.55, t = −1.43, 95% CI = [−19.16; 3.21], p = 0.15) or on IPAQ-walking (B = 5.74, SE = 17.93, t = 0.04, 95% CI = [−28.44; 42.96], p = 0.68) were observed. However, focusing on the mediating effect of activity avoidance, the effect of hopelessness on steps was totally mediated by activity avoidance (B = −5.75, SE = 3.47; 95% CI = [−13.58, −0.05]), while activity avoidance did not have a mediated effect when IPAQ-walking was evaluated as a dependent variable (B = −1.51, SE = 4.90, 95% CI = [−12.21, 8.01]). That is, hopelessness predicted higher activity avoidance, which in turn predicted fewer minutes walked when evaluated by an accelerometer in our sample of women with FM (Figure 1).

3.5. Moderated Mediation Model of Openness to Experience on Activity Acceptance by Positive Effect at Different Levels of Mood Management Goals

Second, a moderated mediation model was conducted to test the indirect effect of hopelessness on physical activity (measured by accelerometer) by activity avoidance at levels of avoidance goals regarding walking and pain as covariates (Figure 2). The results show that the effect of hopelessness on activity avoidance varied at different values of avoidance goals regarding walking (Hayes' algorithm, estimated for physical activity, was ß = −1.67 [95% CI = −4.48/−0.003]), an effect that was maintained when physical activity measured by accelerometer was included as a dependent variable in the model. Particularly, helplessness mediated by activity avoidance was significantly associated with physical activity when levels of avoidance goals regarding walking were medium (Value: 0.48; ß = −5.77, [95% CI = −14.37/−0.01]) and high (Value: 2.48; ß = −9.12, $p < 0.001$, [95% CI = −22.01/−0.36]). This result (Table 3, Figure 2) shows that the strength of the relationship between hopelessness and physical activity (measured by minutes of walking per week by the accelerometer) via activity avoidance increased at higher levels of avoidant goals. Thus, the indirect effect of helplessness on minutes of walking measured by accelerometer via activity avoidance was higher in individuals who placed a higher importance on exercise.

Table 3. Moderate mediation model: regression of hopelessness, activity avoidance (mediator) on minutes walked measured by steps (St), and avoidance goals regarding walking (moderator).

	B (SE)	t	p	[LLCI-ULCI]
VI: Helplessness (H)	0.18 (0.06)	2.97	0.004	[0.05/0.30]
M: Avoidance goals (AG)	0.24 (0.15)	1.61	0.11	[−0.62/0.02]
H × AG (interaction)	0.06 (0.02)	2.51	0.01	[0.01/0.11]

Table 3. *Cont.*

	B (SE)	t	p	[LLCI-ULCI]
* Pain (covariate)	0.13 (0.19)	−0.67	0.50	[−0.40/0.55]
Conditional effects of the focal predictor (H) at values * of the moderator (AG) on positive effect				
−2.51	−0.02 (0.08)	0.30	0.76	[−0.15/0.20]
0.48 *	0.21 (0.06)	3.44	0.001	[0.08/0.33]
2.48 *	0.33 (0.08)	3.88	0.0003	[0.16/0.50]
Regression of helplessness and activity avoidance (AA) on steps (St)				
	B (SE)	t	p	[LLCI-ULCI]
Helplessness (H)	−2.21 (6.13)	−0.36	0.71	[−14.59/10.15]
Activity avoidance (AA)	−26.9 (13.81)	−1.95	0.05	[−54.81/0.88]
* Pain (covariate)	−0.30 (18.12)	−0.01	0.98	[−36.85/36.23]
Model summary	R^2: 0.12			
Indirect effects at values * of AG				
−2.51	−0.74 (3.08)			[−6.82/6.07]
0.48 *	−5.77 (3.74)			[−14.37/−0.01]
2.48 *	−9.12 (5.53)			[−22.01/−0.36]
Indexes of moderated mediation	−1.67 (1.16)			[−4.48/−0.003]
Pairwise contrast between conditional indirect effects (Effect 1 minus Effect2)				
	Effect 1	Effect2	contrast	[LLCI/ULCI]
	−5.77	−0.74	−5.03	[−13.46/−0.009]
	−9.12	−0.74	−8.38	[−22.44/−0.01]
	−9.12	−5.77	−3.35	[−9.97/−0.006]

Notes: Models include controls for age, sex, education level, employment status; conditional effects of the focal predictor at values * of the moderator (AG); indirect effects of helplessness (H) on activity avoidance (AA) at values * of AG. Abbreviations: BootLLCI, bootstrapping lower limit confidence interval; BootULCI, bootstrapping upper limit confidence interval; SE, standard error. Model 7 from Process.

4. Discussion

The present study had two specific objectives. First, based on differences found by researchers between measures related to walking behavior in women with FM [49,69,70], our first objective focused on evaluating the concurrence between two measures related to physical activity—one objective (accelerometer) and one subjective (IPAQ), both selected to evaluate the minutes walked for one week (Table 1). These results are partially in agreement with studies that have shown that physical activity perception in patients with FM is lower compared to activity performed when assessed by objective measures [69,70]. In accordance with recent studies, our results show that, in relation to low-intensity physical activity (walking), both measures show the highest correlation compared to the assessment of sedentary, moderate, or intense activity, assessed using the same measures [22]. It appears that, although our results corroborate this effect for sedentary, moderate, and intense measures of physical activity, the same is not true for walking. Women with FM walk more minutes during a week than they perceive themselves to walk. As previous studies have shown, the perceived physical function may be even worse than the objective physical function among women with fibromyalgia [10]; thus, the impact on the self-confidence about what they are and are not able to do is largely affected, which in turn is related to the concept of self-efficacy. Our objective measurement results may be linked to the fact that women engage in walking behavior as part of their daily routine. However, since this is not undertaken with the specific intention to perform physical exercise, and because they perceive they are not able to exercise (low self-efficacy about physical activity), this activity is not recognized as such [58].

Based on our results and trying to determine how objective and subjective associations differ [70], our second aim focused on the analysis of the differential role of psychological and contextual variables on perception and actual performance. In line with this aim, despite the fact that helplessness, goal conflict, and activity avoidance have been identified as contextual factors to be taken into account in the assessment of physical activity in women with FM, there are no studies to date analyzing these variables together in relation to walking, or aiming to analyze differences when assessing behavior using different measures (objective and subjective). Therefore, following this aim, two models were analyzed. Firstly, one model was focused on analyzing if activity avoidance mediated the relationship between hopelessness and minutes walked during a week, assessed by both measures (Figure 1). Secondly, we analyzed if the mediated effect of activity avoidance between hopelessness and walking was influenced by levels of avoidant goals. The results show interesting data. On the one hand, the mediating role of activity avoidance between hopelessness and minutes walked was corroborated, but only regarding the objective measure of walking behavior assessment. This is in agreement with a recent study where, compared to self-report measures, only step count significantly changed across time, with mean steps peaking at eight weeks [71]. It appears that the effect of helplessness on minutes walked during a week occurs when totally mediated by activity avoidance, and, specifically, when minutes walked are assessed using an accelerometer. Moreover, the fact that higher levels of hopelessness imply greater activity avoidance, which in turn negatively influences minutes walked, is in accordance with a recent study that focused on cognitive variables characterizing FM patients who found pain catastrophizing and, specifically, hopelessness to be a significant predictor of adaptability in a Spanish FM sample [72]. This result shows that pain avoidance is especially dysfunctional in patients with high helplessness. Catastrophizing thoughts about pain are characterized as an exaggerated negative mental stance linked to the real or anticipated experience of pain [30]. As explained above, this notion is empirically structured into three dimensions: magnification, rumination, and helplessness. Magnification is the excessive perception of pain situations and pessimistic expectations regarding the progression of pain, while rumination encompasses repetitive thoughts, worry, and the inability to suppress such thoughts. Finally, helplessness (our focus of study) is the perceived lack of control over these thoughts [56]. Most studies challenge the uniformity of this concept, suggesting that each dimension has distinct effects [24,28]. For instance, it has been noted that shifts in helplessness correlate with improvements across all disease variables, whereas alterations in rumination and magnification have varied impacts on different disease outcomes. On the one hand, these results show that cognitive variables have a basic contextual role when trying to promote exercise, a role that must necessarily consider activity avoidance as a key variable in the promotion of physical activity and, specifically, the promotion of walking with the aim to do exercise in women with FM. This is congruent with studies of the model of fear of movement that have shown that activity avoidance is the highest predictor of FM impact [49,73] and, specifically, that a low level of physical activity is influenced by self-efficacy, mainly through activity avoidance [39]. On the other hand, within the framework of the behavioral activation (BA), if the individual's environment provides contact with reinforcement for unhealthy behavior and lacks reinforcement for healthy behavior, unhealthy behavior will increase and healthy behavior will decrease [50]. Thus, in a clinical context, the prevention of activity avoidance may be a key factor in walking when it deprives women with FM of the opportunity to obtain reinforcement through the walking behavior itself, which in turn may be maintaining the avoidance of activity by promoting the negative perception that women have about their physical activity [74–76]. We can conclude that promoting walking is necessary to improve levels of hopelessness, preventing women from entering an activity avoidance pattern. Women need the opportunity to obtain reinforcement from their own behavior, improving their self-efficacy with regard to their functional capacity.

Secondly, our results show that helplessness plays a significant role in minutes spent walking via the mediated effect of activity avoidance. This result is in concurrence with a recent study in which catastrophizing had a residual importance on physical activity also mediated by a contextual variable, such as psychological flexibility [77]. As Vallejo et al. (2021) have pointed out, contextual variables should be considered for evaluation and early intervention in FM patients. Patients are faced with multiple competing goals, and they should prioritize between those related to avoiding pain and those related to maintaining or incorporating other goals different from pain control [78–81]. Our results show that in women with FM, hopelessness could be another cognitive variable that influences walking via the mediated role of activity avoidance.

This study presents several limitations. Initially, its cross-sectional nature hinders the determination of causality [22]. Additionally, the research focuses solely on women with fibromyalgia (FM), necessitating further studies among males and other pain-affected demographics to confirm the applicability of the results. Although fibromyalgia tends to affect females more frequently (often surpassing 90% prevalence), the correlation between fibromyalgia and gender remains contentious and intricate due to various factors. These factors encompass variances in diagnostic criteria and methodologies, which often results in the underdiagnosis of male patients with fibromyalgia and the overdiagnosis of females in both clinical and research settings [1,2]. Additionally, studies into disparities in symptoms and psychological variables have yielded inconclusive results [5], underscoring the necessity for future studies to separately assess females and males afflicted with fibromyalgia. Lastly, the recruiting method for the participants through mutual-aid pain associations might also skew the sample toward women, potentially not representing the usual cases in secondary care. It is important to note, however, that these types of associations are prevalent among Spanish FM sufferers, and similar clinical and sociodemographic profiles have been observed across various settings [39]. Despite exploring numerous clinical and psychosocial factors, this study does not cover all possible aspects relevant to FM [3].

Nevertheless, considering these factors and recent research indicating that physical activity (PA) affects individual variances in FM symptoms and overall functionality, this study contributes to the evidence supporting interventions that enhance openness to experiences, positive effects, and mood management. These interventions aim to foster pain acceptance, a crucial element in chronic pain management that could significantly improve patient quality of life [82].

In terms of practical application, our findings support a burgeoning field of intervention that utilizes positive psychology in chronic pain populations. This approach seeks to amplify positive emotions, thoughts, and actions [83]. Positive psychology interventions (PPIs) adopt a resource-oriented strategy that emphasizes fortifying the positive traits of individuals, which could be advantageous in the management of chronic pain.

Our findings provide healthcare practitioners with fresh psychological markers that can enhance collaborative care approaches for affected individuals. Considering that there are modern comprehensive pain management programs emphasizing the development of adaptive coping strategies, this study offers a new perspective for healthcare workers, particularly nurses, to tailor their care strategies in fibromyalgia (FM) toward embracing pain, fostering positive emotions, and managing one's mood instead of concentrating solely on diminishing pain sensations. However, further research is essential to definitively determine the cause-and-effect links among these factors.

5. Conclusions

From a clinical point of view, health professionals should consider cognitive and behavioral patterns as psychological variables when encouraging walking behavior. It has been demonstrated that hopelessness does play a role in walking via activity avoidance, specifically in women who consider exercise an important behavior for battling their disease. These results yield significant data within the panorama of FM treatments and, of course, in relation to the adherence, promotion, and prevention of the disease. It appears that helplessness and activity avoidance influence minutes spent walking, as assessed through an objective measure in women who place a high importance on exercise. It seems to be that helplessness has a distinct impact on the behavior of walking as assessed by an objective measure. This influence manifests through the avoidance of activity, particularly in individuals who possess higher levels of hedonic goals, which involves shunning activities due to pain. It can be concluded that promoting exercise among women with fibromyalgia (FM) is crucial, considering not only the amount of exercise but also how it is performed. Helplessness and activity avoidance are measured against the goals women set for their activity levels. Therefore, promoting the work on contextual variables as a preventive measure, and for identifying profiles in women with FM, becomes a successful goal. This is because these variables directly and indirectly influence the ability to exercise and, consequently, the well-being of women with FM.

Author Contributions: Conceptualization, C.E. and C.P.; methodology, C.E.; software, C.E.; validation, C.E, C.P. and L.G.; formal analysis, C.E.; investigation, P.C., L.G., C.E. and C.P.; resources, P.C., C.P., L.G. and C.E.; data curation, P.C., C.P., L.G. and C.E.; writing—original draft preparation, C.E.; writing—review and editing, C.E.; visualization, P.C., C.P., L.G. and C.E.; supervision, C.P., L.G. and P.C.; project administration, P.C., C.P., L.G. and C.E.; funding acquisition, C.P. All authors have read and agreed to the published version of the manuscript.

Funding: This work was funded by the Health Research Fund (Fondo de Investigación en Salud), grant number PI17/00858 from the Instituto de Salud Carlos III (Spain), co-financed by the European Union through the Fondo Europeo de Desarrollo Regional (FEDER).

Institutional Review Board Statement: This study was conducted in accordance with the Declaration of Helsinki and approved by the Institutional Review Board (or Ethics Committee) of Rey Juan Carlos University for studies involving humans [Reference number PI17/00858].

Informed Consent Statement: All participants included in the study provided informed consent. Written consent has been obtained from the patient(s) to publish this paper.

Data Availability Statement: The data presented in this study are available upon request from the corresponding author.

Conflicts of Interest: The authors declare that they have no conflicts of interest.

References

1. Wolfe, F.; Clauw, D.J.; Fitzcharles, M.-A.; Goldenberg, D.L.; Katz, R.S.; Mease, P.; Russell, A.S.; Russell, I.J.; Winfield, J.B.; Yunus, M.B. The American College of Rheumatology Preliminary Diagnostic Criteria for Fibromyalgia and Measurement of Symptom Severity. *Arthrit. Care Res.* **2010**, *62*, 600–610. [CrossRef] [PubMed]
2. Macfarlane, G.J.; Kronisch, C.; Atzeni, F.; Häuser, W.; Choy, E.H.; Amris, K.; Branco, J.; Dincer, F.; Leino-Arjas, P.; Longley, K.; et al. EULAR recommendations for management of fibromyalgia. *Ann. Rheum. Dis.* **2017**, *76*, e54. [CrossRef] [PubMed]
3. Mahgoub, M.Y.; Elnady, B.M.; Abdelkader, H.S.; Abdelhalem, R.A.; Hassan, W.A. Comorbidity of Fibromyalgia in Primary Knee Osteoarthritis: Potential Impact on Functional Status and Quality of Life. *Open Access Rheumatol.* **2020**, *12*, 55–63. [CrossRef] [PubMed]
4. Cane, D.; McCarthy, M.; Mazmanian, D. Obstacles to activity pacing. *Pain* **2016**, *157*, 1508. [CrossRef] [PubMed]
5. Segura-Jiménez, V.; Borges-Cosic, M.; Soriano-Maldonado, A.; Estévez-López, F.; Álvarez-Gallardo, I.C.; Herrador-Colmenero, M.; Delgado-Fernández, M.; Ruiz, J.R. Association of sedentary time and physical activity with pain, fatigue, and impact of fibromyalgia: The al-Ándalus study. *Scand. J. Med. Sci. Sports* **2015**, *27*, 83–92. [CrossRef]
6. Pulido-Martos, M.; Luque-Reca, O.; Segura-Jiménez, V.; Álvarez-Gallardo, I.C.; Soriano-Maldonado, A.; Acosta-Manzano, P.; Gavilán-Carrera, B.; McVeigh, J.G.; Geenen, R.; Delgado-Fernández, M.; et al. Physical and psychological paths toward less severe fibromyalgia: A structural equation model. *Ann. Phys. Rehabil. Med.* **2020**, *63*, 46–52. [CrossRef] [PubMed]
7. Thieme, K.; Mathys, M.; Turk, D.C. Evidenced-Based Guidelines on the Treatment of Fibromyalgia Patients: Are They Consistent and If Not, Why Not? Have Effective Psychological Treatments Been Overlooked? *J. Pain* **2017**, *18*, 747–756. [CrossRef] [PubMed]
8. O'dwyer, T.; Maguire, S.; Mockler, D.; Durcan, L.; Wilson, F. Behaviour change interventions targeting physical activity in adults with fibromyalgia: A systematic review. *Rheumatol. Int.* **2019**, *39*, 805–817. [CrossRef]
9. Ahmed, S.; Aggarwal, A.; Lawrence, A. Performance of the American College of Rheumatology 2016 criteria for fibromyalgia in a referral care setting. *Rheumatol. Int.* **2019**, *39*, 1397–1403. [CrossRef]
10. O'Connor, S.R.; Tully, M.A.; Ryan, B.; Bleakley, C.M.; Baxter, G.D.; Bradley, J.M.; McDonough, S.M. Walking Exercise for Chronic Musculoskeletal Pain: Systematic Review and Meta-Analysis. *Arch. Phys. Med. Rehabil.* **2015**, *96*, 724–734.e3. [CrossRef]
11. Sanz-Baños, Y.; Pastor-Mira, M.; Lledó, A.; López-Roig, S.; Peñacoba, C.; Sánchez-Meca, J. Do women with fibromyalgia adhere to walking for exercise programs to improve their health? Systematic review and meta-analysis. *Disabil. Rehabil.* **2017**, *40*, 2475–2487. [CrossRef] [PubMed]
12. Peñacoba, C.; Pastor, M.Á.; López-Roig, S.; Velasco, L.; Lledo, A. Walking Beliefs in Women with Fibromyalgia: Clinical Profile and Impact on Walking Behavior. *Clin. Nurs. Res.* **2017**, *26*, 632–650. [CrossRef]
13. Bidonde, J.; Boden, C.; Foulds, H.; Kim, S.Y. Physical Activity and Exercise Training for Adults with Fibromyalgia. In *Fibromyalgia Syndrome*; Springer International Publishing: Cham, Switzerland, 2021; pp. 59–72.
14. Andrade, A.; Dominski, F.H.; Sieczkowska, S.M. What we already know about the effects of exercise in patients with fibromyalgia: An umbrella review. *Semin. Arthritis Rheum.* **2020**, *50*, 1465–1480. [CrossRef] [PubMed]

15. Hurley, M.; Dickson, K.; Hallett, R.; Grant, R.; Hauari, H.; Walsh, N.; Stansfield, C.; Oliver, S. Exercise interventions and patient beliefs for people with hip, knee or hip and knee osteoarthritis: A mixed methods review. *Cochrane Database Syst. Rev.* **2018**, *4*, CD010842. [CrossRef] [PubMed]
16. Polaski, A.M.; Phelps, A.L.; Kostek, M.C.; Szucs, K.A.; Kolber, B.J. Exercise-induced hypoalgesia: A meta-analysis of exercise dosing for the treatment of chronic pain. *PLoS ONE* **2019**, *14*, e0210418. [CrossRef]
17. Chiaramonte, R.; Bonfiglio, M.; Chisari, S. Multidisciplinary protocol for the management of fibromyalgia associated with imbalance. Our experience and literature review. *Rev. Assoc. Med. Bras.* **2019**, *65*, 1265–1274. [CrossRef] [PubMed]
18. Vlaeyen, J.W.S.; Linton, S.J. Fear-avoidance and its consequences in chronic musculoskeletal pain: A state of the art. *Pain* **2000**, *85*, 317–332. [CrossRef]
19. Lami, M.J.; Martínez, M.P.; Miró, E.; Sánchez, A.I.; Guzmán, M.A. Catastrophizing, Acceptance, and Coping as Mediators Between Pain and Emotional Distress and Disability in Fibromyalgia. *J. Clin. Psychol. Med. Settings* **2018**, *25*, 80–92. [CrossRef]
20. Racine, M.; Galán, S.; de la Vega, R.; Pires, C.T.; Solé, E.; Nielson, W.R.; Miró, J.; Moulin, D.E.; Jensen, M.P. Pain-related Activity Management Patterns and Function in Patients with Fibromyalgia Syndrome. *Clin. J. Pain* **2018**, *34*, 122–129. [CrossRef]
21. Bernard, P.; Romain, A.-J.; Caudroit, J.; Chevance, G.; Carayol, M.; Gourlan, M.; Dancause, K.N.; Moullec, G. Cognitive behavior therapy combined with exercise for adults with chronic diseases: Systematic review and meta-analysis. *Heal. Psychol.* **2018**, *37*, 433–450. [CrossRef]
22. López-Roig, S.; Ecija, C.; Peñacoba, C.; Ivorra, S.; Nardi-Rodríguez, A.; Lecuona, O.; Pastor-Mira, M.A. Assessing Walking Programs in Fibromyalgia: A Concordance Study between Measures. *Int. J. Environ. Res. Public Health* **2022**, *19*, 2995. [CrossRef] [PubMed]
23. Munguía-Izquierdo, D.; Pulido-Martos, M.; Acosta, F.M.; Acosta-Manzano, P.; Gavilán-Carrera, B.; Rodriguez-Ayllon, M.; Geenen, R.; Delgado-Fernández, M.; Álvarez-Gallardo, I.C.; Segura-Jiménez, V.; et al. Objective and subjective measures of physical functioning in women with fibromyalgia: What type of measure is associated most clearly with subjective well-being? *Disabil. Rehabil.* **2019**, *43*, 1649–1656. [CrossRef] [PubMed]
24. Écija, C.; Luque-Reca, O.; Suso-Ribera, C.; Catala, P.; Peñacoba, C. Associations of Cognitive Fusion and Pain Catastrophizing with Fibromyalgia Impact through Fatigue, Pain Severity, and Depression: An Exploratory Study Using Structural Equation Modeling. *J. Clin. Med.* **2020**, *9*, 1763. [CrossRef] [PubMed]
25. Edwards, R.R.; Cahalan, C.; Mensing, G.; Smith, M.; Haythornthwaite, J.A. Pain, catastrophizing, and depression in the rheumatic diseases. *Nat. Rev. Rheumatol.* **2011**, *7*, 216–224. [CrossRef]
26. Keefe, F.J.; Rumble, M.E.; Scipio, C.D.; Giordano, L.A.; Perri, L.M. Psychological aspects of persistent pain: Current state of the science. *J. Pain* **2004**, *5*, 195–211. [CrossRef]
27. Quartana, P.J.; Campbell, C.M.; Edwards, R.R. Pain catastrophizing: A critical review. *Expert. Rev. Neurother.* **2009**, *9*, 745–758. [CrossRef]
28. Suso-Ribera, C.; García-Palacios, A.; Botella, C.; Ribera-Canudas, M.V. Pain Catastrophizing and Its Relationship with Health Out-comes: Does Pain Intensity Matter? *Pain Res. Manag.* **2017**, *2017*, 1–8. [CrossRef]
29. Whitaker, M.M.; Odell, D.; Deboeck, P.R.; Stefanucci, J.K.; Okifuji, A. Increased Pain Variability in Patients With Chronic Pain: A Role for Pain Catastrophizing. *J. Pain* **2024**, 104494, *in press*. [CrossRef]
30. Sullivan, M.J.L.; Adams, H.; Ellis, T. Targeting Catastrophic Thinking to Promote Return to Work in Individuals with Fibromyalgia. *J. Cogn. Psychother.* **2012**, *26*, 130–142. [CrossRef]
31. Eccleston, C.; Crombez, G. Worry and chronic pain: A misdirected problem solving model. *Pain* **2007**, *132*, 233–236. [CrossRef]
32. Aldrich, S.; Eccleston, C.; Crombez, G. Worrying about chronic pain: Vigilance to threat and misdirected problem solving. *Behav. Res. Ther.* **2000**, *38*, 457–470. [CrossRef]
33. Nijs, J.; Roussel, N.; Van Oosterwijck, J.; De Kooning, M.; Ickmans, K.; Struyf, F.; Meeus, M.; Lundberg, M. Fear of movement and avoidance behaviour toward physical activity in chronic-fatigue syndrome and fibromyalgia: State of the art and implications for clinical practice. *Clin. Rheumatol.* **2013**, *32*, 1121–1129. [CrossRef] [PubMed]
34. McCracken, L.M.; Morley, S. The Psychological Flexibility Model: A Basis for Integration and Progress in Psychological Approaches to Chronic Pain Management. *J. Pain* **2014**, *15*, 221–234. [CrossRef] [PubMed]
35. Murphy, M.H.; Nevill, A.; Murtagh, E.; Holder, R.L. The effect of walking on fitness, fatness and resting blood pressure: A meta-analysis of randomised, controlled trials. *Prev. Med.* **2007**, *44*, 377–385. [CrossRef] [PubMed]
36. Murtagh, E.M.; Nichols, L.; Mohammed, M.A.; Holder, R.; Nevill, A.M.; Murphy, M.H. The effect of walking on risk factors for cardio-vascular disease: An updated systematic review and meta-analysis of randomized control trials. *Prev. Med.* **2015**, *72*, 34–43. [CrossRef]
37. Dima, A.L.; Gillanders, D.T.; Power, M.J. Dynamic pain–emotion relations in chronic pain: A theoretical review of moderation studies. *Heal. Psychol. Rev.* **2013**, *7*, S185–S252. [CrossRef]
38. Ecija, C.; Catala, P.; López-Roig, S.; Pastor-Mira, M.; Gallardo, C.; Peñacoba, C. Are Pacing Patterns Really Based on Value Goals? Exploring the Contextual Role of Pain Acceptance and Pain Catastrophizing in Women with Fibromyalgia. *J. Clin. Psychol. Med. Settings* **2021**, *28*, 734–745. [CrossRef]
39. Pastor-Mira, M.; López-Roig, S.; Toribio, E.; Martínez-Zaragoza, F.; Nardi-Rodríguez, A.; Peñacoba, C. Pain-Related Worrying and Goal Preferences Determine Walking Persistence in Women with Fibromyalgia. *Int. J. Environ. Res. Public Heal.* **2022**, *19*, 1513. [CrossRef] [PubMed]

40. Velasco, L.; López-Gómez, I.; Gutiérrez, L.; Écija, C.; Catalá, P.; Peñacoba, C. Exploring the Preference for Fatigue-avoidance Goals as a Mediator Between Pain Catastrophizing, Functional Impairment, and Walking Behavior in Women with Fibromyalgia. *Clin. J. Pain* **2021**, *38*, 182–188. [CrossRef]
41. Turk, D.C.; Swanson, K.S.; Tunks, E.R. Psychological Approaches in the Treatment of Chronic Pain Patients—When Pills, Scalpels, and Needles are Not Enough. *Can. J. Psychiatry* **2008**, *53*, 213–223. [CrossRef]
42. Hallam, K.T.; Peeters, A.; Gupta, A.; Bilsborough, S. Moving minds: Mental health and wellbeing benefits of a 50-day workplace physical activity program. *Curr. Psychol.* **2022**, *42*, 13038–13049. [CrossRef] [PubMed]
43. Nigg, C.R.; Fuchs, R.; Gerber, M.; Jekauc, D.; Koch, T.; Krell-Roesch, J.; Lippke, S.; Mnich, C.; Novak, B.; Ju, Q.; et al. Assessing physical activity through questionnaires—A consensus of best practices and future directions. *Psychol. Sport. Exerc.* **2020**, *50*, 101715. [CrossRef]
44. Martínez, M.P.; Sánchez, A.I.; Prados, G.; Lami, M.J.; Villar, B.; Miró, E. Fibromyalgia as a heterogeneous condition: Subgroups of patients based on physical symptoms and cognitive-affective variables related to pain. *Span. J. Psychol.* **2021**, *24*, e33. [CrossRef] [PubMed]
45. Ecija, C.; Catala, P.; Sanroman, L.; Lopez-Roig, S.; Pastor-Mira, M.Á.; Peñacoba, C. Is Perfectionism Always Dysfunctional? Looking into Its Interaction with Activity Patterns in Women with Fibromyalgia. *Clin. Nurs. Res.* **2020**, *30*, 567–578. [CrossRef] [PubMed]
46. Suso-Ribera, C.; Catala, P.; Ecija, C.; Sanromán, L.; López-Gómez, I.; Pastor-Mira, Á.; Peñacoba-Puente, C. Exploring the contextual role of pain severity as a moderator of the relationship between activity patterns and the physical and mental functioning of women with fibromyalgia. *Eur. J. Pain* **2020**, *25*, 257–268. [CrossRef] [PubMed]
47. Collado-Mateo, D.; Lavín-Pérez, A.; Peñacoba, C.; Del Coso, J.; Leyton-Román, M.; Luque-Casado, A.; Gasque, P.; Fernández-Del-Olmo, M.; Amado-Alonso, D. Key Factors Associated with Adherence to Physical Exercise in Patients with Chronic Diseases and Older Adults: An Umbrella Review. *Int. J. Environ. Res. Public Health* **2021**, *18*, 2023. [CrossRef] [PubMed]
48. Luthi, F.; Vuistiner, P.; Favre, C.; Hilfiker, R.; Léger, B. Avoidance, pacing, or persistence in multidisciplinary functional rehabilitation for chronic musculoskeletal pain: An observational study with cross-sectional and longitudinal analyses. *PLoS ONE* **2018**, *13*, e0203329. [CrossRef] [PubMed]
49. López-Roig, S.; Pastor-Mira, M.Á.; Núñez, R.; Nardi, A.; Ivorra, S.; León, E.; Peñacoba, C. Assessing Self-Efficacy for Physical Activity and Walking Exercise in Women with Fibromyalgia. *Pain Manag. Nurs.* **2021**, *22*, 571–578. [CrossRef]
50. Hopko, D.R.; Lejuez, C.; Ruggiero, K.J.; Eifert, G.H. Contemporary behavioral activation treatments for depression: Procedures, principles, and progress. *Clin. Psychol. Rev.* **2003**, *23*, 699–717. [CrossRef]
51. Yu, L.; Norton, S.; McCracken, L.M. Change in "Self-as-Context" ("Perspective-Taking") Occurs in Acceptance and Commitment Therapy for People with Chronic Pain and Is Associated with Improved Functioning. *J. Pain* **2017**, *18*, 664–672. [CrossRef]
52. Van Damme, S.; Kindermans, H. A Self-Regulation Perspective on Avoidance and Persistence Behavior in Chronic Pain. *Clin. J. Pain* **2015**, *31*, 115–122. [CrossRef]
53. Wolfe, F.; Clauw, D.J.; Fitzcharles, M.A.; Goldenberg, D.L.; Häuser, W.; Katz, R.L.; Mease, P.J.; Russell, A.S.; Russell, I.J.; Walitt, B. 2016 Revisions to the 2010/2011 fibromyalgia diagnostic criteria. *Semin. Arthritis Rheum.* **2016**, *46*, 319–329. [CrossRef] [PubMed]
54. Wolfe, F.; Walitt, B.; Perrot, S.; Rasker, J.J.; Häuser, W. Fibromyalgia diagnosis and biased assessment: Sex, prevalence and bias. *PLoS ONE* **2018**, *13*, e0203755. [CrossRef] [PubMed]
55. García Campayo, J.; Rodero, B.; Alda, M.; Sobradiel, N.; Montero, J.; Moreno, S. Validation of the Spanish version of the Pain Catastrophizing Scale in fibromyalgia. *Med. Clin.* **2008**, *131*, 487–492. [CrossRef] [PubMed]
56. Sullivan, M.J.L.; Thorn, B.; Haythornthwaite, J.A.; Keefe, F.; Martin, M.; Bradley, L.A.; Lefebvre, J.C. Theoretical Perspectives on the Relation Between Catastrophizing and Pain. *Clin. J. Pain* **2001**, *17*, 52–64. [CrossRef]
57. Esteve, R.; Ramírez-Maestre, C.; Peters, M.L.; Serrano-Ibáñez, E.R.; Ruíz-Párraga, G.T.; López-Martínez, A.E. Development and Initial Validation of the Activity Patterns Scale in Patients with Chronic Pain. *J. Pain* **2015**, *17*, 451–461. [CrossRef]
58. Estévez-López, F.; Álvarez-Gallardo, I.C.; Segura-Jiménez, V.; Soriano-Maldonado, A.; Borges-Cosic, M.; Pulido-Martos, M.; Aparicio, V.A.; Carbonell-Baeza, A.; Delgado-Fernández, M.; Geenen, R. The discordance between subjectively and objectively measured physical function in women with fibromyalgia: Association with catastrophizing and self-efficacy cognitions. The al-Ándalus project. *Disabil. Rehabil.* **2016**, *40*, 329–337. [CrossRef]
59. Karsdorp, P.A.; Vlaeyen, J.W. Goals matter: Both achievement and pain-avoidance goals are associated with pain severity and disability in patients with low back and upper extremity pain. *Pain* **2011**, *152*, 1382–1390. [CrossRef]
60. Cleeland, C.S.; Ryan, K.M. Pain assessment: Global use of the Brief Pain Inventory. *Ann. Acad. Med. Singap.* **1994**, *23*, 129–138.
61. Jensen, M.P.; Turner, L.R.; Turner, J.A.; Romano, J.M. The use of multiple-item scales for pain intensity measurement in chronic pain patients. *Pain* **1996**, *67*, 35–40. [CrossRef]
62. de Andrés Ares, J.; Cruces Prado, L.M.; Canos Verdecho, M.A.; Penide Villanueva, L.; del Valle Hoyos, M.; Herdman, M.; Traseira Lugilde, S.; Velázquez Rivera, I. Validation of the Short Form of the Brief Pain Inventory (BPI-SF) in Spanish Patients with Non-Cancer-Related Pain. *Pain Pract.* **2014**, *15*, 643–653. [CrossRef]
63. Benítez-Porres, J.; Delgado, M.; Ruiz, J.R. Comparison of physical activity estimates using International Physical Activity Questionnaire (IPAQ) and accelerometry in fibromyalgia patients: The Al-Andalus study. *J. Sports Sci.* **2013**, *31*, 1741–1752. [CrossRef]

64. Kop, W.J.; Lyden, A.; Berlin, A.A.; Ambrose, K.; Olsen, C.; Gracely, R.H.; Williams, D.A.; Clauw, D.J. Ambulatory monitoring of physical activity and symptoms in fibromyalgia and chronic fatigue syndrome. *Arthritis Rheum.* **2005**, *52*, 296–303. [CrossRef]
65. De Cocker, K.; De Bourdeaudhuij, I.; Brown, W.; Cardon, G. The pedometer-based community intervention "10,000 Steps Ghent": Who used a pedometer and who increased their steps? *J. Sci. Med. Sport* **2010**, *12*, e159. [CrossRef]
66. Iacobucci, D.; Schneider, M.J.; Popovich, D.L.; Bakamitsos, G.A. Mean centering, multicollinearity, and moderators in multiple re-gression: The reconciliation redux. *Behav. Res. Methods* **2017**, *49*, 403–404. [CrossRef]
67. Aiken, L.S.; West, S.G.; Reno, R.R. *Multiple Regression: Testing and Interpreting Interactions*; Sage: Thousand Oaks, CA, USA, 1991.
68. Hayes, A.F. An Index and Test of Linear Moderated Mediation. *Multivar. Behav. Res.* **2015**, *50*, 1–22. [CrossRef]
69. Deegan, O.; Fullen, B.M.; Casey, M.B.; Segurado, R.; Hearty, C.; Doody, C.M. Protocol: Combined online interactive mindfulness and exercise programme (MOVE-Online) compared with a self-management guide for adults with chronic pain: Protocol for a randomised controlled feasibility trial. *BMJ Open* **2022**, *12*, e058265. [CrossRef]
70. Asad-Cabrera, I.; Borrueco-Sánchez, J.; López-Sánchez, C.; Lopez-Moral, A.; Munguía-izquierdo, D.; Bueno-Antequera, J. Behavioral Change Techniques to Increase Adherence to Physical Activity in Severe Mental Disorders: The Psychiactive Project. In *Combining Exercise and Psychotherapy to Treat Mental Health*; IGI Global: Hershey, PA, USA, 2024; pp. 239–264.
71. Grunberg, V.A.; Greenberg, J.; Mace, R.A.; Bakhshaie, J.; Choi, K.W.; Vranceanu, A.-M. Fitbit Activity, Quota-Based Pacing, and Physical and Emotional Functioning Among Adults with Chronic Pain. *J. Pain* **2022**, *23*, 1933–1944. [CrossRef]
72. Angarita-Osorio, N.; Pérez-Aranda, A.; Feliu-Soler, A.; Andrés-Rodríguez, L.; Borràs, X.; Suso-Ribera, C.; Slim, M.; Herrera-Mercadal, P.; Fernández-Vergel, R.; Blanco, M.E.; et al. Patients with Fibromyalgia Reporting Severe Pain but Low Impact of the Syndrome: Clinical and Pain-Related Cognitive Features. *Pain Pr.* **2019**, *20*, 255–261. [CrossRef]
73. Ecija, C.; Catala, P.; Lopez-Gomez, I.; Bedmar, D.; Peñacoba, C. What Does the Psychological Flexibility Model Contribute to the Relationship Between Depression and Disability in Chronic Pain? The Role of Cognitive Fusion and Pain Acceptance. *Clin. Nurs. Res.* **2022**, *31*, 217–229. [CrossRef]
74. Sitthipornvorakul, E.; Klinsophon, T.; Sihawong, R.; Janwantanakul, P. The effects of walking intervention in patients with chronic low back pain: A meta-analysis of randomized controlled trials. *Musculoskelet. Sci. Pr.* **2018**, *34*, 38–46. [CrossRef] [PubMed]
75. Cheng, S.-T.; Leung, C.M.C.; Chan, K.L.; Chen, P.P.; Chow, Y.F.; Chung, J.W.Y.; Law, A.C.B.; Lee, J.S.W.; Leung, E.M.F.; Tam, C.W.C. The relationship of self-efficacy to catastrophizing and depressive symptoms in community-dwelling older adults with chronic pain: A moderated mediation model. *PLoS ONE* **2018**, *13*, e0203964. [CrossRef]
76. Munguía-Izquierdo, D.; Segura-Jiménez, V.; Camiletti-Moirón, D.; Pulido-Martos, M.; Alvarez-Gallardo, I.C.; Romero, A.; Aparicio, V.A.; Carbonell-Baeza, A.; Delgado-Fernández, M. Multi-dimensional fatigue inventory: Spanish adaptation and psychometric properties for fibromyalgia patients. The Al-andalus study. *Clin. Exp. Rheumatol.* **2012**, *30* (Suppl. S74), 94–102. [PubMed]
77. Vallejo, M.A.; Vallejo-Slocker, L.; Offenbaecher, M.; Hirsch, J.K.; Toussaint, L.L.; Kohls, N.; Sirois, F.; Rivera, J. Psychological Flexibility Is Key for Reducing the Severity and Impact of Fibromyalgia. *Int. J. Environ. Res. Public Health* **2021**, *18*, 7300. [CrossRef] [PubMed]
78. Crombez, G.; Eccleston, C.; Van Damme, S.; Vlaeyen, J.W.; Karoly, P. Fear-Avoidance Model of Chronic Pain. *Clin. J. Pain* **2012**, *28*, 475–483. [CrossRef]
79. Meulders, A. From fear of movement-related pain and avoidance to chronic pain disability: A state-of-the-art review. *Curr. Opin. Behav. Sci.* **2019**, *26*, 130–136. [CrossRef]
80. Tabor, A.; Van Ryckeghem, D.M.L.; Hasenbring, M.I. Pain Unstuck. *Clin. J. Pain* **2020**, *36*, 143–149. [CrossRef]
81. Van Damme, S.; De Waegeneer, A.; Debruyne, J. Do Flexible Goal Adjustment and Acceptance Help Preserve Quality of Life in Patients with Multiple Sclerosis? *Int. J. Behav. Med.* **2016**, *23*, 333–339. [CrossRef] [PubMed]
82. Dwarswaard, J.; Bakker, E.J.; van Staa, A.; Boeije, H.R. Self-management support from the perspective of patients with a chronic con-dition: A thematic synthesis of qualitative studies. *Health Expect.* **2016**, *19*, 194–208. [CrossRef]
83. Braunwalder, C.; Müller, R.; Glisic, M.; Fekete, C. Are positive psychology interventions efficacious in chronic pain treatment? A systematic review and meta-analysis of randomized controlled trials. *Pain Med.* **2022**, *23*, 122–136. [CrossRef]

pharmacy

MDPI

Article

Explaining Correlates of Cervical Cancer Screening among Minority Women in the United States

Manoj Sharma [1], Kavita Batra [2], Christopher Johansen [1,*] and Siddharth Raich [1]

[1] Department of Social and Behavioral Health, School of Public Health, University of Nevada, Las Vegas, NV 89119, USA; manoj.sharma@unlv.edu (M.S.); raichs2@unlv.nevada.edu (S.R.)
[2] Office of Research, Kirk Kerkorian School of Medicine, University of Nevada, Las Vegas, NV 89102, USA; kavita.batra@unlv.edu
* Correspondence: christopher.johansen@unlv.edu

Abstract: Globally, cervical cancer is the fourth leading cause of death among women. While overall cervical cancer rates have decreased over the last few decades, minority women continue to be disproportionately affected compared to White women. Given the paucity of theory-based interventions to promote Pap smear tests among minority women, this cross-sectional study attempts to examine the correlates of cervical cancer screening by Pap test using the Multi-theory Model (MTM) as a theoretical paradigm among minority women in the United States (U.S.). Structural Equation Modelling (SEM) was done for testing the construct validity of the survey instrument. Data were analyzed through bivariate and multivariate tests. In a sample of 364 minority women, nearly 31% (n = 112) of women reported not having received a Pap test within the past three years compared to the national rate (20.8%) for all women. The MTM constructs of participatory dialogue, behavioral confidence, and changes in the physical environment explained a substantial proportion of variance (49.5%) in starting the behavior of getting Pap tests, while the constructs of emotional transformation, practice for change, and changes in the social environment, along with lack of health insurance and annual household income of less than $25,000, significantly explained the variance (73.6%) of the likelihood to sustain the Pap test behavior of getting it every three years. Among those who have had a Pap smear (n = 252), healthcare insurance, emotional transformation, practice for change, and changes in the social environment predicted nearly 83.3% of the variance in sustaining Pap smear test uptake behavior (adjusted $R^2 = 0.833$, $F = 45.254$, $p < 0.001$). This study validates the need for health promotion interventions based on MTM to be implemented to address the disparities of lower cervical cancer screenings among minority women.

Keywords: Multi-theory Model; cervical cancer; screening; minority women

1. Introduction

Cervical cancer is the fourth leading cause of death in the world among women [1]. It was estimated that, worldwide, 570,000 women were diagnosed with cervical cancer and approximately 311,000 women died due to cervical cancer in 2018 [1]. While there has been a decrease in cervical cancer mortality in the United States (U.S.), approximately 13,800 women are diagnosed and approximately 4290 women die per year [2,3]. These rates have decreased over the past few decades, yet cervical cancer disparities in the U.S. continue to affect minority women, (i.e., women who are not of White/European heritage such as African American, Hispanic/Latino, Asian American, Pacific Islander, American Indian, etc.) [4].

The Papanicolaou (Pap) test is an effective cervical cancer screening tool to decrease the rates of cervical cancer [5]. The American Cancer Society (ACS) recommends cervical cancer screening with an HPV test alone every 5 years for everyone with a cervix from age 25 until age 65 [6]. Rates of cervical cancer screening (Pap testing) in the U.S. were

81.7% for women 21–44 years old and 79.2% from women 45–64 years old [7], but the rates of cervical cancer screening are lower for Pap testing among minorities in the U.S. and disparities still exist for African Americans, Hispanics/Latina, Asians, and American Indians compared to White women [2,3,8–11].

Cervical cancer occurs primarily in low-resource, underserved areas and is typically associated with poverty, race/ethnicity, and/or other health disparities [3,11–14]. Outside the U.S., researchers found that in Norway, immigrant women reported lower adherence to cervical cancer uptake compared to native Norwegian women [15]. Similar associations have been found among Non-European Union and European Union migrants compared to German women [16], Middle Eastern women from Asian and Middle-Eastern countries [17], and Syrian refugees in Greece [18]. West African migrant women reported lower knowledge related to the importance of cervical cancer screening [19] and in China, uptake of cervical cancer screening services in Chinese migrant workers is lower than non-migrant workers in China [20].

Two determinants of cervical cancer incidence are carcinogenic HPV infection and lack of access to cervical cancer screening [3,12]. Other possible important correlates of cervical cancer screening include lack of adequate access to preventive services and not utilizing these services (e.g., lack of transportation, fear of results, and mistrust of the health care system) [12,15–27].

Interventions to increase Pap testing among minority women have had some success and, in some cases, self-sampling for HPV has performed well [28–31]. For example, a culturally tailored randomized control trial (RCT) cervical cancer screening intervention among Latinas reported that women in the intervention arm had increased Pap test screening compared to those in the control group [32]. Another culturally tailored RCT intervention among North American Chinese women reported that women in the intervention arms (i.e., community outreach or direct mail) increased Pap test screening compared to women in the control group, suggesting that culturally and linguistically appropriate interventions may increase Pap test levels [33]. Another study among African American women reported that African immigrant women reported lower knowledge of cervical cancer and lower Pap test screening rates compared to African American women [34]. Yet, more studies focusing specifically on minority women in the U.S. are needed to promote Pap testing.

Few interventions among minority women utilized health behavior theories. For example, in a review, Brevik (2020) found that four RCTs of culturally tailored intervention materials were associated with a 54% increase in Pap testing [32,35–38]. However, many of these studies did not use theory in their interventions. Those that did use theory drew from social cognitive theory, the health belief model, the transtheoretical model, the social support model, elaboration theory, or multiple theories [39–42]. In sum, there are limited studies to increase cervical cancer screening among minority women and only a few of these interventions among minority women utilized theory.

There is a need to focus on newer models, such as the fourth-generation Multi-theory Model (MTM) of health behavior, to explain correlates of cervical cancer screening among minority women in the U.S. The MTM has been used in previous health behavior studies, such as for COVID-19, sleep, HPV vaccination, mammography, and melanoma, but to date, researchers have not tested the MTM on cervical cancer screening [43–48]. The purpose of this study was to examine the correlates of cervical cancer screening by Pap test using MTM as a theoretical paradigm in U.S. minority women.

2. Materials and Methods

2.1. *Study Design, Setting, and Sampling*

Data for this cross-sectional, descriptive, and U.S. based study were collected from 7 October to 12 October through actively managed, double-opt-in market panels recruited by the Qualtrics team. The Qualtrics utilize high-quality research panels and quota sampling to meet the specific requirements of the sample requested by researchers. Previous literature described the differences between traditional survey and market-based or commercial research panels [35]. As described by Qualtrics (more information available at https://www.qualtrics.com/research-services/online-sample/, accessed on 10 February 2022), the company uses multiple strategies (e.g., dynamic surveys in a dashboard style, app-based recruitment, or through online/mobile games and social media) to recruit eligible participants through convenience sampling. Respondents can self-select to participate in the survey if they satisfy the eligibility criteria. Given the use of multiple avenues, response rate is difficult to compute. The recruitment of the sample is based on the quota constraints and screening opted by researchers who signed a contractual agreement with Qualtrics. In addition, Qualtrics ensures the quality of data by checking for bots, duplicates, speeders, and fraudulent responses before providing a complete and high-quality dataset to the researchers. Participants could be screened out due to multiple reasons: (1) if they did not qualify for the inclusion criteria; (2) if the quota was already filled during fielding; and (3) if participants took significantly less time (less than half the median time) to complete the survey, which would indicate lack of thoughtfulness to answer the questions.

2.2. Participants' Selection Criteria

Women belonging to racial minority groups, aged between 21 and 65 years, living in the U.S., who had the ability to understand the English language, and provided voluntary informed consent were eligible to participate in this study. If participants opted to take the survey, they were asked to answer a few screening questions without revealing the original objective of the study. This was done to prevent self-selection and response bias. Eligible participants who thoughtfully completed the survey were compensated through incentives per terms and conditions set forth by Qualtrics and its data collection partners.

2.3. Ethical Considerations

The study (protocol #1804208-1) was deemed "exempt" by the institutional review board in accordance with the Federal regulatory statutes. Detailed information about study's objective and significance was provided in an information sheet, which helped participants to make informed decisions about participating in the study. In other words, participation in this survey was completely voluntary. All methods were performed in accordance with the relevant guidelines and regulations.

2.4. Data Integrity

Qualtrics used multiple ways, such as digital fingerprinting and 'prevent ballot box stuffing option', to prevent multiple responses from the same participant. No identifying information was collected during the survey and responses were anonymized to prevent the collection of IP address, location data, and contact information. Data were provided to the researchers in an encrypted file.

2.5. Survey Tool

A 48-item questionnaire including 18 items related to sociodemographic factors and the remaining 30 items related to MTM constructs was developed based on the fourth-generation behavioral theory proposed by Sharma and Petosa in 2014 [36]. The MTM offered a robust approach to explain several health-related behaviors in the past [29–34]. This tool to explain the correlates of the Pap test underwent a series of iterations to check its face and content validity by a group of Subject Matter Experts (SMEs). Experts in behavioral theories, health promotion, and cancer-related research areas were randomly selected to participate in a blinded review of the tool. Their feedback and comments were addressed in a series of revisions before the final version of the tool was obtained. Once finalized, this tool was assessed for its construct validity using structural equation modelling described in detail in the methodology section. For the initiation model, except "changes in physical environment" (measured by 2 items), the subscales of perceived advantages, perceived disadvantages, and behavioral confidence (surety to overcome external and internal barriers) were measured by 5 items measured on a 5-point Likert scale. The "advantages" and "disadvantages" were measured on a frequency scale which included the following response options: never (0), almost never (1), sometimes (2), fairly often (3), and very often (4). Participatory dialogue was a difference derivative of "advantages" and "disadvantages", and the score could range from −20 units to +20 units. For "change in physical environment" and "behavioral confidence", a scale of surety was used which ranged from "not at all sure" to "completely sure." For sustenance, "emotional transformation" and "practice for change" scales were measured on 3 items each. However, "changes in social environment" was measured through 5 items. Emotional transformation is the ability to transform emotional distress into a positive emotional state. Practice of change entails actions to maintain the behavior initiated despite the challenges and "changes in social environment" considers the role of the social support system (family and friends) to help change a particular behavior. A detailed description of the components (initiation and sustenance) of the survey is provided in Figure 1.

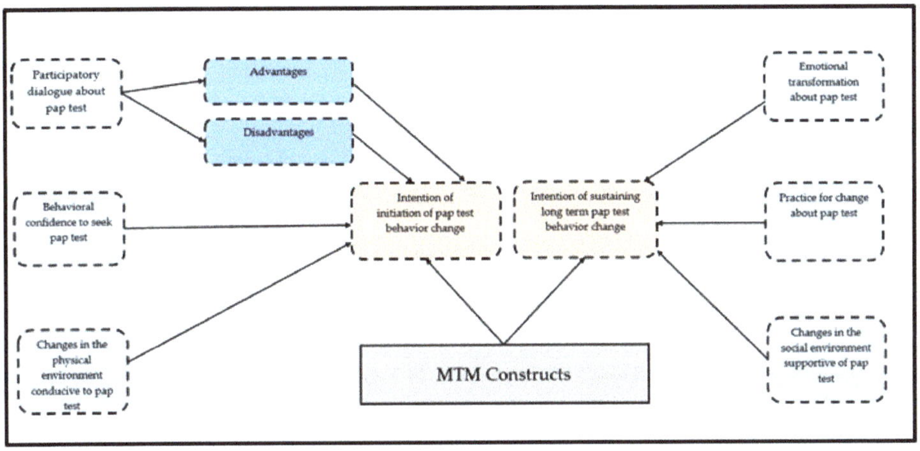

Figure 1. MTM theoretical framework for a survey tool used to explain Pap test behavior among racial minority groups.

2.6. Minimum Sample Size Calculation

Referring to the G*power 3.1.9.7 software (linear multiple regression: fixed model, R^2 increase), a minimal number of 154 participants was required to reach significance when considering the following statistical parameters: type I error $\alpha = 5\%$, power $1\text{-}\beta = 95\%$, a moderate effect size $f^2 = 0.15$, and a total number of variables $N = 15$ to be integrated in the multivariable regression analysis [37,38]. Given the lack of consensus in the sample size recommendations for the Structural Equation Modelling (SEM), we used Kline (2015) criteria that had 20 observations (participants) for each estimated parameter in the model, with a typical size of $N = 200$, among models using the maximum likelihood method [39]. However, recently, several studies recommended a sample size which would vary from 50 to 400 participants [40–42]. Our study sample meets the minimum requirements to yield hypothesized effects.

2.7. Data Analyses

The SPSS software v.26 (Armonk, NY, USA: IBM Corp.) was used to conduct the descriptive and inferential statistical analysis. All assumptions were tested prior to the application of statistical models. Comparison between groups for the normally distributed numeric data was conducted using the independent samples test, whereas the chi-squared test was used to compare categorical data among groups. The Pearson correlation test was used to correlate two continuous variables. Hierarchical regression was conducted by taking initiation and sustenance scores as dependent variables. Polytomous variables used in the regression were dummy-coded. The statistical significance was denoted as $p < 0.05$. Missing data analysis was not warranted as a complete dataset and was obtained from Qualtrics.

The SPSS AMOS software v.24 [43] was utilized to perform the Structural Equation Modelling (SEM) for testing the MTM model. All items of the main constructs of the MTM instrument were used as indicators of the latent variables of initiation and sustenance (described elsewhere in the text). A fair pair of items with similar contents were allowed correlation measurement errors. The maximum likelihood method was used for estimation. Multiple indices of goodness-of-fit were used: the relative chi-square ($\chi 2/df$; cut-off values: <2–5), the Root Mean Square Error of Approximation (RMSEA; close and acceptable fit are considered for values <0.05 and <0.11, respectively), the Tucker Lewis Index (TLI), and the Comparative Fit Index (CFI; acceptable values are $\geq$0.90) [44,45]. For each model, the overall fit, significance of structural paths, and amount of variability of the latent variables accounted for by the observed variables were assessed [39,45,46]. Standardized estimates for path coefficients, interpreted as regression coefficients, were calculated for all proposed relationships in the model. Reliability diagnostics were also performed.

3. Results

In a sample of a total of 364 participants, two hundred and fifty-two (69.2%) participants reported having the Pap smear test and nearly 31% had not had the Pap test over the past 3 years (Table 1). Among those who had a Pap smear test, the majority of the participants had it normally. The median age of both groups were comparable. The majority of the respondents from both groups were non-Hispanics, Christians, and African Americans, and had comorbidities of non-psychological in origin (Table 1). Upon comparing the socio-economic and healthcare access factors, participants who had not had a Pap smear test were less educated (5.4% vs. 0.8%; $p < 0.001$), uninsured (28.6% vs. 5.2%; $p < 0.01$), and unemployed (59.8% vs. 38.9%; $p < 0.001$), and had a lower income (27.7% vs. 19.8%; $p = 0.004$; Table 2). Among the participants with no Pap smear test, only 31.3% reported being recommended by their healthcare providers for a Pap test as opposed to the 58.3% of participants with a Pap test (Table 2). As indicated in Table 3, participants with a Pap test had higher overall initiation (3.02 ± 0.99 vs. 1.69 ± 1.41; $p < 0.001$) and sustenance mean scores (2.98 ± 1.06 vs. 1.50 ± 1.34; $p < 0.001$; Table 3) as opposed to those who had not had a Pap smear test in the past. Except for the subscale "perceived disadvantages", the mean scores of "perceived advantages", "participatory dialogue", "behavioral confidence", and "changes in physical environment" were significantly higher among participants who had a Pap smear test in the past than those who had not had a Pap smear test (Table 3). The mean scores of "perceived disadvantages" were not statistically different among both groups. For sustenance, the scores of all the subscales, namely "emotional transformation", "practice for change", and "changes in social environment", were higher among participants with a Pap smear test, with statistically significant mean differences compared to the participants who had not had a Pap smear test in the past (Table 3).

Table 1. Demographic characteristics of the sample ($N = 364$).

Variable	Categories	Participants Who Had Pap Smear 252, 69.2%	Participants Who Had Not Had Pap Smear 112, 30.8%	*p*-Value
Was the Pap smear normal	Yes	234 (93.0)	Not applicable	-
	No	18 (7.0)	Not applicable	-
Had hysterectomy	Yes	44 (17.5)	26 (23.2)	0.2
	No	208 (82.5)	86 (76.8)	
Age (M ± SD)	-	44.79 ± 13.3	44.1 ± 14.6	0.6

Table 1. *Cont.*

Variable	Categories	Participants Who Had Pap Smear 252, 69.2%	Participants Who Had Not Had Pap Smear 112, 30.8%	*p*-Value
Hispanic or Latina	Yes	113 (44.8)	49 (43.8)	0.8
	No	139 (55.2)	63 (56.3)	
Religion	Christianity	178 (70.6)	70 (62.5)	0.1
	Non-Christianity	74 (29.4)	42 (37.5)	
Marital status	Married	105 (41.7)	34 (30.4)	0.2
	Never married	68 (27.0)	38 (33.9)	
	Divorced/Separated	41 (16.3)	24 (21.4)	
	Other	38 (15.1)	16 (14.3)	
Ethnicity	African American	93 (36.9)	38 (33.9)	0.2
	Hispanic–White	62 (24.6)	28 (25.0)	
	Asian	44 (17.5)	12 (10.7)	
	Others including multiethnic origin	53 (21.0)	34 (30.4)	
Comorbidities	Psychological	94 (37.3)	36 (32.1)	0.3
	Non-psychological	158 (62.7)	76 (67.9)	
Duration of U.S. residency (M ± SD)	-	39.7 ± 16.3	39.3 ± 16.5	0.8
Residence	Rural	49 (19.4)	15 (13.4)	0.2
	Suburban	105 (41.7)	44 (39.3)	
	Urban	98 (38.9)	53 (47.9)	
Encouraged Pap test by family/friends	Yes	107 (42.5)	43 (38.4)	0.5
	No	145 (57.5)	69 (61.6)	

Table 2. Socio-economic and healthcare access characteristics of the sample (N = 364).

Variable	Categories	Participants Who Had Pap Smear	Participants Who Had Not Had Pap Smear	*p*-Value
Education	Less than high school diploma	2 (0.8)	6 (5.4)	<0.001 *
	High school graduate	49 (19.4)	24 (21.4)	
	Some college but no degree	64 (25.4)	43 (38.4)	
	Associate/Bachelor	99 (39.3)	31 (27.7)	
	Graduate's degree	38 (15.1)	8 (7.1)	
Healthcare insurance	Yes	239 (94.8)	80 (71.4)	<0.001 *
	No	13 (5.2)	32 (28.6)	
Employed	Yes	154 (61.1)	45 (40.2)	<0.001 *
	No	98 (38.9)	67 (59.8)	
Hours worked/week	-	35.7 ± 10.5	Not applicable	-
Income	<$25,000	50 (19.8)	31 (27.7)	0..004 *
	$25,000–$50,000	85 (33.7)	41 (36.6)	
	$50,001–$75,000	54 (21.4)	16 (14.3)	

Table 2. *Cont.*

Variable	Categories	Participants Who Had Pap Smear	Participants Who Had Not Had Pap Smear	*p*-Value
	\$75,001–\$100,000	33 (13.1)	8 (7.1)	
	\$100,001–\$125,000	10 (4.0)	1 (0.9)	
	\$125,001–\$150,000	6 (2.4)	3 (2.7)	
	>\$150,001	11 (4.4)	3 (2.7)	
Visited healthcare provider	Yes	210 (83.3)	63 (56.3)	0.2
	No	42 (16.7)	49 (43.8)	
Recommended Pap test by healthcare providers	Yes	147 (58.3)	35 (31.3)	<0.001 *
	No	105 (41.7)	77 (68.8)	

* Significant *p*-values.

Table 3. Comparison of Multi-theory Model (MTM) constructs of participants who had Pap test and those who did not have Pap test (*N* = 364).

MTM Construct	Had Pap Smear Test		*p*-Value
	Yes (*n* = 252)	No (*n* = 112)	
Overall initiation score	3.02 ± 0.99	1.69 ± 1.41	<0.001 *
Subscales			
Perceived advantages	15.62 ± 3.84	13.01 ± 5.65	<0.001 *
Perceived disadvantages	10.36 ± 4.55	10.99 ± 5.07	0.3
Participatory dialogue	5.55 ± 1.12	2.29 ± 146	<0.001 *
Behavioral confidence	14.01 ± 4.64	9.35 ± 5.53	<0.001 *
Changes in the physical environment	6.16 ± 1.85	4.59 ± 2.65	<0.001 *
Overall sustenance	2.98 ± 1.06	1.50 ± 1.34	<0.001 *
Subscales			
Emotional transformation	9.03 ± 2.85	5.31 ± 3.95	<0.001 *
Practice for change	8.68 ± 2.71	5.27 ± 4.02	<0.001 *
Changes in social environment	13.2 ± 4.65	8.18 ± 5.56	<0.001 *

* Significant *p*-values.

Table 4 shows the Pearson correlation coefficient matrix of all the observed variables. Perceived advantages are directly correlated with perceived disadvantages (r = 0.26, $p < 0.01$), behavioral confidence (r = 0.58, $p < 0.01$), changes in physical environment (r = 0.50, $p < 0.01$), emotional transformation (r = 0.47, $p < 0.01$), practice for change (r = 0.46, $p < 0.01$), and changes in social environment (r = 0.49, $p < 0.01$). Changes in physical environment is strongly and directly correlated with behavioral confidence (r = 0.75, $p < 0.01$), emotional transformation (r = 0.73, $p < 0.01$), and changes in social environment (r = 0.64, $p < 0.01$). Changes in social environment is directly correlated with practice for change (r = 0.82, $p < 0.01$) and emotional transformation (r = 0.78, $p < 0.01$, Table 4). The reliability of the entire scale was 0.94, with individual scales' reliability ranging from 0.81 to 0.94 (Table 4).

All goodness-of-fit indices suggest that the presented models (Figures 2 and 3) reasonably fit the data. For the initiation model, the relative chi-square ($\chi 2/df = 2.51$; cut-off values: <2–5), the Root Mean Square Error of Approximation (RMSEA = 0.064 (LCL 0.056; UCL 0.073); close and acceptable fit are considered for values <0.05 and <0.11, respectively), the Tucker Lewis Index (TLI = 0.94), and the Comparative Fit Index (CFI = 0.95; acceptable values are ≥0.90) were reasonable to indicate model fit. The estimates of each structural relationship between the MTM subscales and initiation are shown in Figure 2. Upon observing the standardized effects of latent variables on factor loadings, statistically significant effects that ranged from moderate to large were found. Except for "perceived disadvantages", all other latent variables, including "perceived advantages" (β = 0.55 to 0.90), "behavioral confidence" (β =0.73 to 0.88), and "changes in physical environment" (β = 0.82 to 0.91), had large effects on their reflective indicators, which is suggestive of the valid measurements of the constructs used (Figure 2). Behavioral confidence had a moderate direct effect on initiating Pap smear behavior (β = 0.62, $p < 0.001$), whereas disadvantages had a small direct negative effect (β = −0.11, $p = 0.02$). Effects of advantages and change in physical activity were insignificant.

Table 4. Pearson correlations and reliability estimates for study variables in the sample population ($n = 364$).

Variables	1	2	3	4	5	6	7
1. Advantages	-	0.26 **	0.58 **	0.50 **	0.47 **	0.46 **	0.49 **
2. Disadvantages	0.26 **	1	0.04	0.05	−0.03	−0.06	−0.03
3. Behavioral confidence	0.58 **	0.04	1	0.75 **	0.81 **	0.78 **	0.72 **
4. Changes in the physical environment	0.50 **	0.05	0.75 **	1	0.73 **	0.73 **	0.64 **
5. Emotional transformation	0.47 **	−0.03	0.81 **	0.73 **	1	0.87 **	0.77 **
6. Practice for change	0.46 **	−0.07	0.79 **	0.73 **	0.87 **	1	0.82 **
7. Changes in social environment	0.49 **	−0.03	0.72 **	0.64 **	0.78 **	0.82 **	1
Cronbach's alpha values	0.85	0.81	0.90	0.86	0.94	0.92	0.86

** $p < 0.01$. The Cronbach's alpha value of the entire scale is 0.94.

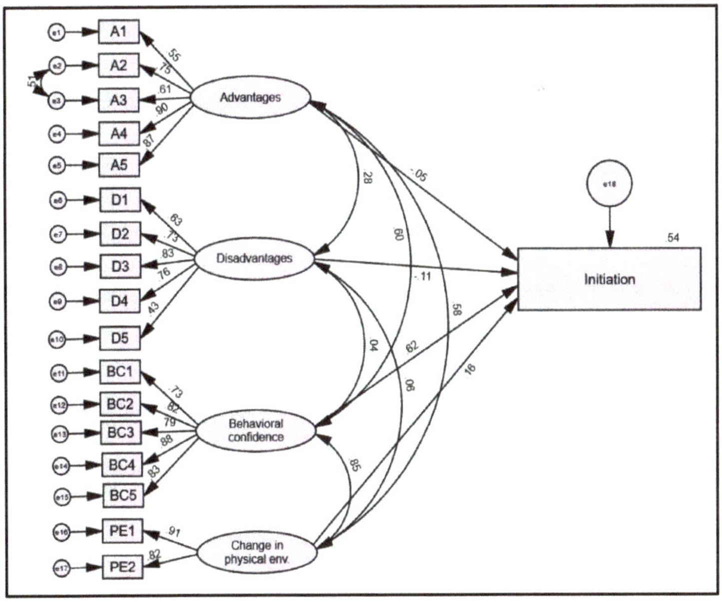

Figure 2. Model diagram of the four-factor model of the initiation. Legend: e1–17 = error terms 1–17; A = advantages; D = disadvantages; BC = behavioral confidence; and PE = change in the physical environment. Latent variables/factors are represented with ovals. Measured/manifest variables are represented with squares. Single-headed arrows indicate a hypothesized direct relationship between two variables. Double-headed arrows demonstrate the bi-directional relationship (i.e., covariance).

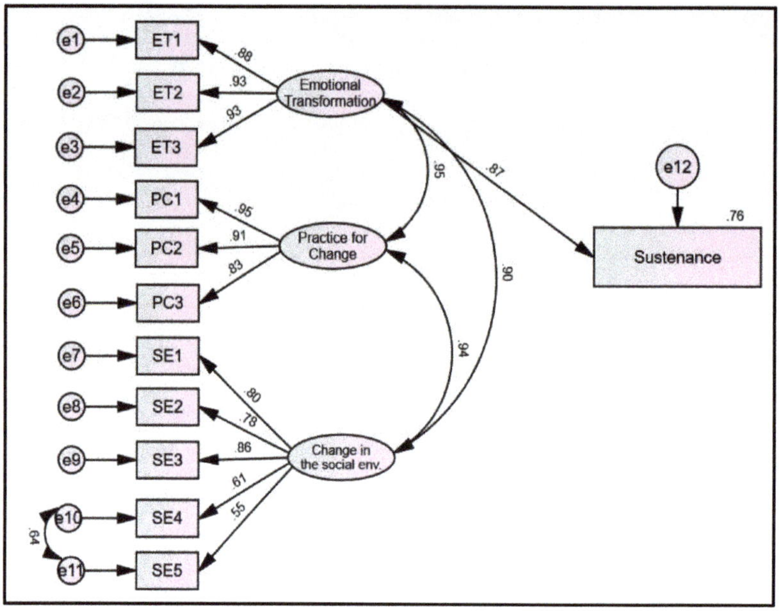

Figure 3. Model diagram of the three-factor model of the sustenance. Legend: e1–11 = error terms 1–11; ET = emotional transformation; PC = practice for change; BC = behavioral confidence; and SE = change in the social environment. Latent variables/factors are represented with ovals. Measured/manifest variables are represented with squares. Single-headed arrows indicate a hypothesized direct relationship between two variables. Double-headed arrows demonstrate the bi-directional relationship (i.e., covariance).

Similarly, for the sustenance model, the relative chi-square ($\chi2/df = 2.44$), the Root Mean Square Error of Approximation (RMSEA = 0.063 (LCL 0.049; UCL 0.077)), the Tucker Lewis Index (TLI = 0.97), and the Comparative Fit Index (CFI = 0.98) were calculated. The estimates of each structural relationship between the MTM subscales and sustenance are shown in Figure 3. All latent variables, including "emotional transformation" (β = 0.88 to 0.93), "practice for change" (β = 0.83 to 0.95), and "changes in social environment" (β = 0.55 to 0.86), had moderate–large effects on their reflective indicators, which is suggestive of the valid measurements of the constructs used (Figure 3). Emotional transformation had a large direct effect on the sustenance of Pap smear behavior ($\beta = 0.87$, $p < 0.001$), as shown Figure 3.

In a multilevel regression model of initiation, Model 4 (final model) predicted nearly 50% of the variance in initiating Pap smear test uptake behavior among participants who had not had it over the past 3 years (adjusted $R^2 = 0.495$, $F = 30.66$, $p < 0.001$, Table 5). With each unit increment in the subscales of initiation (i.e., participatory dialogue, behavior confidence, and changes in physical environment), the conditional mean for initiating Pap smear uptake behavior increased by 0.021, 0.117, and 0.106 units, respectively (Model 4, Table 5). None of the slopes of socio-economic and healthcare access variables were significant, which indicates no significant differences in the conditional mean changes in initiating Pap smear test uptake behavior among participants who had not had this test done over the past 3 years.

In a multilevel regression model of sustenance, Model 4 (final model) predicted nearly 74% of the variance in initiating Pap smear test uptake behavior among participants who had not had it before (adjusted $R^2 = 0.736$, $F = 85.338$, $p < 0.001$, Table 6). With each unit increment in the subscales of sustenance (i.e., emotional transformation, practice for change, and changes in social environment), the conditional mean for sustaining Pap smear uptake behavior increased by 0.184, 0.097, and 0.032 units, respectively (Model 4, Table 6). Except for healthcare insurance and lower income, none of the slopes of socio-economic and healthcare access variables were significant, which indicates no significant differences in the conditional mean changes in the sustenance of Pap smear test uptake behavior among participants who had not had this test done over the past 3 years.

Table 5. Multilevel modelling to predict likelihood for initiation of Pap test behavior among participants who had not had the Pap test over the past 3 years (n = 112).

Variables	Model 1		Model 2		Model 3		Model 4	
	B	β	B	β	B	β	B	β
INITIATION MODEL								
Constant	3.292 **	-	2.766 **	-	0.878 **	-	0.673 *	
Socio-economic factors								
Health insurance (ref: yes)	−0.899 **	−0.229	−0.696 **	−0.177	−0.275	−0.070	−0.276	−0.070
Employed (ref: yes)	−0.151	−0.058	−0.160	−0.062	−0.158	−0.061	−0.153	−0.059
Encouraged by HCW (ref: yes)	−0.313	−0.121	−0.211	−0.081	−0.132	−0.051	−0.113	−0.044
Income (ref: >$150,000)								
<$25,000	−0.263	−0.085	−0.135	−0.043	0.089	0.028	0.095	0.031
$25,000–$50,000	−0.498	−0.183	−0.401	−0.147	−0.158	−0.058	−0.150	−0.055
$50,001–$75,000	−0.197	−0.060	−0.098	−0.030	−0.074	−0.023	−0.038	−0.012
$75,001–$100,000	−0.429	−0.105	−0.139	−0.034	−0.034	−0.008	−0.055	−0.014
$100,001–$125,000	−0.697	−0.092	−0.560	−0.074	−0.293	−0.039	−0.327	−0.043
$125,001–$150,000	−0.207	−0.025	−0.170	−0.020	−0.204	−0.024	−0.219	−0.026
Participatory dialogue (advantages–disadvantages)	-	-	0.079 **	0.346	0.023 *	0.102	0.021 *	0.092
Behavioral confidence	-	-	-	-	0.149 **	0.617	0.117 **	0.484
Changes in the physical environment	-	-	-	-	-	-	0.106 *	0.184
R^2	0.096	-	0.209	-	0.498	-	0.512	-
F	4.173 **	-	9.301 **	-	31.708 **	-	30.667 **	-
ΔR^2	0.096	-	0.113	-	0.289	-	0.014	-
ΔF	4.173 **	-	50.236 **	-	202.64 **	-	10.149 *	-

* p-value < 0.05; ** p-value < 0.001; income variable was dummy-coded; and adjusted R^2 = 0.495.

Table 6. Multilevel modelling to predict likelihood for sustenance of Pap test behavior among participants who had not had the Pap test over the past 3 years (n = 112).

Variables	Model 1		Model 2		Model 3		Model 4	
	B	β	B	β	B	β	B	β
SUSTENANCE MODEL								
Constant	2.847 **	-	0.046	-	−0.135	-	−0.216	-
Socio-economic factors								
Health insurance (ref: yes)	−1.018 **	−0.249	−0.458 **	−0.112	−0.365 *	−0.089	−0.353 *	−0.087
Employed (ref: yes)	−0.055	−0.020	0.053	0.020	0.056	0.021	0.070	0.026
Encouraged by HCW (ref: yes)	−0.388 *	−0.144	−0.138	−0.051	−0.128	−0.048	−0.093	−0.035

Table 6. *Cont.*

Variables	Model 1		Model 2		Model 3		Model 4	
	B	β	B	β	B	β	B	β
Income (ref: >$150,000)								
<$25,000	0.122	0.038	0.384 *	0.119	0.396 *	0.123	0.390 *	0.121
$25,000–$50,000	−0.071	−0.025	0.197	0.070	0.251	0.089	0.249	0.088
$50,001–$75,000	0.180	0.053	0.211	0.062	0.212	0.062	0.193	0.057
$75,001–$100,000	−0.037	−0.009	0.247	0.058	0.230	0.054	0.225	0.053
$100,001–$125,000	−0.267	−0.034	0.120	0.015	0.077	0.010	0.088	0.011
$125,001–$150,000	−0.008	−0.001	0.076	0.009	0.082	0.010	0.067	0.008
MTM constructs								
Emotional transformation	-	-	0.299 **	0.812	0.195 **	0.529	0.184 **	0.500
Practice for change	-	-	-	-	0.126 **	0.333	0.097 **	0.256
Changes in social environment	-	-	-	-	-	-	0.032 *	0.129
R^2	0.097	-	0.714	-	0.740	-	0.745	-
F	4.247 **	-	88.00 **	-	90.998 **	-	85.338 **	-
ΔR^2	0.097	-	0.616	-	0.026	-	0.005	-
ΔF	4.247	-	759.83 **	-	35.347 **	-	6.744 *	-

* *p*-value < 0.05; ** *p*-value < 0.001; income variable was dummy-coded; and adjusted $R^2 = 0.736$.

In a multilevel regression model of sustenance among those who had a Pap smear ($n = 252$), Model 4 (final model) predicted nearly 83.3% of the variance in sustaining Pap smear test uptake behavior (adjusted $R^2 = 0.833$, $F = 45.254$, $p < 0.001$, Table 7). With each unit increment in the subscales of sustenance (i.e., emotional transformation, practice for change, and changes in social environment), the conditional mean for sustaining Pap smear uptake behavior increased by 0.168, 0.111, and 0.032 units, respectively (Model 4, Table 7). Except for healthcare insurance, none of the slopes of socio-economic and healthcare access variables were significant, which indicates no significant differences in the conditional mean changes in the sustenance of Pap smear test uptake behavior among participants who had this test done over the past 3 years.

Table 7. Multilevel modelling to predict likelihood for sustenance of Pap test behavior among participants who had the Pap test over the past 3 years ($n = 252$).

Variables	Model 1		Model 2		Model 3		Model 4	
	B	β	B	β	B	β	B	β
SUSTENANCE MODEL								
Constant	2.973 **	-	0.192	-	0.005	-	−0.037	-
Socio-economic factors								
Health insurance (ref: yes)	−0.674 *	−0.140	−0.423 *	−0.088	−0.436 *	−0.090	−0.398 *	−0.083
Employed (ref: yes)	0.235	0.107	0.123	0.056	0.120	0.055	0.141	0.065
Encouraged by HCW (ref: yes)	−0.066	−0.030	−0.126	−0.058	−0.114	−0.053	−0.090	−0.042
Income (ref: >$150,000)								
<$25,000	0.060	0.022	0.292	0.109	0.250	0.093	0.226	0.084
$25,000–$50,000	−0.151	−0.067	0.115	0.051	0.101	0.045	0.091	0.040
$50,001–$75,000	0.146	0.056	0.170	0.066	0.102	0.039	0.086	0.033

Table 7. *Cont.*

Variables	Model 1		Model 2		Model 3		Model 4	
	B	β	B	β	B	β	B	β
$75,001–$100,000	−0.003	−0.001	0.247	0.078	0.182	0.058	0.169	0.054
$100,001–$125,000	−0.447	−0.082	0.051	0.009	−0.053	−0.010	−0.044	−0.008
$125,001–$150,000	0.321	0.046	0.092	0.013	0.010	0.001	0.014	0.002
MTM constructs								
Emotional transformation	-	-	0.293 **	0.784	0.180 **	0.482	0.168 **	0.450
Practice for change	-	-	-	-	0.144 **	0.366	0.111 **	0.282
Changes in social environment	-	-	-	-	-	-	0.032 *	0.141
R^2	0.052	-	0.645	-	0.687	-	0.694	-
F	1.479	-	43.849 **	-	47.952 **	-	45.254 **	-
ΔR^2	0.052	-	0.593	-	0.042	-	0.007	-
ΔF	1.479	-	403.072 **	-	32.208 **	-	5.557 *	-

* *p*-value < 0.05; ** *p*-value < 0.001; income variable was dummy-coded; and Model 4 adjusted R^2 = 0.833.

4. Discussion

The study aimed to utilize the contemporary Multi-theory Model (MTM) of health behavior change to explain the determinants of cervical cancer in minority women in the U.S. In our sample, 30.8% of the minority women had not received a Pap test within the past three years, which is much higher than the national statistics for all women of 20.8% [7,24]. This finding points at the continued disparities for Pap test screening among minority women in comparison to their White counterparts.

In our study, all three constructs of MTM, namely participatory dialogue (advantages of getting cervical cancer screening outweighing the disadvantages), behavioral confidence (futuristic surety emanating from self, powerful others, Almighty, etc.), and changes in the physical environment (support from the surroundings), were significantly associated with the intent to initiate cervical cancer screening among women who had not received a Pap test over the past three years and together they accounted for 49.5% of the variance in explaining the dependent variable. This is a substantial proportion of the variance in behavioral and social sciences [49]. Likewise, all three constructs of MTM, namely emotional transformation (directing emotions into goals), practice for change (persistent reflection on behavior change), and changes in the social environment (support from family, friends, etc.), as well as lack of health insurance and annual household income less of than $25,000, significantly explained 73.6% of the variance in the likelihood to sustain the Pap test behavior of getting it every three years.

The results of our study align with the previous literature as well as they provide newer insights into the correlates for developing interventions to promote cervical cancer screening through Pap tests. The finding in this study that poverty (annual household income of less than $25,000) and lack of insurance are barriers to cervical cancer screening among minority women is supported by the previous literature [12–14,24,26]. Structural policy efforts must be undertaken to address these root causes.

Our study found that educational tools, such as motivation through participatory dialogue, in which advantages of getting a Pap test and building the behavioral confidence of minority women are attributed, when coupled with changes in the physical environment, such as availability and accessibility of Pap test, can contribute substantially to women's ability to start getting the Pap test at regularly prescribed intervals. The concepts of value expectancy and self-efficacy, which are similar to participatory dialogue and behavioral confidence with subtle differences, have been used in the past for promoting cervical cancer screening among Hispanic American women [41,42]. The MTM constructs should be the foundational pillars of educational interventions. The advantages of getting a Pap test, such as early detection, having peace of mind for self and family, getting early treatment, and reduction in mortality due to cervical cancer, need to be underscored through educational interventions. The feelings of anxiety, physical discomfort/pain, invasion of modesty, embarrassment, and fear of misdiagnosis should be reduced in educational interventions through dialogue. Efforts to combat barriers in getting the Pap test must be undertaken to build the confidence of minority women through educational activities such as role-plays, psychodramas, or simulations. The construct of changes in the physical environment has not yet been used in the literature and our study lends support to the utilization of this dimension in future interventions. It is imperative that access and availability of Pap tests be increased for minority women at all locations in the U.S., especially for those without insurance and those who are indigent.

Our study found that in order to sustain the behavior of getting regular Pap tests, several correlates are essential. For sustenance of the behavior of getting regular Pap tests in both those who were not getting Pap tests and those who were getting Pap tests, all three constructs of MTM were significant and accounted for a substantial proportion of the variance. The construct of social support, which, in MTM, is more broadly referred to as changes in the social environment, has been used in the literature in the context of maintaining the behavior of getting Pap tests [39]. In many minority cultures, family and friends play an important role in the decision-making process for an individual. People are easily influenced by what others say or think of them. This aspect can be used as a potential advantage in health promotion interventions directed toward minority women for enhancing screening through Pap tests. Besides the traditional use of family, friends, and health professionals, in this regard, social media and advertisements are also gaining popularity and must be utilized more strategically in educational interventions. The constructs of emotional transformation and practice for change are unique to MTM and have not been tapped into in the past in the context of promoting the maintenance of Pap tests. Emotions or feelings are a powerful determinant of our behavior. If these can be harnessed into goals, then we can achieve our goals more effectively while combating self-doubt and fostering self-motivation. Educational interventions directed toward promoting Pap tests for minority women should facilitate participants to recognize their emotions, modulate these emotions, self-motivate themselves, and guide these emotions toward the goal of scheduling appointments with a physician and getting the Pap tests done on time. Likewise, a constant awareness of the importance of getting the Pap test done every three years can feed into building the practice for changing the construct of MTM.

While examining the socio-economic and healthcare access variables, as expected, less education, lack of health insurance, being unemployed, having less income, and not getting a recommendation from a healthcare provider were all significantly higher in the participants who did not receive the Pap test in the past three years. Influencing the socio-economic factors are under the purview of making structural policy changes but the lack of recommendation by healthcare providers is amendable through better education and training of healthcare providers that must be doggedly pursued.

Strengths and Limitations

This study was the first to utilize a contemporary, fourth-generation Multi-theory Model in explaining the correlates of cervical cancer screening among minority women. The instrument used in the study had very good psychometric properties. The sample used in the study was nationally representative. The study had an adequate power and sample size to discern medium effect sizes. The study also provided support to MTM, an upcoming theoretical framework. However, there were some limitations to this study. First, the cross-sectional nature of the design precludes making temporal causal inferences between the independent and dependent variables. Future studies must utilize longitudinal experimental designs to provide more definitive evidence. Second, the study did not collect direct data in the form of medical records of Pap tests and relied only on self-reports, which are subject to biases. While some variables such as attitudes can only be measured through self-reports, future studies must utilize more objective data for variables that can have other means of measurement. Another limitation concerns the conducting of this survey only in English, which limited our sample to only those who could read and speak English. Future studies should offer other languages, e.g., Spanish, Chinese, Japanese, etc., to potentially capture more minority women. Finally, the study did not measure the stability of the instrument by test–retest reliability coefficients. Future studies, especially those undertaking interventional research, must test the stability of the instrument.

5. Conclusions

In the U.S., minority women have lower rates of cervical cancer screening through Pap tests. Efforts must be undertaken to increase these rates. The study identified contemporary theory-based correlates of cervical cancer screening among minority women using the framework of MTM and found that all constructs of this theory were significant predictors. The constructs of participatory dialogue, behavioral confidence, and changes in the physical environment explained a substantial proportion of the variance in starting the behavior of getting Pap tests, while the constructs of emotional transformation, practice for change, and changes in the social environment, along with lack of health insurance and annual household income of less than $25,000, significantly explained the likelihood to sustain the Pap test behavior of getting it every three years. Health promotion interventions based on MTM must be implemented to address the disparities of lower cervical cancer screenings among minority women.

Author Contributions: Conceptualization, M.S. and K.B.; methodology, M.S. and K.B.; software, K.B.; validation, K.B. and M.S.; formal analysis, K.B.; investigation, K.B., M.S. and S.R.; resources, M.S.; data curation, K.B.; writing—original draft preparation, C.J., K.B. and M.S.; writing—review and editing, all; visualization, K.B.; supervision, M.S.; project administration, M.S. and K.B.; funding acquisition, M.S. All authors have read and agreed to the published version of the manuscript.

Funding: This research study was funded by the School of Public Health, University of Nevada, Las Vegas, internal grant number PG03008.

Institutional Review Board Statement: This study was conducted according to the guidelines of the Declaration of Helsinki and approved by the Institutional Review Board (or Ethics Committee) of the University of Nevada, Las Vegas (protocol #1804208-1/09-08-2021).

Informed Consent Statement: Written informed consent has been obtained from the patient(s) to publish this paper.

Data Availability Statement: The data presented in this study are available upon request from the corresponding author. The data are not publicly available due to ethical reasons.

Acknowledgments: Authors of this paper would like to acknowledge Kiara Batra for her assistance in creating the visualizations.

Conflicts of Interest: The authors declare no conflict of interest.

References

1. Bray, F.; Ferlay, J.; Soerjomataram, I.; Siegel, R.L.; Torre, L.A.; Jemal, A. Global Cancer Statistics 2018: GLOBOCAN Estimates of Incidence and Mortality Worldwide for 36 Cancers in 185 Countries. *CA Cancer J. Clin.* **2018**, *68*, 394–424. [CrossRef] [PubMed]
2. Siegel, R.L.; Miller, K.D.; Jemal, A. Cancer Statistics, 2020. *CA Cancer J. Clin.* **2020**, *70*, 7–30. [CrossRef]
3. Buskwofie, A.; David-West, G.; Clare, C.A. A Review of Cervical Cancer: Incidence and Disparities. *J. Natl. Med. Assoc.* **2020**, *112*, 229–232. [CrossRef]
4. Yu, L.; Sabatino, S.A.; White, M.C. Rural-Urban and Racial/Ethnic Disparities in Invasive Cervical Cancer Incidence in the United States, 2010–2014. *Prev. Chronic Dis.* **2019**, *16*, E70. [CrossRef]
5. Pierce Campbell, C.M.; Menezes, L.J.; Paskett, E.D.; Giuliano, A.R. Prevention of Invasive Cervical Cancer in the United States: Past, Present, and Future. *Cancer Epidemiol. Biomark. Prev.* **2012**, *21*, 1402–1408. [CrossRef] [PubMed]
6. Fontham, E.T.H.; Wolf, A.M.D.; Church, T.R.; Etzioni, R.; Flowers, C.R.; Herzig, A.; Guerra, C.E.; Oeffinger, K.C.; Shih, Y.T.; Walter, L.C.; et al. Cervical Cancer Screening for Individuals at Average Risk: 2020 Guideline Update from the American Cancer Society. *CA Cancer J. Clin.* **2020**, *70*, 321–346. [CrossRef] [PubMed]

7. Centers for Disease Control and Prevention. Special Feature on Racial and Ethnic Health Disparities. In *Health United States*; U.S. Government Printing Office: Hyattsville, MD, USA, 2015.
8. Akinlotan, M.; Bolin, J.N.; Helduser, J.; Ojinnaka, C.; Lichorad, A.; McClellan, D. Cervical Cancer Screening Barriers and Risk Factor Knowledge Among Uninsured Women. *J. Community Health* **2017**, *42*, 770–778. [CrossRef]
9. Yu, T.C.; Chou, C.F.; Johnson, P.J.; Ward, A. Persistent Disparities in Pap Test Use: Assessments and Predictions for Asian Women in the U.S., 1982–2010. *J. Immigr. Minority Health* **2010**, *12*, 445–453. [CrossRef] [PubMed]
10. Ogunwale, A.N.; Sangi-Haghpeykar, H.; Montealegre, J.; Cui, Y.; Jibaja-Weiss, M.; Anderson, M.L. Non-Utilization of the Pap Test Among Women with Frequent Health System Contact. *J. Immigr. Minority Health* **2016**, *18*, 1404–1412. [CrossRef]
11. Beavis, A.L.; Gravitt, P.E.; Rositch, A.F. Hysterectomy-Corrected Cervical Cancer Mortality Rates Reveal a Larger Racial Disparity in the United States. *Cancer* **2017**, *123*, 1044–1050. [CrossRef] [PubMed]
12. Scarinci, I.C.; Garcia, F.A.R.; Kobetz, E.; Partridge, E.E.; Brandt, H.M.; Bell, M.C.; Dignan, M.; Ma, G.X.; Daye, J.L.; Castle, P.E. Cervical Cancer Prevention: New Tools and Old Barriers. *Cancer* **2010**, *116*, 2531–2542. [CrossRef]
13. Orji, A.F.; Yamashita, T. Racial Disparities in Routine Health Checkup and Adherence to Cancer Screening Guidelines among Women in the United States of America. *Cancer Causes Control* **2021**, *32*, 1247–1256. [CrossRef] [PubMed]
14. Nardi, C.; Sandhu, P.; Selix, N. Cervical Cancer Screening Among Minorities in the United States. *J. Nurse Pract.* **2016**, *12*, 675–682. [CrossRef]
15. Leinonen, M.K.; Campbell, S.; Ursin, G.; Tropé, A.; Nygård, M. Barriers to Cervical Cancer Screening Faced by Immigrants: A Registry-Based Study of 1.4 Million Women in Norway. *Eur. J. Public Health* **2017**, *27*, 873–879. [CrossRef]
16. Brzoska, P.; Aksakal, T.; Yilmaz-Aslan, Y. Utilization of Cervical Cancer Screening among Migrants and Non-Migrants in Germany: Results from a Large-Scale Population Survey. *BMC Public Health* **2020**, *20*, 5. [CrossRef] [PubMed]
17. Aminisani, N.; Armstrong, B.K.; Canfell, K. Cervical Cancer Screening in Middle Eastern and Asian Migrants to Australia: A Record Linkage Study. *Cancer Epidemiol.* **2012**, *36*, e394–e400. [CrossRef] [PubMed]
18. Dalla, V.; Panagiotopoulou, E.K.; Deltsidou, A.; Kalogeropoulou, M.; Kostagiolas, P.; Niakas, D.; Labiris, G. Level of Awareness Regarding Cervical Cancer Among Female Syrian Refugees in Greece. *J. Cancer Educ.* **2020**. [CrossRef]
19. Ogunsiji, O.; Wilkes, L.; Peters, K.; Jackson, D. Knowledge, Attitudes and Usage of Cancer Screening among West African Migrant Women. *J. Clin. Nurs.* **2013**, *22*, 1026–1033. [CrossRef]
20. Holt, H.K.; Zhang, X.; Hu, S.Y.; Zhao, F.H.; Smith, J.S.; Qiao, Y.L. Inequalities in Cervical Cancer Screening Uptake Between Chinese Migrant Women and Local Women: A Cross-Sectional Study. *Cancer Control* **2021**, *28*. [CrossRef]
21. Mojica, C.M.; Morales-Campos, D.Y.; Carmona, C.M.; Ouyang, Y.; Liang, Y. Breast, Cervical, and Colorectal Cancer Education and Navigation: Results of a Community Health Worker Intervention. *Health Promot. Pract.* **2016**, *17*, 353–363. [CrossRef]
22. Kessler, T.A. Cervical Cancer: Prevention and Early Detection. *Semin. Oncol. Nurs.* **2017**, *33*, 172–183. [CrossRef]
23. Ramondetta, L.M.; Meyer, L.A.; Schmeler, K.M.; Daheri, M.E.; Gallegos, J.; Scheurer, M.; Montealegre, J.R.; Milbourne, A.; Anderson, M.L.; Sun, C.C. Avoidable Tragedies: Disparities in Healthcare Access among Medically Underserved Women Diagnosed with Cervical Cancer. *Gynecol. Oncol.* **2015**, *139*, 500–505. [CrossRef] [PubMed]
24. Tsui, J.; Saraiya, M.; Thompson, T.; Dey, A.; Richardson, L. Cervical Cancer Screening among Foreign-Born Women by Birthplace and Duration in the United States. *J. Women's Health* **2007**, *16*, 1447–1457. [CrossRef] [PubMed]
25. Marlow, L.A.V.; Waller, J.; Wardle, J. Barriers to Cervical Cancer Screening among Ethnic Minority Women: A Qualitative Study. *J. Fam. Plan. Reprod. Health Care* **2015**, *41*, 248–254. [CrossRef] [PubMed]
26. Grimm, B.; Alnaji, N.; Watanabe-Galloway, S.; Leypoldt, M. Cervical Cancer Attitudes and Knowledge in Somali Refugees in Nebraska. *Pedagog. Health Promot.* **2017**, *3*, 81S–87S. [CrossRef]
27. Marques, P.; Nunes, M.; Antunes, M.D.L.; Heleno, B.; Dias, S. Factors Associated with Cervical Cancer Screening Participation among Migrant Women in Europe: A Scoping Review. *Int. J. Equity Health* **2020**, *19*, 1–15. [CrossRef]
28. Inturrisi, F.; Aitken, C.A.; Melchers, W.J.G.; van den Brule, A.J.C.; Molijn, A.; Hinrichs, J.W.J.; Niesters, H.G.M.; Siebers, A.G.; Schuurman, R.; Heideman, D.A.M.; et al. Clinical Performance of High-Risk HPV Testing on Self-Samples versus Clinician Samples in Routine Primary HPV Screening in the Netherlands: An Observational Study. *Lancet Reg. Health—Eur.* **2021**, *11*, 100235. [CrossRef]
29. Enerly, E.; Bonde, J.; Schee, K.; Pedersen, H.; Lönnberg, S.; Nygård, M. Self-Sampling for Human Papillomavirus Testing among Non-Attenders Increases Attendance to the Norwegian Cervical Cancer Screening Programme. *PLoS ONE* **2016**, *11*, e0151978. [CrossRef]
30. Acera, A.; Manresa, J.M.; Rodriguez, D.; Rodriguez, A.; Bonet, J.M.; Trapero-Bertran, M.; Hidalgo, P.; Sànchez, N.; de Sanjosé, S. Increasing Cervical Cancer Screening Coverage: A Randomised, Community-Based Clinical Trial. *PLoS ONE* **2017**, *12*, e0170371. [CrossRef]
31. Aranda Flores, C.E.; Gomez Gutierrez, G.; Ortiz Leon, J.M.; Cruz Rodriguez, D.; Sørbye, S.W. Self-Collected versus Clinician-Collected Cervical Samples for the Detection of HPV Infections by 14-Type DNA and 7-Type MRNA Tests. *BMC Infect. Dis.* **2021**, *21*, 504. [CrossRef]
32. Byrd, T.L.; Wilson, K.M.; Smith, J.L.; Coronado, G.; Vernon, S.W.; Fernandez-Esquer, M.E.; Thompson, B.; Ortiz, M.; Lairson, D.; Fernandez, M.E. AMIGAS: A Multicity, Multicomponent Cervical Cancer Prevention Trial among Mexican American Women. *Cancer* **2013**, *119*, 1365–1372. [CrossRef] [PubMed]

33. Taylor, V.M.; Hislop, T.G.; Jackson, J.C.; Tu, S.P.; Yasui, Y.; Schwartz, S.M.; Teh, C.; Kuniyuki, A.; Acorda, E.; Marchand, A.; et al. A Randomized Controlled Trial of Interventions to Promote Cervical Cancer Screening among Chinese Women in North America. *J. Natl. Cancer Inst.* **2002**, *94*, 670–677. [CrossRef]
34. Amuta-Jimenez, A.O.; Smith, G.P.A.; Brown, K.K. Patterns and Correlates of Cervical Cancer Prevention Among Black Immigrant and African American Women in the USA: The Role of Ethnicity and Culture. *J. Cancer Educ.* **2020**. [CrossRef] [PubMed]
35. Brevik, T.B.; Laake, P.; Bjørkly, S. Effect of Culturally Tailored Education on Attendance at Mammography and the Papanicolaou Test. *Health Serv. Res.* **2020**, *55*, 457–468. [CrossRef] [PubMed]
36. Jandorf, L.; Bursac, Z.; Pulley, L.; Trevino, M.; Castillo, A.; Erwin, D.O. Breast and Cervical Cancer Screening among Latinas Attending Culturally Specific Educational Programs. *Prog. Community Health Partnersh. Res. Educ. Action* **2008**, *2*, 195–204. [CrossRef]
37. Maxwell, A.E.; Bastani, R.; Vida, P.; Warda, U.S. Results of a Randomized Trial to Increase Breast and Cervical Cancer Screening among Filipino American Women. *Prev. Med.* **2003**, *37*, 102–109. [CrossRef]
38. O'Brien, M.J.; Halbert, C.H.; Bixby, R.; Pimentel, S.; Shea, J.A. Community Health Worker Intervention to Decrease Cervical Cancer Disparities in Hispanic Women. *J. Gen. Intern. Med.* **2010**, *25*, 1186–1192. [CrossRef]
39. Liu, D.; Schuchard, H.; Burston, B.; Yamashita, T.; Albert, S. Interventions to Reduce Healthcare Disparities in Cancer Screening Among Minority Adults: A Systematic Review. *J. Racial Ethn. Health Disparities* **2021**, *8*, 107–126. [CrossRef]
40. Mosavel, M.; Genderson, M.W. Daughter-Initiated Cancer Screening Appeals to Mothers. *J. Cancer Educ.* **2016**, *31*, 767–775. [CrossRef]
41. Fernández, M.E.; Gonzales, A.; Tortolero-Luna, G.; Williams, J.; Saavedra-Embesi, M.; Chan, W.; Vernon, S.W. Effectiveness of Cultivando La Salud: A Breast and Cervical Cancer Screening Promotion Program for Low-Income Hispanic Women. *Am. J. Public Health* **2009**, *99*, 936–943. [CrossRef]
42. Nuño, T.; Martinez, M.E.; Harris, R.; García, F. A Promotora-Administered Group Education Intervention to Promote Breast and Cervical Cancer Screening in a Rural Community along the U.S.-Mexico Border: A Randomized Controlled Trial. *Cancer Causes Control* **2011**, *22*, 367–374. [CrossRef] [PubMed]
43. Sharma, A.; Jain, M.; Nahar, V.K.; Sharma, M. Predictors of Behaviour Change for Unhealthy Sleep Patterns among Indian Dental Students. *Int. J. Adolesc. Med. Health* **2020**. [CrossRef] [PubMed]
44. Penny, K.; Sharma, M.; Flischel, A.E.; Brodell, R.T.; Nahar, V.K. Atopic Dermatitis: Preventing and Managing the Itch That Rashes, and a Case for the Multi-Theory Model (MTM) for Health Behavior Change for Educational Interventions. *SKIN J. Cutan. Med.* **2021**, *5*, 462–473. [CrossRef]
45. Sharma, M.; Dai, C.-L.; Batra, K.; Chen, C.-C.; Pharr, J.R.; Coughenour, C.; Awan, A.; Catalano, H. Using the Multi-Theory Model (MTM) of Health Behavior Change to Explain the Correlates of Mammography Screening among Asian American Women. *Pharmacy* **2021**, *9*, 126. [CrossRef]
46. Sharma, M.; Asare, M.; Largo-Wight, E.; Merten, J.; Binder, M.; Lakhan, R.; Batra, K. Testing Multi-Theory Model (Mtm) in Explaining Sunscreen Use among Florida Residents: An Integrative Approach for Sun Protection. *Healthcare* **2021**, *9*, 1343. [CrossRef]
47. Sharma, M.; Batra, K.; Batra, R. A Theory-Based Analysis of Covid-19 Vaccine Hesitancy among African Americans in the United States: A Recent Evidence. *Healthcare* **2021**, *9*, 1273. [CrossRef]
48. Asare, M.; Agyei-Baffour, P.; Lanning, B.A.; Owusu, A.B.; Commeh, M.E.; Boozer, K.; Koranteng, A.; Spies, L.A.; Montealegre, J.R.; Paskett, E.D. Multi-Theory Model and Predictors of Likelihood of Accepting the Series of HPV Vaccination: A Cross-Sectional Study among Ghanaian Adolescents. *Int. J. Environ. Res. Public Health* **2020**, *17*, 571. [CrossRef]
49. Sharma, M.; Petosa, R.L. *Measurement and Evaluation for Health Educators*; Jones & Bartlett Learning: Burlington, MA, USA, 2014.

pharmacy

MDPI

Article

Using the Multi-Theory Model (MTM) of Health Behavior Change to Explain the Correlates of Mammography Screening among Asian American Women

Manoj Sharma [1], Chia-Liang Dai [2], Kavita Batra [3,*], Ching-Chen Chen [4], Jennifer R. Pharr [1], Courtney Coughenour [1], Asma Awan [5] and Hannah Catalano [6]

1 Department of Environmental and Occupational Health, School of Public Health, University of Nevada, Las Vegas, NV 89119, USA; manoj.sharma@unlv.edu (M.S.); Jennifer.pharr@unlv.edu (J.R.P.); courtney.coughenour@unlv.edu (C.C.)
2 Department of Teaching and Learning, College of Education, University of Nevada, Las Vegas, NV 89154, USA; chia-liang.dai@unlv.edu
3 Office of Research, Kirk Kerkorian School of Medicine, University of Nevada, Las Vegas, NV 89102, USA
4 Department of Counselor Education, School Psychology, and Human Services, College of Education, University of Nevada, Las Vegas, NV 89154, USA; ching-chen.chen@unlv.edu
5 Department of Health Informatics, School of Health Sciences, Purdue University, West Lafayette, IN 47906, USA; asmaawan@student.purdueglobal.edu
6 School of Health and Applied Human Sciences, University of North Carolina Wilmington, Wilmington, NC 28403, USA; catalanoh@uncw.edu
* Correspondence: Kavita.batra@unlv.edu

Abstract: Globally, breast cancer is the most common malignancy affecting women. The incidence of breast cancer has been growing among Asian American women. Mammography is a screening procedure that provides early diagnosis for the timely treatment to reduce premature mortality due to breast cancer. However, there are no national data available that summarize the rates of mammography screening among Asian American women. Some small-scale studies have reported low rates of mammography uptake among Asian American women. This cross-sectional study utilized the fourth-generation, multi-theory model (MTM) of health behavior change to explain the correlates of mammography screening among Asian American women between the ages of 45–54 years. A 44-item instrument was evaluated for face, content, and construct validity (using structural equation modeling) and reliability (Cronbach's alpha) and administered electronically to a nationally representative sample of Asian American women (n = 374). The study found that Asian American women who have had received mammograms in the past 12 months as per recommendations, all three constructs of MTM, namely, participatory dialogue ($\beta = 0.156, p < 0.05$), behavioral confidence ($\beta = 0.236, p < 0.001$), and changes in the physical environment ($\beta = 0.426, p < 0.001$) were statistically significant and crucial in their decision to initiate getting a mammogram, accounting for a substantial 49.9% of the variance in the decision to seek mammography. The study also found that the MTM constructs of emotional transformation ($\beta = 0.437, p < 0.001$) and practice for change ($\beta = 0.303, p < 0.001$) were significant for maintaining the repeated behavior of getting annual mammograms and were responsible for 53.9% of the variance. This evidence-based study validates the use of MTM in designing and evaluating mammography screening promotion programs among Asian American women aged 45–54 years.

Keywords: mammography; multi-level theory; screening; behavior; Asian American

1. Introduction

Globally, cancer is the second leading cause of mortality accounting for approximately 9.6 million deaths [1]. Breast cancer is the most common malignancy affecting women worldwide [2]. In the United States (U.S.), breast cancer is the most commonly diagnosed cancer after skin cancers, with one in eight (13%) women being diagnosed with an invasive type of breast cancer during their lifetime [3]. According to the American Cancer Society's [4] recent projected estimates, there will be approximately 284,200 new cases and 44,130 deaths attributed to breast cancer in the U.S. in 2021. The differential risk of breast cancer by nativity, racial, and ethnic characteristics was also reported with Asian American women bearing a disproportionate burden [5,6].

The incidence of breast cancer has been growing with a rate of 94 cases per 100,000 among Asian American women residing in the U.S. [5,7]. Previous reports confirmed that the odds of survival were associated with the Asian ethnicity overall [8]. An analysis of this limited SEER registry data from 2019 indicated that there was a total of 47,401 Asian/Pacific Islander women diagnosed with invasive breast cancer between 2012 and 2016 [3]. With regard to the nativity of Asian American women, 132 cases of women with diagnosed breast cancer were compared with 438 Asian American without breast cancer diagnosis [6]. The results of the study suggested that the breast cancer risk is higher among immigrant Asian American women compared with their US-born counterparts or those who have lived less than 50% of their life in the U.S. [6]. The rate of survival also varied across racial and ethnic groups, which highlights the need of detecting breast cancers at an early stage with the help of primary and secondary levels of prevention, including awareness and screening.

Mammography is a screening procedure that provides early diagnosis, which can lead to treatment and reduced premature mortality due to breast cancer (Centers for Disease Control & Prevention (CDC)) [9]. However, the use of mammograms as a screening method is still a debatable issue due to the problems of false positives, over-diagnosis, and over-treatment [10]. Additionally, health authorities differ in their stances on mammography recommendations across age groups. Four primary authorities in the U.S. proposed guidelines on mammography: American College of Obstetricians and Gynecologists (ACOG), U.S. Preventive Services Task Force, American Cancer Society (ACS), and National Comprehensive Cancer Network (NCCN) [11]. There seems to be some general agreement in these four sets of guidelines that women ages 45–54 years should undergo annual mammograms, and this guideline was used for our study.

To our best knowledge, there are no national data available that summarize the rates of mammography screening among Asian American women through a country-wide population-based survey. However, some small-scale studies have reported low rates of mammography uptake [12]. For instance, a study of Korean American women reported that 22.2% of women ages 45–49 years and 29% of women ages 50–54 years had a mammogram in the past year [12]. According to a 2008 Behavioral Risk Factor Surveillance System (BRFSS) data-based study, 60.3% of Asian American women over the age of 40 years had mammograms in the past year, which was the lowest among all the groups studied [13]. However, the estimates of mammography uptake or utilization are not yet available. Some studies reported regional differences across the U.S. for the mammography screening rates among Asian American women. For instance, a pooled weighted data analysis from five cycles of the California Health Interview Survey conducted between 2001 and 2009, reported an increase in mammograms across all ages in Asian American women from 76–82% from 2001 to 2009 [14]. There is a caveat to this finding; the response rate to this survey was quite low (17.7% to 37.7% in different cycles), which emphasizes the need to conduct additional research pertaining to mammography screening utilization among Asian American women. The Asian American community is increasing rapidly in the U.S. and the present healthcare system and health research are not catering to the needs of this diverse community [13]. In order to meet the growing needs and address the gap in the literature for this underserved minority group, this study is being undertaken [13]. The findings of this study will help in designing behavior change interventions to increase mammography uptake or utilization among Asian American women.

Several factors were known to affect the utilization of mammography screening among Asian American women. Some determinants that are associated with increased rates of mammography screening in Asian American women are having (1) U.S. citizenship [15], (2) longer residency in the U.S. [14,16], (3) a college education [14,17], (4) knowledge of the guidelines [16], (5) health insurance [13,14], (6) a primary care provider who recommended a mammogram [17–19], (7) a routine health check-up in the past year [13], and (8) knowing someone with a history of breast cancer and/or having undergone mammography [16]. Some factors that are barriers to getting mammograms among Asian American women are (1) being of Muslim religion [19,20], (2) perceived religious discrimination [19], (3) impingement on modesty [19], (4) being less acculturated [21], and (5) logistical barriers [22]. It is important to note that not all Asian Americans are a monolithic entity and there are variations among the determinants based on national origin.

There are few interventions that promote mammography among Asian American women. Some of the intervention approaches that have been used are the patient navigator care management model [23], community workshops [24], medical interpretation services for limited English proficiency patients [25], use of primary care providers [26], religiously tailored interventions [27,28], store-based education [29], web-based education delivery [30] among others. Further, very few studies have used behavioral theories as a basis for these interventions. For instance, Boxwala and colleagues [17] and Lee and colleagues [30] used the health belief model, Wu and West [31] used the transtheoretical model, and Sun and colleagues [32] used the prospect theory. Non-theory-based approaches and utilization of older theories do not improve the predictability of the health behavior change. Such approaches lead to doing "same old same old" without advancement of the scientific discipline of health behavior research (HBR). Furthermore, most of the older approaches were about behavior acquisition and newer fourth-generation approaches have been developed that promote behavior "change" instead of mere acquisition and lead to development of precision interventions [33,34]. The first-generation models were about knowledge transfer, the second-generation models were about skill acquisition, third generation models were about behavior acquisition, and the fourth-generation models are about behavior change utilizing constructs from multiple evidence-based theories [33,34]. Therefore, there is a need to utilize recent fourth-generation health behavior change models to explain the correlates of mammography screening and design precise interventions to promote mammography in this understudied and underserved population of Asian American women.

One emerging fourth-generation model is the multi-theory model (MTM) of health behavior change [33,34]. This model breaks down the complex health behavior change into two components of initiation and maintenance with three explanatory constructs for each of the two components (Figure 1). This model has been used in qualitative [35,36], cross-sectional [37–40], and experimental studies [41–43] with a variety of behaviors in different priority populations but has not been applied to understanding mammography screening behaviors. Therefore, the current study aims to utilize the multi-theory model (MTM) of health behavior change to explain the correlates of mammography screening in a sample of Asian American women between the ages of 45–54 years.

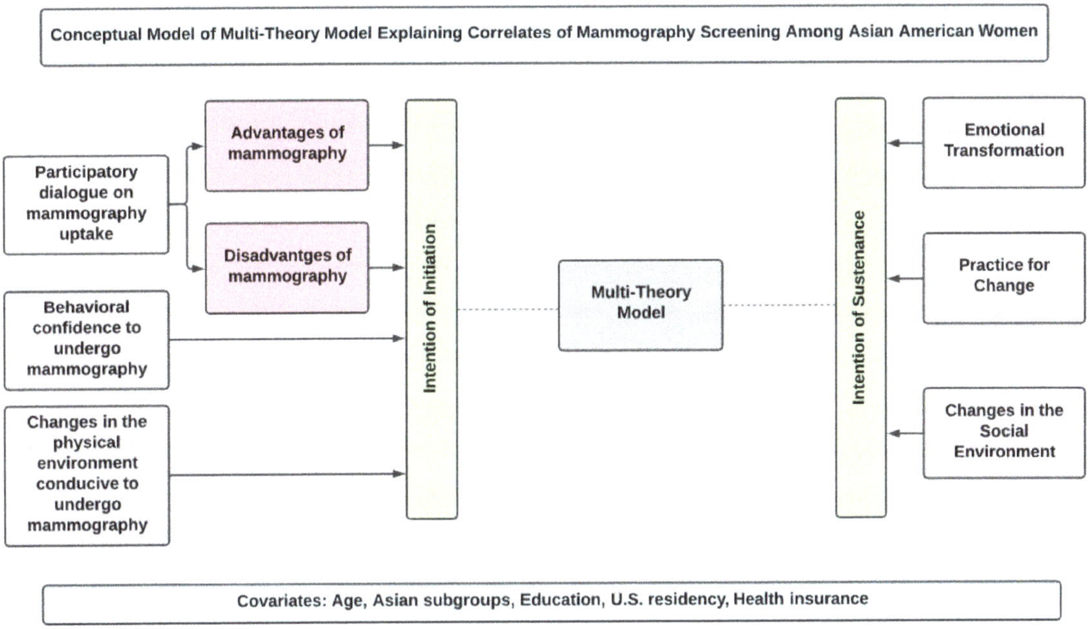

Figure 1. Conceptual model of Multi-Theory Model.

2. Materials and Methods

2.1. Study Design and Data Collection

The data collection for this cross-sectional study was conducted from 10 March 2021 through 18 March 2021, utilizing a research panel of participants facilitated by the market research firm Qualtrics [44]. Qualtrics® (the world's leading enterprise survey technology solution and XM platform) has been providing samples for over a decade now. Qualtrics partners with over 20 online sample providers to recruit a research panel of participants, which has been created via convenience sampling to build samples from multiple sources. This enable researchers with the diverse and representative datasets. The sample partners randomly select respondents, who are likely to qualify. The majority of the samples come from traditional, actively managed, panel portals. Occasionally, social media is used to gather respondents. For inaccessible groups, Qualtrics utilizes niche panels via special recruitment campaigns [45]. The survey invitations are intentionally kept general to prevent the self-selection bias. Depending upon the study's inclusion criteria, Qualtrics adds screening questions in the beginning of the survey to ensure inclusion of eligible participants. All qualifying participants who complete the survey are compensated in accordance with Qualtrics® panel agreement. The agreement varies and may include cash, airline miles, charitable donations, sweepstakes entrance, vouchers, gift certificate, etc. Additional information about ethical, methodological, and regulatory guidelines can be found at www.esomar.org (accessed on 8 July 2021). Previous studies have provided the detailed information related to the use of Qualtrics® research panel platforms [45].

2.2. Ethical Considerations

The study (protocol #1727672-1, dated 4 March 2021) was considered an exempt research study by the Institutional Review Board (IRB). Participation in the study was completely voluntary, and detailed information about the study's objectives and significance were provided to participants in an informed consent attached with the web-based survey. Personal identifiers, including name and email address, were not collected to preserve anonymity. Only one response per participant was allowed. We used the "Prevent Ballot Box Stuffing" feature in the Qualtrics to restrict multiple responses from the same participant. This feature is driven by a strong algorithm to ensure data integrity and unique responses. Additionally, Qualtrics utilizes digital fingerprinting technology to preserve integrity of the survey.

2.3. *Data Intergrity*

Data for this study were collected by Qualtrics Research Services as a part of the contractual agreement. As an essential part of the contract, all data privacy laws and regulations were followed to preserve data integrity. Qualtrics database does not hold confidential information of the respondents or panelists. Qualtrics® provided deidentified data to the researchers in an excel sheet, which was stored on a password protected desktop computer in a locked office. Only the principal investigator and statistician of this study had access to the deidentified data files.

2.4. *Survey Questionnaire*

Based on MTM, a 44-item survey questionnaire was developed to determine the correlates of mammography screening uptake among Asian American women aged 45–54 years. The survey was composed of 13 demographic questions and mammography history, and 31 items for the two primary MTM theoretical constructs (initiation and sustenance). A panel of eight subject matter experts (SMEs), investigated face and content validity of the questionnaire in several rounds of review. The reviews were blinded to prevent observer bias. Several revisions were performed to enhance readability and content of the questionnaire. A detailed description of the instrument's domains and constructs is provided in Table 1.

Table 1. Domains and constructs of MTM theoretical framework.

Domain	Constructs		Definition (s) and Examples from This Study	Number of Items	Possible Range (Min–Max)
Intention of Initiation	Participatory dialogue (Derived after subtracting summative score of disadvantages from advantages)	Advantages	Perception of advantages following the specific behavior initiation, e.g., early detection, peace of mind, etc.	5	0–20 units
		Disadvantages	Perception of disadvantages following the specific behavior initiation, e.g., invasion of modesty, inconvenience, etc.	5	0–20 units
	Behavior confidence		Surety of behavior despite external and internal driving factors, e.g., overcoming cost, overcoming discomfort, etc.	5	0–20 units
	Changes in the physical environment		Overcoming enabling factors for behavior initiation, e.g., easy access to a place, ability to get it when one wants it, etc.	3	0–12 units
Intention of Sustenance	Emotional transformation		Converting emotions into intention, e.g., directing feelings into goal, self-motivation, etc.	3	0–12 units
	Practice for change		Continuous adaptation for behavior changes, e.g., monitoring, overcoming barriers, etc.	3	0–12 units
	Changes in the social environment		Using social cues for behavior change, e.g., support from family, friends, etc.	5	0–20 units

2.4.1. Intention of Initiation

Constructs of advantages and disadvantages of intention of initiation were measured on a 5-point Likert scale, which ranges from "strongly disagree" to "strongly agree."

The score of Participatory dialogue was derived by subtracting the summative score of disadvantages from advantages. The other two constructs of intention to initiation were behavioral confidence and changes in the physical environment. These were also measured on 5-point Likert scale of surety, which had the response options of Not at all sure (0), slightly sure (1), moderately sure (2), very sure (3), completely sure (4). A high score was associated with the likelihood of initiation of behavior change.

2.4.2. Intention of Sustenance

Constructs of emotional transformation, practice for change, and changes in the social environment were measured on a 5-point Likert scale of surety, which has the response options of Not at all sure (0), slightly sure (1), moderately sure (2), very sure (3), completely sure (4). A high score was associated with the likelihood of sustenance of behavior change. Additionally, two items were used to model initiation and sustenance, which were measured as scale variables.

2.5. Statistical Analysis

We used IBM SPSS version 27.0 (IBM Corp. Armonk, NY, USA), Mplus 7.11, and G* Power software packages for the analyses. Minimum sample size was estimated using the Cohen's effect sizes conventions (based on the type of statistical test) corresponding to 99% power [46,47]. The significance level was set at 0.05, and 95% confidence intervals were reported wherever appropriate. Data normality assumptions were assessed through visual inspection of normal Q-Q plots and histograms. An independent-samples t-test was utilized to compare the mean scores of MTM constructs across groups who have had mammography and those who have not. Categorical variables were expressed as counts and proportions, whereas continuous variables were represented as means and standard deviations. Two separate Hierarchical Regression Models (HRM) were built to predict the variance in the likelihood of initiation and sustenance of mammography behavior by multiple factors, such as demographic characteristics and MTM constructs.

For construct validation, Structural Equation Modelling (SEM) was utilized to determine the structural relationship between measured variables and latent constructs. Weighted least squares approach (WLSMV estimator) and the 0.05 alpha level were used to test our two hypothesized structural models among the samples. Drawing upon the theory and prior research, our hypothesized model included participatory dialogue (advantages and disadvantages), behavioral confidence, changes in physical environment, changes in social environment, practice for change, and emotional transformation as independent variables; and initiation and sustenance of health behavior change as dependent variables. We hypothesized that (1) the variables of participatory dialogue (advantages and disadvantages), behavioral confidence, and changes in physical environment constructs would impact the initiation of mammography screening behavior change, and (2) the changes in social environment, practice for change, and emotional transformation constructs would impact the sustenance of mammography screening behaviors. This study used a variety of fit indices because they provide different information about model fit. We considered the substantive meaningfulness of the model, significant χ^2 statistics as evidence that models did not fit the data exactly [48], Tucker–Lewis (TLI) and comparative fit (CFI) indices greater than 0.95 evidence of good fit [48–50], and root means square error of approximation (RMSEA) values of less than 0.05 to be acceptable [51]. To estimate the sample size for testing hypothesized models, we first sought to meet the conventional 10 subjects per variable ratio [52–54]. Next, sample size calculation for Structural Equation Modeling [55] recommended a minimum of 137 participants were required to achieve a statistical power level of 0.8 at an alpha level of 0.05 with 0.3 (medium) anticipated effect size and number of variables in the models. Finally, previous studies suggested that, for confirmatory factor analysis, this sample size was sufficiently powered to evaluate the hypothesized models [56–58].

3. Results

A total of 374 participants completed this study. The mean age of the study sample was 49.25 (SD: 2.68) years. Chinese Americans represented 41.2% of the sample. The majority of participants (69.3%) were employed, working 34.9 average hours per week. The percentage of participants with health insurance coverage was 93%, over 60% of the population had a household income under $100,000 and lived in suburban neighborhoods. Forty percent of participants reported their religious affiliation as Christianity and 68.7% of the women were married (Table 2).

Table 2. Demographic characteristics of the sample population (n = 374) of Asian American women collected in March 2021.

Variable	n (%)
Years of residency in the U.S.	
Less than 30 years	166 (44.4)
More than 30 years	208 (55.6)
Asian sub-groups	
Chinese American	154 (41.2)
Korean American	22 (5.9)
Filipino American	59 (15.8)
South Asian American	51 (13.6)
Japanese American	40 (10.7)
Others [1]	36 (9.6)
Prefer not to answer	12 (3.2)
Religion affiliation	
Christianity	162 (43.3)
Buddhism	48 (12.8)
Atheist	45 (12)
Hinduism	31 (8.3)
Others including Islam, Judaism and other categories	88 (23.6)
Residence	
Rural	28 (7.5)
Urban	110 (29.4)
Suburban	236 (63.1)
Educational attainment	
High school graduate or less	15 (4.0)
Some college or trade school	36 (9.6)
Associate's degree	46 (12.3)
Bachelor's degree	175 (46.8)
Master's degree or above	102 (27.3)
Health insurance status	
Yes	348 (93)
No	26 (7)
Household income (USD)	
<25,000	24 (6.4)
25,000–50,000	65 (17.4)
50,001–75,000	72 (19.3)
75,001–100,000	65 (17.4)
>100,000	148 (39.5)

Table 2. *Cont.*

Variable	n (%)
Marital status	
Married	257 (68.7)
Never married	52 (13.9)
Divorced/separated/widowed	51 (13.6)
Others [2]	14 (3.8)
Employment status	
Yes	259 (69.3)
No	115 (30.7)

[1]. Others Asian subgroups include Vietnamese American, Middle East American, and other South East Asian American.; [2]. Others in marital status include those in a civil union or registered domestic partnership and a member of an unmarried couple.

There were significant differences in the mean scores for all constructs of initiation and sustenance among those who have had mammography compared with those who have not had mammography. Mammography users had a statistically significant higher mean scores for initiation (3.24 ± 0.90 vs. 1.63 ± 1.2, $p < 0.001$) and sustenance (3.13 ± 1.0 vs. 1.23 ± 1.1, $p < 0.001$) compared to mammography non-users (Table 3).

Table 3. Comparing mean scores of multi-theory model constructs of behavior change across groups of survey respondents of Asian American women.

Groups	Women Who Have Had Mammography (n = 199)			Women Who Have Not Had Mammography (n = 175)			
Constructs	**Possible Score Range**	**Observed Score Range**	**Mean ± SD**	**Possible Score Range**	**Observed Score Range**	**Mean ± SD**	**p-Value ***
Initiation	0–4	0–4	3.24 ± 0.90	0–4	0–4	1.63 ± 1.2	<0.001
Participatory dialogue: advantages	0–20	4–20	17.11 ± 2.96	0–20	2–20	14.48 ± 3.7	<0.001
Participatory dialogue: disadvantages	0–20	0–20	9.07 ± 3.78	0–20	0–20	10.62 ± 3.46	<0.001
Participatory dialogue **	−20–[+20]	−13–[+20]	8.04 ± 5.3	−20–[+20]	−12–[+20]	3.86 ± 5.36	<0.001
Behavior confidence	0–20	1–20	14.91 ± 3.98	0–20	0–20	10.05 ± 4.95	<0.001
Changes in the physical environment	0–12	2–12	10.12 ± 2.23	0–12	0–12	8.01 ± 3.09	<0.001
Sustenance	0–4	0–4	3.13 ± 1.0	0–4	0–4	1.23 ± 1.1	<0.001
Emotional transformation	0–12	0–12	9.42 ± 2.65	0–12	0–12	5.02 ± 3.26	<0.001
Practice for change	0–12	1–12	8.85 ± 2.55	0–12	0–12	4.82 ± 3.14	<0.001
Changes in the social environment	0–20	0–20	13.16 ± 4.71	0–20	0–20	8.69 ± 4.40	<0.001

* p values less than 0.05 are considered statistically significant; ** Participatory dialogue is computed by subtracting disadvantages from advantages.

3.1. Asian American Women Following Recommendations on Routine Mammography Screening

Hierarchical multiple regression was performed to determine if the sequential addition of participatory dialogue, behavioral confidence, and changes in the physical environment improved the likelihood of initiation over the demographic variables of age, Asian subgroups, education, duration of U.S. residency and health insurance (Model 1). The addition of participatory dialogue to the prediction of initiation led to a statistically significant increase in R^2 of 0.207, F (1, 191) = 12.113, $p < 0.001$ (Model 2). The addition of behavioral confidence to the prediction of initiation led to a statistically significant increase in R^2 of 0.139, F (1, 190) = 19.198, $p < 0.001$ (Model 3). Among participants following mammography screening recommendations, the full model containing demographic variables and all three constructs to predict initiation was statistically significant, R^2 = 0.519, F (1, 189) = 25.490, $p < 0.001$; adjusted R^2 = 0.499 (Model 4). All model results can be found in Table 4.

Table 4. Hierarchical Multiple Regression (HRM) predicting likelihood for initiation and sustenance of mammogram behavior among survey respondents of Asian American women following recommendations on routine mammography screening (*n* = 199).

Variables	Model 1		Model 2		Model 3		Model 4	
	B	*β*	B	*β*	B	*β*	B	*β*
The Likelihood for initiation as a dependent variable								
Constant	1.936		0.281		−0.099		−1.042	
Age	0.005	0.015	0.020	0.065	0.013	0.043	0.019	0.063
Asian subgroups	−0.008	−0.021	−0.020	−0.054	−0.012	−0.034	−0.012	−0.032
Education	−0.041	−0.071	−0.006	−0.011	−0.007	−0.012	−0.016	−0.028
U.S. Residency	0.011 **	0.188	0.009 *	0.157	0.003	0.055	0.001	0.024
Health Insurance	1.008 *	0.163	1.195 **	0.194	0.921 **	0.149	0.784 *	0.127
Participatory dialogue			0.076 **	0.465	0.043 **	0.261	0.026 *	0.156
Behavioral confidence					0.096 **	0.439	0.051 **	0.236
Changes in the physical environment							0.166 **	0.426
R^2	0.069		0.276		0.414		0.519	
F	2.840 *		12.113 **		19.198 **		25.490 **	
Δ R^2	0.069		0.207		0.139		0.105	
Δ F	2.840 *		54.521 **		44.971 **		41.145 **	
The Likelihood for sustenance as a dependent variable								
Constant	0.937		−0.210		−0.277		−0.368	
Age	0.024	0.069	0.014	0.039	0.012	0.033	0.013	0.037
Asian subgroups	−0.004	−0.010	−0.021	−0.051	−0.019	−0.046	−0.020	−0.047
Education	−0.010	−0.016	0.012	0.019	0.008	0.011	0.008	0.013
U.S. Residency	0.015 **	0.221	0.001	0.016	0.002	0.025	0.002	0.025
Health Insurance	0.578	0.082	0.111	0.016	0.080	0.011	0.103	0.014
Emotional transformation			0.267 **	0.707	0.168 **	0.447	0.164 **	0.437
Practice for change					0.129 **	0.327	0.119 **	0.303
Changes in the social environment							0.010	0.047
R^2	0.066		0.517		0.557		0.558	
F	2.694 *		34.119 **		34.128 **		29.844 **	
Δ R^2	0.066		0.452		0.040		0.001	
Δ F	2.694 *		178.773 **		17.014 **		0.493	

B (Unstandardized coefficient); β (Standardized coefficient), * *p*-value < 0.05; ** *p*-value < 0.001; Adjusted R^2 of initiation = 0.499; Adjusted R^2 of sustenance = 0.539.

Hierarchical multiple regression was performed to determine if the sequential addition of emotional transformation and practice for change improved the likelihood of sustenance over the demographic variables of age, Asian subgroups, education, duration of U.S. residency and health insurance (Model 1). In the hierarchical regression with sustenance as the dependent variable, the addition of emotional transformation to the prediction of sustenance led to a statistically significant increase in R^2 of 0.452, F (1, 191) = 34.119, $p < 0.001$ (Model 2). The addition of practice for change to the prediction of sustenance led to a statistically significant increase in R^2 of 0.040, F (1, 190) = 34.128, $p < 0.001$ (Model 3). The full model containing preselected demographic variables and three MTM constructs to predict sustenance was statistically significant, R^2 = 0.558, F (1, 189) = 29.844, $p < 0.001$; adjusted R^2 = 0.539 (Model 4). All model results can be found in Table 4.

3.2. Asian American Women Not Following Recommendations on Routine Mammography Screening

Among participants not following mammography screening recommendations, hierarchical multiple regression was performed to determine if the sequential addition of participatory dialogue, behavioral confidence, and changes in the physical environment improved the likelihood of initiation over the demographic variables of age, Asian subgroups, education, duration of U.S. residency and health insurance (Model 1). The addition of participatory dialogue to the prediction of initiation led to a statistically significant increase in R^2 of 0.202, F (1, 168) = 8.185, $p < 0.001$ (Model 2). The addition of behavior confidence to the prediction of initiation led to a statistically significant increase in R^2 of 0.090, F (1, 167) = 11.014, $p < 0.001$ (Model 3). The full model containing demographic variables and all three constructs to predict initiation was statistically significant, $R^2 = 0.319$, F (1, 166) = 9.709, $p < 0.001$; adjusted $R^2 = 0.286$ (Model 4). All model results can be found in Table 5.

Table 5. Hierarchical Multiple Regression (HRM) predicting likelihood for initiation and sustenance of mammogram behavior among survey respondents of Asian American women not following recommendations on routine mammography screening (*n* = 175).

Variables	Model 1		Model 2		Model 3		Model 4	
	B	*β*	B	*β*	B	*β*	B	*β*
The Likelihood for initiation as a dependent variable								
Constant	1.679		1.298		1.196		1.028	
Age	−0.013	−0.029	−0.015	−0.033	−0.020	−0.043	−0.018	−0.039
Asian subgroups	0.030	0.067	0.042	0.096	0.056	0.126	0.054	0.121
Education	0.031	0.040	0.045	0.058	0.037	0.047	0.031	0.039
U.S. Residency	−0.002	−0.025	0.000	0.004	−0.007	−0.081	−0.007	−0.086
Health Insurance	0.444	0.127	0.318	0.091	0.161	0.046	0.173	0.050
Participatory dialogue			0.098 **	0.452	0.066 **	0.304	0.064 **	0.294
Behavioral confidence					0.082 **	0.350	0.073 **	0.310
Changes in the physical environment							0.026	0.071
R^2	0.025		0.226		0.316		0.319	
F	0.852		8.185 **		11.014 **		9.709 **	
ΔR^2	0.025		0.202		0.090		0.003	
ΔF	0.852		43.772 **		21.885 **		0.704	
The Likelihood for sustenance as a dependent variable								
Constant	0.608		−1.312		−1.418		−1.205	
Age	0.013	0.027	0.026	0.055	0.028	0.060	0.022	0.047
Asian subgroups	0.041	0.091	0.035	0.078	0.030	0.066	0.024	0.054
Education	−0.032	−0.040	0.013	0.016	0.003	0.004	−0.006	−0.007
U.S. Residency	−0.006	−0.078	−0.016 **	−0.192	−0.016 **	−0.199	−0.166 **	−0.188
Health Insurance	0.265	0.074	0.268	0.075	0.276	0.077	0.213	0.060
Emotional transformation			0.270 **	0.742	0.184 **	0.507	0.174 **	0.478
Practice for change					0.106 **	0.280	0.072 *	0.192
Changes in the social environment							0.044 *	0.165
R^2	0.024		0.557		0.580		0.594	
F	0.847		35.205 **		32.920 **		30.341 **	
ΔR^2	0.024		0.533		0.023		0.014	
ΔF	0.847		201.956 **		9.067 **		5.744 *	

B (Unstandardized coefficient); β (Standardized coefficient), * *p*-value < 0.05; ** *p*-value < 0.001; Adjusted R^2 of initiation = 0.286; Adjusted R^2 of sustenance = 0.574.

Hierarchical multiple regression was performed to determine if the sequential addition of emotional transformation and practice for change improved the likelihood of sustenance over the demographic variables of age, Asian subgroups, education, duration of U.S. residency and health insurance (Model 1). In the hierarchical regression with sustenance as a dependent variable, the addition of emotional transformation led to a statistically significant increase in R^2 of 0.533, F (1, 168) = 35.205, $p < 0.001$ (Model 2). The addition of practice for change to the prediction of sustenance led to a statistically significant increase in R^2 of 0.023, F (1, 167) = 32.920, $p < 0.001$ (Model 3). The full model containing demographic variables and three MTM constructs to predict sustenance was statistically significant, $R^2 = 0.594$, F (1, 166) = 30.341, $p < 0.001$; adjusted $R^2 = 0.574$ (Model 4). All model results can be found in Table 5.

3.3. *Structural Equation Modelling*

We examined two hypothesized models. The results of the initiation model indicated the model fits the data well (e.g., χ^2 [142] = 304.56 [$p < 0.01$], CFI = 0.96, TLI= 0.95, and RMSEA = 0.06) (Table A1). We observed the standardized effects of latent variables on their reflective indicators (i.e., factor loadings) and found an overall pattern of statistically significant loadings for advantages, disadvantages, behavioral confidence, and changes in the physical environment. The advantages had large effects (e.g., β ranging from 0.68 to 0.91) on its five indicators; the disadvantages had moderate effects (e.g., β ranging from 0.34 to 0.79) on its five indicators; the behavioral confidence had large effects (e.g., β ranging from 0.74 to 0.92) on its five indicators; and the changes in the physical environment had large effects (e.g., β ranging from 0.82 to 0.93) on its three indicators (Figure 2, Table A2). These effects suggested that our scale scores provided valid measurement of their constructs. Next, we examined between construct correlations and standardized regression coefficients. We found advantages, behavioral confidence, and changes in the physical environment had small to moderate positive direct effects on the initiation of mammography behavior (e.g., β ranging from.16 to 0.37, $p < 0.001$), while disadvantages had small negative direct effects on the initiation of mammography behavior (β = −0.13, $p < 0.001$).

For the sustenance model, the fit of the model was excellent (e.g., χ^2 [48] = 152.98 [$p < 0.01$], CFI = 0.97, TLI = 0.95, and RMSEA = 0.08) (Table A1). We observed the standardized effects of latent variables on their reflective indicators (i.e., factor loadings) and found an overall pattern of statistically significant loadings for emotional transformation, practice for change, and changes in the social environment. The emotional transformation had large effects (e.g., β ranging from 0.89 to 0.95) on its three indicators; the practice for change had large effects (e.g., β ranging from 0.88 to 0.93) on its three indicators; and the changes in the social environment had moderate to large effects (e.g., β ranging from 0.56 to 0.85) on its five indicators (Figure 3, Table A3). These effects also suggested that our scale scores provided valid measurement of their constructs. We then examined between construct correlations and standardized regression coefficients for the sustenance model. We found emotional transformation had moderate direct effects on the sustenance of mammography behavior (β = 0.61, $p < 0.001$). However, both practice for change and changes in the social environment did not have any significant effects on the sustenance of mammography behavior.

We found an overall pattern of statistically significant ($p < 0.05$) relationships among the constructs. The negative correlation between disadvantages and other factors was observed (Table 6). The Cronbach's alphas for all subscales were greater than 0.70 (ranging from 0.72 to 0.95).

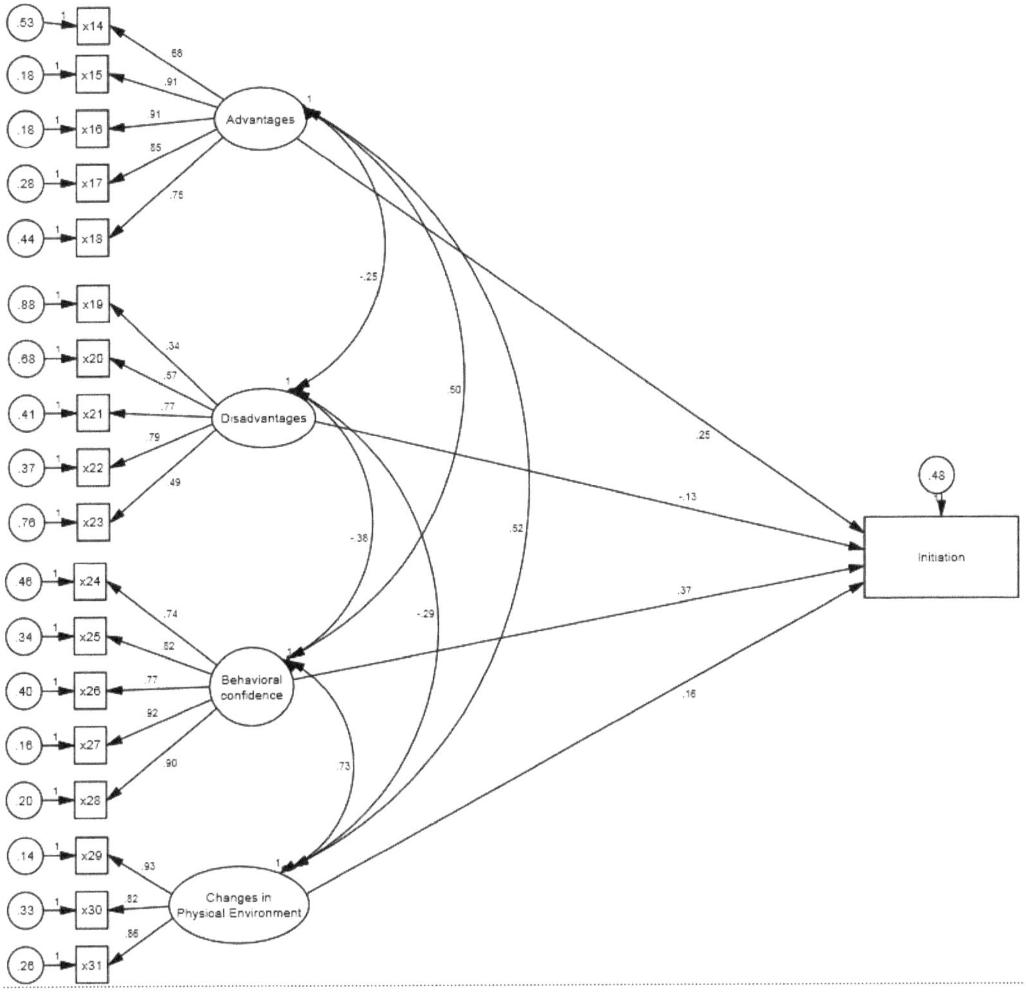

Figure 2. Structural Equation Modeling for Initiation of Mammogram Behavior among Survey Respondents of Asian American women.

Table 6. Summary of bivariate correlations, means, standard deviations, and internal consistency estimates for study variables using data from Asian American women.

Variables	1	2	3	4	5	6	7
1. Advantages	-						
2. Disadvantages	−0.23 *	-					
3. Behavioral Confidence	0.46 *	−0.37 *	-				
4. Physical Environment	0.48 *	−0.28 *	0.68 *	-			
5. Emotional Transformation	0.52 *	−0.32 *	0.72 *	0.61 *	-		
6. Practice for Change	0.53 *	−0.32 *	0.75 *	0.64 *	0.88 *	-	
7. Changes in Social Environment	0.53 *	−0.30 *	0.65 *	0.64 *	0.69 *	0.74 *	-
M	15.88	9.79	12.64	9.13	7.36	6.97	11.07
SD	3.57	3.71	5.08	2.87	3.68	3.48	5.08
α	0.91	0.72	0.92	0.90	0.95	0.93	0.87

Note. $n = 374$, * $p < 0.05$.

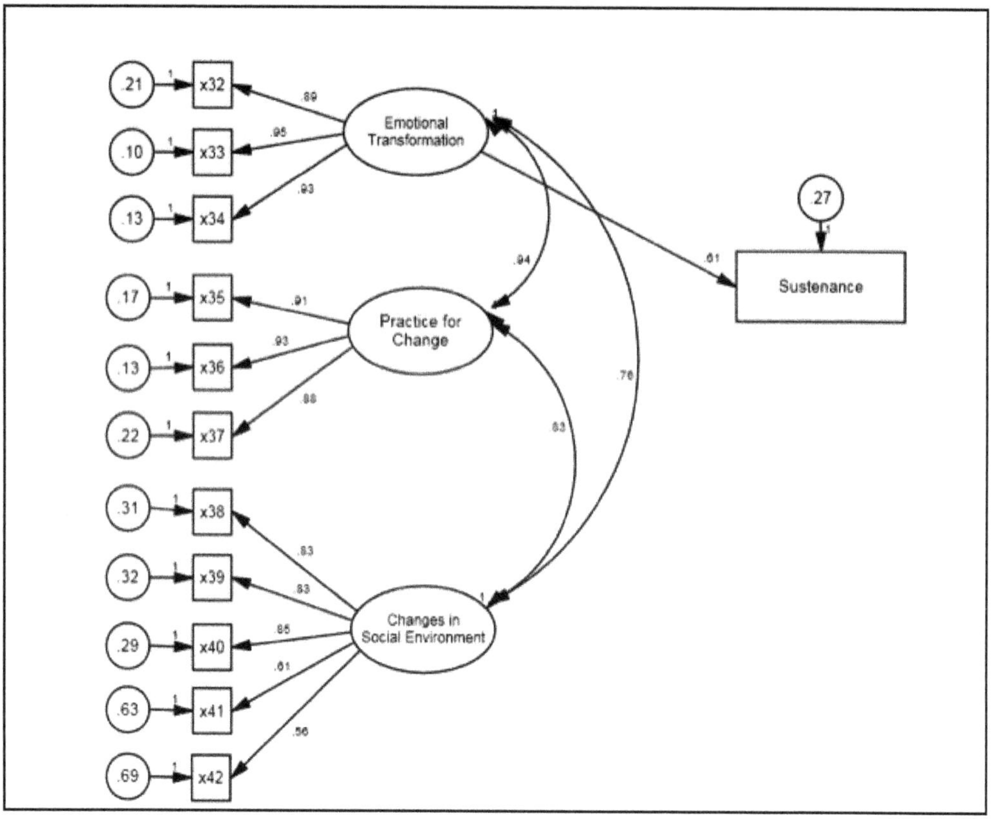

Figure 3. Structural Equation Modeling for Sustenance Model.

4. Discussion

The aim of this study was to explain the correlates of mammography screening using the paradigm of MTM in a nationally representative sample of Asian American women aged 45–54 years. The study found that for Asian American women

Who had received mammograms in the past 12 months as per recommendations, all three constructs of the MTM, namely, participatory dialogue ($\beta = 0.156$, $p < 0.05$), behavioral confidence ($\beta = 0.236$, $p < 0.001$), and changes in the physical environment ($\beta = 0.426$, $p < 0.001$) were statistically significant and crucial in their decision to initiate getting the mammogram. In addition, health insurance status ($\beta = 0.127$, $p < 0.05$) was also a significant contributor which is also supported by previous literature [13,14]. However, age, Asian subgroups, education, and U.S. residency were not significant contributors in the final model. The final model accounted for a substantial proportion of variance (49.9%) in explaining the decision to receive mammography, which is considered high in social and behavioral sciences [33,34]. While this analysis was not necessary because this group of women were indeed adhering to the guidelines, it was conducted to confirm that the putative MTM constructs are indeed crucial in achieving the starting of the behavior. The study also found that the MTM constructs of emotional transformation ($\beta = 0.437$, $p < 0.001$) and practice for change ($\beta = 0.303$, $p < 0.001$) were significant for maintaining the repeated behavior of getting mammograms and were responsible for 53.9% of the variance, which again is substantial [33,34]. Similar significant correlates of MTM were observed in the group of Asian American women who had not received a mammogram in the past 12 months, where participatory dialogue ($\beta = 0.294$, $p < 0.001$) and behavior confidence ($\beta = 0.310$, $p < 0.001$) accounted for 28.6% of the variance in the intention to get mammograms. It is worth noting that the construct of changes in physical environment which was significant for those following mammography recommendations was not significant for those not following the recommendations which is indicative of the barriers that this group may be encountering. These need to be addressed by interventions that promote mammography in Asian American women. Regarding the intention for getting repeat annual mammograms (sustenance), all MTM constructs of sustenance emotional transformation ($\beta = 0.478$, $p < 0.001$), practice for change ($\beta = 0.192$, $p < 0.05$) changes in the social environment ($\beta = 0.165$, $p < 0.05$) were significant contributors accounting for 57.4% of the variance, which is quite considerable [33,34]. It is important to note that all the constructs of MTM are significant in their putative role of explaining continuation of mammography behavior for those Asian American women not following recommendations thus underscoring the relevance of the MTM in designing interventions to promote mammography.

It is worth noting that in this nationally representative sample of Asian American women aged 45–54 years, 46.8% of them had not received a mammogram as per the recommendations of getting one every year [11]. These findings are similar to those from the BRFSS data that found that 39.7% of Asian American women over 40 years had not received mammograms [13]. This is a sizable number of Asian American women who are not following the recommendations, underscoring the need for educational and policy efforts in promoting mammography screening to this subgroup of the population.

On close examination of each construct of MTM in its role associated with mammography screening among Asian American women aged 45–54 years old, we found several important outcomes. First, the participatory dialogue had, as expected, a significantly higher mean score (8.04 ± 5.3) among those who had received a mammogram as per recommendations compared to those who had not (3.86 ± 5.36) ($p < 0.001$). Clearly, those who were convinced of the advantages of getting a mammography screening were motivated to get it. This is also supported by previous studies on determinants of mammography in Asian American women [14–19]. However, on hierarchical regression, the construct was found to be significant among those who were adhering to the recommendations but was not significant for those who were not adhering, after adding the construct of changes in the physical environment. This may point to the relative importance of changes in the physical environment construct which has also been supported in the literature in the form of access to health insurance [13,14] or the recommendations from health care providers [17–19].

The second construct of MTM, behavioral confidence for initiating mammography screening, had the mean score that was significantly higher for those who had mammograms (14.91 ± 3.98) compared with those who had not had mammograms (10.05 ± 4.95) ($p < 0.001$). It was also a significant predictor in the regression models. Previous studies have not examined the extent of the role of this construct, as most of the studies have not utilized behavioral theories for studying determinants of mammography screening among Asian American women [17–19]. However, other studies, with other behaviors and other target populations, lend support to this construct of behavioral confidence as playing a significant role in the decision whether to seek mammograms or not [38–40].

The third MTM construct of changes in the physical environment for initiating the mammography screening had a mean score that was significantly higher for those who had mammograms (10.12 ± 2.23) compared with those who had not had mammograms (8.01 ± 3.09) ($p < 0.001$). It was also a significant predictor in regression models. As discussed earlier, there is evidence from previous research that aspects of the physical environment are very important for Asian American women to seek mammography [13,14,17–19]. There is clearly a need to help Asian American women overcome logistical barriers that prevent them from seeking mammography screening [22].

For getting repeated annual mammograms (sustenance), the first MTM construct that was significant was emotional transformation. The mean score for this construct was significantly higher for those who had mammograms (9.42 ± 2.65) compared to those who had not had mammograms (5.02 ± 3.26) ($p < 0.001$). It was also a significant predictor in the regression models. Previous studies have not examined the extent of the role of this construct in improving adherence to mammography screening recommendations among Asian American women because this is a relatively new conceptualization where feelings are purported to be used for goal setting in behavior change [33,34]. However, its role has shown to be important with other behaviors and with other target populations [37–40] so there is a need to use this construct in planning educational interventions that promote mammography screening among Asian American women.

The mean score on the construct for practice for change, which is another construct that predicts maintenance of behavior, was significantly higher for those who had mammograms (8.85 ± 2.55) compared with those who had not had mammograms (4.82 ± 3.14) ($p < 0.001$). However, on hierarchical regression, the construct was found to be significant among those who were adhering to the recommendations but was not significant for those who were not adhering, after adding the construct of changes in the social environment. This may point to the relative importance of changes in the social environment construct which may play a greater role in the Asian American culture. The role of friends and family members and what they think is an important influence in the lives of Asian Americans. This phenomenon has not been studied extensively in relation to mammography screening among Asian American women, but Somanchi and colleagues [16] found that knowing someone with a history of breast cancer and/or having undergone mammography was a determinant in getting a mammogram for Asian American women. Therefore, this provides support to our conjecture about changes in the social environment playing a greater role. As predictable based on MTM, the mean score of the construct of changes in the social environment was also significantly higher for those who had mammograms (13.16 ± 4.71) compared with those who had not had mammograms (8.69 ± 4.40) ($p < 0.001$). The role of this MTM construct is also supported from research with other behaviors in other target populations [38,39]. There is a need to garner support from social influences in educational programs that promote mammograms among Asian American women.

Since the Asian American community is not a monolithic entity, we collected data on the Asian subgroups. In our sample, the largest representation was from Chinese Americans (41.2%) followed by Filipino Americans (15.8%), followed by South Asian Americans (13.6%) which is more or less representative of the distribution of Asian Americans in the U.S. However, we did not find any significant explanatory potential of these subgroup classifications on predicting potential utilization of mammography screening when MTM constructs are included in the modeling. Future researchers may want to reexamine it more carefully. Previous studies have noted religion, especially being a Muslim, as being a deterrent for getting mammography screening [19,20]. In our sample only nine (2.4%) Asian American women practiced Islam, so we could not analyze this subgroup given the constraints of the small sample size. Future researchers may want to oversample this subgroup to discern if religion indeed is a putative determinant of mammography screening when MTM constructs are taken into consideration.

4.1. Implications for Practice

There is a need for both theory-based educational interventions and policy measures that promote mammography screening among Asian American women particularly in the 45–54 age group. The educational interventions can be delivered in primary care settings, OBGYN clinics, community organizations with which Asian American women are associated, faith-based organizations specific to various religions embraced by the Asian American women community, social media, and directed mHealth interventions specifically geared toward this subgroup. MTM can serve as a promising theoretical paradigm in designing and evaluating such interventions. The construct of participatory dialogue in educational interventions can be built by underscoring advantages such as early detection of breast cancer, having peace of mind for self and family, possibility of early treatment, and reduction in premature mortality. Potential barriers such as discomfort, invasion on modesty, inconvenience, and fear of getting a false positive must be discussed and reduced to the extent possible in educational interventions. The construct of behavioral confidence can be fostered through exploration of sources of confidence, using role models, and using stepwise strategies in overcoming barriers. The construct of changes in the physical environment can be mobilized through resources support and reminders. The construct of emotional transformation can be channelized in educational interventions by appealing to the feelings of Asian American women and harnessing these into concrete goals of getting timely mammograms, helping overcome self-doubt, and remaining motivated. The construct of practice for change can be operationalized by encouraging Asian American women to keep records and have reminder systems, overcoming barriers, and making alternate plans if faced with obstacles. Finally, the construct of changes in the social environment must be used by educational programs where family, friends, and healthcare providers should be encouraged to promote, remind, and help with mammography screening.

4.2. Strengths and Limitations

This study is among the few studies that are based on a behavioral theory to decipher determinants of mammography screening in the high-risk Asian American women community. The study collected data on a nationally representative adequately powered sample representing all subgroups of Asian American women aged 45–54 years. The study utilized a contemporary fourth-generation paradigm of MTM. The psychometric validation of the tool used in the study was done meticulously. However, there were also some limitations to this study. Self-reports were utilized to collect information about mammography. Objective data using medical records could have been used to provide more accuracy. The cross-sectional nature of the design always limits causal inferences because the data on the independent variables (MTM constructs) and dependent variables (intentions) are collected at the same point in time. Future research must look into longitudinal designs. Finally, as mentioned earlier, we did not have adequate representation of the Muslim Asian American women in our sample, so we could not examine the role of MTM constructs while controlling for religion.

5. Conclusions

MTM is a fourth-generation behavioral theory that is gaining popularity and accumulating empirical evidence. This study is among one of those burgeoning studies that provide support to MTM. The Asian American women lag behind their White counterparts in getting screened for breast cancer and availing mammography screening, as verified by this study where almost 47% had not received the recommended mammogram in the past year. MTM-based educational and policy interventions can help Asian American women, particularly those 45–54 years old, meet the recommendations of annual mammograms thereby reducing disparities for this high-risk subgroup in the U.S. population.

Author Contributions: Conceptualization, M.S.; methodology, M.S.; K.B., C.-L.D., C.-C.C.; software, K.B., C.-L.D., C.-C.C.; validation, M.S.; K.B., C.-L.D., C.-C.C.; formal analysis, C.-L.D., C.-C.C., K.B.; investigation, M.S.; K.B., C.-L.D., C.-C.C., J.R.P., C.C., A.A., H.C.; resources, M.S., K.B., C.-L.D., C.-C.C.; data curation, M.S., K.B.; writing— M.S.; K.B., C.-L.D., C.C.C., J.P., C.C., A.A., H.C.; writing—review and editing, M.S., K.B., C.-L.D., C.-C.C., J.R.P., C.C., A.A., H.C.; visualization, K.B., C.-L.D., C.-C.C.; supervision, M.S.; project administration, M.S., K.B. All authors have read and agreed to the published version of the manuscript.

Funding: Funding for data collection was provided by the School of Public Health, University of Nevada, Las Vegas.

Institutional Review Board Statement: The study was conducted according to the guidelines of the Declaration of Helsinki and approved by the Institutional Review Board (or Ethics Committee) of the University of Nevada, Las Vegas (1727672-1 dated 4 March 2021).

Informed Consent Statement: Informed consent was obtained from all subjects involved in the study.

Data Availability Statement: The data presented in this study are available on request from the corresponding author. The data are not publicly available due to ethical reasons.

Conflicts of Interest: The authors declare no conflict of interest.

Appendix A

Table A1. Values of Selected Fit Statistics for Hypothesized Measurement and Full Structural Models.

Hypothesis/Model	χ^2	*df*	RMSEA (90% CI)	CFI	TLI
Initiation model	304.56 **	142	0.06(0.05–0.06)	0.96	0.95
Sustenance Model	152.98 **	48	0.08(0.06–0.09)	0.97	0.95

** $p < 0.01$.

Table A2. Unstandardized and Standardized Parameter Estimates of Initiation Model.

			b	*SE*	*p* *	*β*
Initiation Model						
x14	←	Advantages	1.000	-	-	0.682
x15	←	Advantages	1.326	0.122	<0.001	0.907
x16	←	Advantages	1.310	0.118	<0.001	0.907
x17	←	Advantages	1.319	0.127	<0.001	0.847
x18	←	Advantages	1.221	0.115	<0.001	0.750
x19	←	Disadvantages	1.000	-	-	0.344
x20	←	Disadvantages	1.623	0.301	<0.001	0.565
x21	←	Disadvantages	2.292	0.393	<0.001	0.766
x22	←	Disadvantages	2.284	0.399	<0.001	0.793
x23	←	Disadvantages	1.212	0.234	<0.001	0.486
x24	←	Behavioral Confidence	1.000	-	-	0.737
x25	←	Behavioral Confidence	1.072	0.065	<0.001	0.815
x26	←	Behavioral Confidence	1.060	0.065	<0.001	0.773
x27	←	Behavioral Confidence	1.180	0.071	<0.001	0.915
x28	←	Behavioral Confidence	1.150	0.065	<0.001	0.895
x29	←	Physical Environment	1.000	-	-	0.925
x30	←	Physical Environment	0.965	0.048	<0.001	0.818
x31	←	Physical Environment	1.014	0.047	<0.001	0.862
Initiation	←	Advantages	0.594	0.135	<0.001	0.249
Initiation	←	Disadvantages	−0.446	0.169	<0.001	−0.130
Initiation	←	Behavioral Confidence	0.545	0.113	<0.001	0.371
Initiation	←	Physical Environment	0.223	0.102	<0.001	0.156
Advantages	↔	Disadvantages	−0.052	0.019	<0.001	−0.248
Behavioral Confidence	↔	Advantages	0.243	0.033	<0.001	0.500
Behavioral Confidence	↔	Disadvantages	−0.128	0.036	<0.001	−0.380
Physical Environment	↔	Advantages	0.257	0.032	<0.001	0.515
Physical Environment	↔	Disadvantages	−0.099	0.031	<0.001	−0.286
Physical Environment	↔	Behavioral Confidence	0.592	0.060	<0.001	0.730

* Marker variable *p* values are from tests of standardized effect significance. ← represents connections between nodes (variables). ↔ indicates covariance of residuals between sets of variables.

Table A3. Unstandardized and Standardized Parameter Estimates for Sustenance Model.

			b	*SE*	*p* *	*β*
Sustenance Model						
x32	←	Emotional Transformation	1.000	-	-	0.888
x33	←	Emotional Transformation	1.126	0.032	<0.001	0.947
x34	←	Emotional Transformation	1.045	0.035	<0.001	0.931
x35	←	Practice for Change	1.000	-	-	0.909
x36	←	Practice for Change	1.007	0.035	<0.001	0.932
x37	←	Practice for Change	0.935	0.042	<0.001	0.884
x38	←	Social Environment	1.000	-	-	0.831
x39	←	Social Environment	1.150	0.061	<0.001	0.827
x40	←	Social Environment	1.048	0.071	<0.001	0.845
x41	←	Social Environment	0.897	0.082	<0.001	0.610
x42	←	Social Environment	0.840	0.084	<0.001	0.557
Sustenance	←	Emotional Transformation	0.785	0.173	<0.001	0.612
Emotional Transformation	↔	Practice for Change	1.204	0.087	<0.001	0.937
Emotional Transformation	↔	Social Environment	0.784	0.073	<0.001	0.761
Practice for Change	↔	Social Environment	0.863	0.074	<0.001	0.826

* Marker variable *p* values are from tests of standardized effect significance. ← represents connections between nodes (variables). ↔ indicates covariance of residuals between sets of variables.

References

1. World Health Organization. Cancer. 2021. Available online: https://www.who.int/health-topics/cancer#tab=tab_1 (accessed on 1 May 2021).
2. Ghoncheh, M.; Pournamdar, Z.; Salehiniya, H. Incidence and mortality and epidemiology of breast cancer in the world. *Asian Pac. J. Cancer Prev.* **2016**, *17*, 43–46. [CrossRef] [PubMed]
3. DeSantis, C.E.; Ma, J.; Gaudet, M.M.; Newman, L.A.; Miller, K.D.; Goding Sauer, A.; Jemal, A.; Siegel, R.L. Breast cancer statistics, 2019. *CA Cancer J. Clin.* **2019**, *69*, 438–451. [CrossRef] [PubMed]
4. American Cancer Society. *Cancer Facts & Figures 2021*; American Cancer Society: Atlanta, GA, USA, 2021; Available online: https://www.cancer.org/content/dam/cancer-org/research/cancer-facts-and-statistics/annual-cancer-facts-and-figures/2021/cancer-facts-and-figures-2021.pdf (accessed on 1 May 2021).
5. Iqbal, J.; Ginsburg, O.; Rochon, P.A.; Sun, P.; Narod, S.A. Differences in breast cancer stage at diagnosis and cancer-specific survival by race and ethnicity in the United States. *JAMA* **2015**, *313*, 165–173. [CrossRef]
6. Morey, B.N.; Gee, G.C.; von Ehrenstein, O.S.; Shariff-Marco, S.; Canchola, A.J.; Yang, J.; Gomez, S.L. Higher breast cancer risk among immigrant Asian American women than among US-born Asian American women. *Prev. Chronic Dis.* **2019**, *16*, E20. [CrossRef] [PubMed]
7. Wu, T.Y.; Ronis, D. Correlates of recent and regular mammography screening among Asian-American women. *J. Adv. Nurs.* **2009**, *65*, 2434–2446. [CrossRef] [PubMed]
8. Parise, C.; Caggiano, V. Breast Cancer Mortality among Asian-American Women in California: Variation according to Ethnicity and Tumor Subtype. *J. Breast Cancer* **2016**, *19*, 112–121. [CrossRef]
9. Centers for Disease Control and Prevention. What Is Breast Cancer Screening? 2020. Available online: https://www.cdc.gov/cancer/breast/basic_info/screening.htm (accessed on 1 May 2021).
10. Løberg, M.; Lousdal, M.L.; Bretthauer, M.; Kalager, M. Benefits and harms of mammography screening. *Breast Cancer Res.* **2015**, *17*, 63. [CrossRef] [PubMed]
11. American College of Obstetricians and Gynecologists. Breast cancer risk assessment and screening in average-risk women. Practice Bulletin Number 179. *Obstet. Gynecol.* **2017**, *130*, e1–e16. [CrossRef] [PubMed]
12. Lee, M.H.; Merighi, J.R.; Lee, H.Y. Factors associated with mammogram use in Korean American immigrant women. *Am. J. Health Behav.* **2019**, *43*, 1075–1085. [CrossRef]
13. Oh, K.M.; Zhou, Q.P.; Kreps, G.L.; Ryu, S.K. Breast cancer screening practices among Asian Americans and Pacific Islanders. *Am. J. Health Behav.* **2012**, *36*, 711–722. [CrossRef]
14. Chawla, N.; Breen, N.; Liu, B.; Lee, R.; Kagawa-Singer, M. Asian American women in California: A pooled analysis of predictors for breast and cervical cancer screening. *Am. J. Public Health* **2015**, *105*, e98–e109. [CrossRef]
15. De Alba, I.; Hubbell, F.A.; McMullin, J.M.; Sweningson, J.M.; Saitz, R. Impact of U.S. citizenship status on cancer screening among immigrant women. *J. Gen. Intern. Med.* **2005**, *20*, 290–296. [CrossRef]

16. Somanchi, M.; Juon, H.S.; Rimal, R. Predictors of screening mammography among Asian Indian American women: A cross-sectional study in the Baltimore-Washington metropolitan area. *J. Womens Health* **2010**, *19*, 433–441. [CrossRef]
17. Boxwala, F.I.; Bridgemohan, A.; Griffith, D.M.; Soliman, A.S. Factors associated with breast cancer screening in Asian Indian women in metro-Detroit. *J. Immigr. Minor. Health* **2010**, *12*, 534–543. [CrossRef]
18. Kagawa-Singer, M.; Pourat, N.; Breen, N.; Coughlin, S.; Abend McLean, T.; McNeel, T.S.; Ponce, N.A. Breast and cervical cancer screening rates of subgroups of Asian American women in California. *Med. Care Res. Rev.* **2007**, *64*, 706–730. [CrossRef]
19. Padela, A.I.; Murrar, S.; Adviento, B.; Liao, C.; Hosseinian, Z.; Peek, M.; Curlin, F. Associations between religion-related factors and breast cancer screening among American Muslims. *J. Immigr. Minor. Health* **2015**, *17*, 660–669. [CrossRef] [PubMed]
20. Padela, A.I.; Vu, M.; Muhammad, H.; Marfani, F.; Mallick, S.; Peek, M.; Quinn, M.T. Religious beliefs and mammography intention: Findings from a qualitative study of a diverse group of American Muslim women. *Psychooncology* **2016**, *25*, 1175–1182. [CrossRef] [PubMed]
21. Pourat, N.; Kagawa-Singer, M.; Breen, N.; Sripipatana, A. Access versus acculturation: Identifying modifiable factors to promote cancer screening among Asian American women. *Med. Care* **2010**, *48*, 1088–1096. [CrossRef] [PubMed]
22. Miller, B.C.; Bowers, J.M.; Payne, J.B.; Moyer, A. Barriers to mammography screening among racial and ethnic minority women. *Soc. Sci. Med.* **2019**, *239*, 112494. [CrossRef]
23. Battaglia, T.A.; Roloff, K.; Posner, M.A.; Freund, K.M. Improving follow-up to abnormal breast cancer screening in an urban population. A patient navigation intervention. *Cancer* **2007**, *109*, 359–367. [CrossRef]
24. Berger, S.; Huang, C.C.; Rubin, C.L. The role of community education in increasing knowledge of breast health and cancer: Findings from the Asian Breast Cancer Project in Boston, Massachusetts. *J. Cancer Educ.* **2017**, *32*, 16–23. [CrossRef]
25. Dang, J.; Lee, J.; Tran, J.H.; Kagawa-Singer, M.; Foo, M.A.; Nguyen, T.U.; Valdez-Dadia, A.; Thomson, J.; Tanjasiri, S.P. The role of medical interpretation on breast and cervical cancer screening among Asian American and Pacific Islander women. *J. Cancer Educ.* **2010**, *25*, 253–262. [CrossRef] [PubMed]
26. Keshinro, A.; Hatzaras, I.; Rifkind, K.; Dhage, S.; Joseph, K.A. The impact of primary care providers on patient screening mammography and initial presentation in an underserved clinical setting. *Ann. Surg. Oncol.* **2017**, *24*, 692–697. [CrossRef] [PubMed]
27. Padela, A.I.; Malik, S.; Ally, S.A.; Quinn, M.; Hall, S.; Peek, M. Reducing Muslim mammography disparities: Outcomes from a religiously tailored mosque-based intervention. *Health Educ. Behav.* **2018**, *45*, 1025–1035. [CrossRef] [PubMed]
28. Padela, A.I.; Malik, S.; Din, H.; Hall, S.; Quinn, M. Changing mammography-related beliefs among American Muslim women: Findings from a religiously tailored mosque-based intervention. *J. Immigr. Minor. Health* **2019**, *21*, 1325–1333. [CrossRef]
29. Sadler, G.R.; Beerman, P.R.; Lee, K.; Hung, J.; Nguyen, H.; Cho, J.; Huang, W. Promoting breast cancer screening among Asian American women: The Asian grocery store-based cancer education program. *J. Cancer Educ.* **2012**, *27*, 612–617. [CrossRef] [PubMed]
30. Lee, E.E.; Brecht, M.L.; Park, H.; Lee, J.; Oh, K.M. Web-based study for improving mammography among Korean American women. *J. Cancer Educ.* **2017**, *32*, 257–263. [CrossRef] [PubMed]
31. Wu, T.Y.; West, B.T. Mammography stage of adoption and decision balance among Asian Indian and Filipino American women. *Cancer Nurs.* **2007**, *30*, 390–398. [CrossRef]
32. Sun, Y.; Sarma, E.A.; Moyer, A.; Messina, C.R. Promoting mammography screening among Chinese American women using a message-framing intervention. *Patient Educ. Couns.* **2015**, *98*, 878–883. [CrossRef]
33. Sharma, M. Multi-theory model (MTM) for health behavior change. *WebmedCentral Behav.* **2015**, *6*, WMC004982. Available online: http://www.webmedcentral.com/article_view/4982 (accessed on 6 April 2021).
34. Sharma, M. *Theoretical Foundations of Health Education and Health Promotion*, 4th ed.; Jones and Bartlett: Burlington, MA, USA, 2021; pp. 250–262. ISBN 978-1284208627.
35. Agyei-Baffour, P.; Asare, M.; Lanning, B.; Koranteng, A.; Millan, C.; Commeh, M.E.; Montealegre, J.R.; Mamudu, H.M. Human papillomavirus vaccination practices and perceptions among Ghanaian healthcare providers: A qualitative study based on multi-theory model. *PLoS ONE* **2020**, *15*, e0240657. [CrossRef]
36. Mousali, A.; Moradveisi, L.; Barati, M.; Moeini, B.; Bashirian, S.; Sharma, M.; Mohammadi, Y. Male addicts' experiences on predictors of relapse to drug use: A directed qualitative content analysis. *Addicta Turk. J. Addict.* **2020**, *7*, 166–173. [CrossRef]
37. Asare, M.; Agyei-Baffour, P.; Lanning, B.A.; Owusu, A.B.; Commeh, M.E.; Boozer, K.; Koranteng, A.; Spies, L.A.; Montealegre, J.R.; Paskett, E.D. Multi-theory model and predictors of likelihood of accepting the series of HPV vaccination: A cross-sectional study among Ghanaian adolescents. *Int. J. Environ. Res. Public Health* **2020**, *17*, 571. [CrossRef] [PubMed]
38. Sharma, M.; Largo-Wight, E.; Kanekar, A.; Kusumoto, H.; Hooper, S.; Nahar, V.K. Using the multi-theory model (MTM) of health behavior change to explain intentional outdoor nature contact behavior among college students. *Int. J. Environ. Res. Public Health* **2020**, *17*, 6104. [CrossRef]
39. Sharma, M.; Batra, K.; Davis, R.; Wilkerson, A. Explaining handwashing behavior among college students during COVID-19 pandemic using the multi-theory model (MTM) of health behavior change. *Healthcare* **2021**, *9*, 55. Available online: https://www.mdpi.com/2227-9032/9/1/55 (accessed on 1 May 2021). [CrossRef]
40. Williams, J.L.; Sharma, M.; Mendy, V.L.; Leggett, S.; Akil, L.; Perkins, S. Using multi theory model (MTM) of health behavior change to explain intention for initiation and sustenance of the consumption of fruits and vegetables among African American men from barbershops in Mississippi. *Health Promot. Perspect.* **2020**, *10*, 200–206. [CrossRef]

41. Bashirian, S.; Barati, M.; Sharma, M.; Abasi, H.; Karami, M. Water pipe smoking reduction in the male adolescent students: An educational intervention using multi-theory model. *J. Res. Health Sci.* **2019**, *19*, e00438.
42. Brown, L.; Sharma, M.; Leggett, S.; Sung, J.H.; Bennett, R.L.; Azevedo, M. Efficacy testing of the SAVOR (Sisters Adding Fruits and Vegetables for Optimal Results) intervention among African American women: A randomized controlled trial. *Health Promot. Perspect.* **2020**, *10*, 270–280. [CrossRef]
43. Hayes, T.; Sharma, M.; Shahbazi, M.; Sung, J.H.; Bennett, R.; Reese-Smith, J. The evaluation of a fourth-generation multi-theory model (MTM) based intervention to initiate and sustain physical activity in African American women. *Health Promot. Perspect.* **2019**, *9*, 13–23. [CrossRef]
44. Qualtrics Market Research Panel Survey. 2021. Available online: https://www.qualtrics.com/market-research/ (accessed on 1 May 2021).
45. Miller, C.A.; Guidry, J.P.D.; Dahman, B.; Thomson, M.D. A tale of two diverse Qualtrics samples: Information for online survey researchers. *Cancer Epidemiol. Biomark. Prev.* **2020**, *29*, 731–735. [CrossRef]
46. Cohen, J. *Statistical Power Analysis for the Behavioral Sciences*, 2nd ed.; Lawrence Erlbaum Associates: Mahwah, NJ, USA, 1988; ISBN 0-8058-0283-5. Available online: http://utstat.toronto.edu/~{}brunner/oldclass/378f16/readings/CohenPower.pdf (accessed on 1 May 2021).
47. Faul, F.; Erdfelder, E.; Buchner, A.; Lang, A.G. Statistical power analyses using G*Power 3.1: Tests for correlation and regression analyses. *Behav. Res. Methods* **2009**, *41*, 1149–1160. [CrossRef]
48. Bollen, K.A. A new incremental fit index for general structural equation models. *Socio. Methods. Res.* **1989**, *17*, 303–316. [CrossRef]
49. Byrne, B.M. *Structural Equation Modeling with AMOS: Basic Concepts, Applications, and Programming*, 2nd ed.; Routledge Taylor & Francis Group: New York, NY, USA, 2001; ISBN 978-0-8058-6372-7.
50. Hu, L.; Bentler, P.M. Cutoff criteria for fit indexes in covariance structure analysis: Conventional criteria versus new alternatives. *Struc. Equ. Model. Multidiscp. J.* **1999**, *6*, 1–55. [CrossRef]
51. Browne, M.W.; Cudeck, R. Alternative Ways of Assessing Model fit. In *Testing Structural Equation Models*; Bollen, K.A., Long, J.S., Eds.; SAGE Publications: Newbury Park, UK, 1993; pp. 136–162. ISBN 978-0803945074.
52. Nunnally, J.C. *Psychometric Theory*; McGraw-Hill: New York, NY, USA, 1967.
53. Lipsey, M.W.; Wilson, D.B. The efficacy of psychological, educational, and behavioral treatment: Confirmation from meta-analysis. *Am. Psychol.* **1993**, *48*, 1181–1209. [CrossRef]
54. Sharma, M.; Petosa, R.L. *Measurement and Evaluation for Health Educators*, 1st ed.; Jones & Bartlett Learning: Burlington, MA, USA, 2014.
55. Soper, D.S. A-Priori Sample Size Calculator for Structural Equation Models [Software]. 2021. Available online: https://www.danielsoper.com/statcalc (accessed on 3 April 2021).
56. Hoyle, R.H.; Gottfredson, N.C. Sample Size Considerations in Prevention Research Applications of Multilevel Modeling and Structural Equation Modeling. *Prev. Sci.* **2015**, *16*, 987–996. [CrossRef] [PubMed]
57. Muthén, L.K.; Muthén, B.O. How to use a Monte Carlo study to decide on sample size and determine power. *Struct. Equ. Modeling APA PsycNet.* **2002**, *9*, 599–620. [CrossRef]
58. Wolf, E.J.; Harrington, K.M.; Clark, S.L.; Miller, M.W. Sample Size Requirements for Structural Equation Models: An Evaluation of Power, Bias, and Solution Propriety. *Educ. Psychol. Meas.* **2013**, *76*, 913–934. [CrossRef]

pharmacy

MDPI

Article

Adherence to and Persistence with Adalimumab Therapy among Swedish Patients with Crohn's Disease

Yifei Liu [1,*], Joakim Söderberg [2] and Jingdong Chao [3]

[1] Division of Pharmacy Practice and Administration, The University of Missouri–Kansas City School of Pharmacy, Kansas City, MO 64108, USA
[2] Health Solutions, 118 26 Stockholm, Sweden; joakim.soderberg@healthsolutions.se
[3] Regeneron Pharmaceuticals, Inc., Tarrytown, NY 10591, USA; jingdong.chao@regeneron.com
* Correspondence: liuyif@umkc.edu

Abstract: Objectives: (1) to determine the adherence and persistence rates of adalimumab therapy among Swedish patients with Crohn's disease (CD), and (2) to compare self-administration devices to predict the medication adherence and persistence. Methods: We conducted a retrospective analysis of the Swedish National Board of Health and Welfare database during a unique time period, when both the pen and the syringe were available. The pen was proposed to indicate a larger extent of internal control, according to health locus of control. Medication adherence was defined as a medication possession ratio (MPR) ≥ 0.8. A patient was considered nonpersistent if the time between any two dispensing records, minus the days of supply dispensed exceeded 180 days. The predictors of adherence were evaluated using a logistic regression, and the predictors of persistence were evaluated using a Cox proportional hazards model. Results: Among the 1083 patients studied, 89% were adherent and 77% were persistent. The patients using the pen and the patients treated in gastroenterology centers were more likely to be adherent and less likely to be nonpersistent. Conclusions: The adherence rate to adalimumab therapy was 89% and the one-year persistence rate was 70%. The pen and treatment in a gastroenterology center had a positive impact on the adherence and persistence among Swedish patients with CD.

Keywords: medication adherence; medication persistence; health locus of control; adalimumab

1. Introduction

Crohn's disease (CD), a common type of inflammatory bowel disease (IBD), has become a global disease [1]. In Europe, the direct health care costs are approximately EUR 3500 for CD per patient per year [2]. Additionally, there is a clear north–south gradient for CD incidence rates, with European countries in the north having a much higher rate [3]. In Sweden, the CD incidence rate was 8.1 per 100,000 person–years from 1990 to 2014 [4], and the prevalence of CD was 0.19% in 2010 [5].

Medication adherence and persistence have important implications for the long-term management of CD, because the ultimate goal of therapy is to induce and maintain remission. Medication adherence is "the extent to which a patient acts in accordance with the prescribed interval and dose of a dosing regimen," whereas medication persistence is "the duration of time from initiation to discontinuation of therapy" [6].

Health locus of control distinguishes the dimensions of internal and external control [7,8]. The former is the belief that health is under one's own control, whereas the latter is the belief that health is under the control of external factors. Health locus of control has an impact on medication adherence [9,10]. In general, internal control is associated with better medication adherence [9], although occasionally opposite findings are demonstrated [10]. Nevertheless, in terms of predicting health outcomes, while plenty of studies have compared the impact of internal vs. external control factors, fewer have examined the varying extent of control within the same dimension of either internal or external control.

For patients with moderate to severe CD who do not respond to glucocorticoids or immunomodulators, tumor necrosis factor (TNF) inhibitors including adalimumab therapy, are recommended to induce and maintain remission [11,12]. There was a time period in Sweden when two types of self-administration devices for adalimumab therapy were available at the same time. One was a single-use, prefilled auto-injection pen, and the other was a single-use, prefilled glass syringe. Compared with the syringe, the pen was relatively new and had an improved design enclosing a syringe with protective caps and an activator button [13].

According to health locus of control, the self-administration of either device would be under a patient's internal control. Yet, with its improved design to help patients carry and administer the medication, the pen would indicate a larger extent of internal control than the syringe. We hypothesized that a larger extent of internal control would yield better health outcomes. Namely, the pen would lead to better adherence to and persistence with adalimumab therapy than the syringe. The objectives of our study were to (1) determine the adherence and persistence rates of adalimumab therapy among Swedish patients with CD, and (2) compare the pen vs. the syringe to predict the medication adherence and persistence in this population.

2. Methods

This was a retrospective cohort study of adalimumab dispensing records, among Swedish patients with CD. We focused on the time period from 6 July 2005 to 30 September 2009, because of the availability of 2 self-administration devices in Sweden during this period, and also because of data access. The Swedish National Board of Health and Welfare is a government agency that maintains data in the areas of health, medical care, and social services [14]. Study subjects were all patients with CD in the Swedish National Board of Health and Welfare database. The dispensing records contained the following information: patient age group, sex, days of supply associated with a dispensing activity, self-administration device (pen or syringe), prescriber specialty (gastroenterologist or other), and prescriber practice setting (gastroenterology, internal medicine, or other).

Utilizing health locus of control, as mentioned earlier, we proposed that the self-administration device would be a proxy of the varying extent of internal control (Figure 1), and the pen would be associated with a larger extent. In addition, we proposed that prescriber characteristics such as specialty and practice setting would be factors of external control. Furthermore, the health outcomes would include both medication adherence and persistence. Of note, owing to secondary data, we were unable to directly measure the variables of health locus of control with survey items. Instead, we used the self-administration device as a proxy for the varying extent of internal control, and prescriber characteristics as factors of external control.

The index date was the date of the first adalimumab dispensing record. If a patient did not switch self-administration device or prescriber (either specialty or practice setting), the censoring date was 30 September 2009. If a patient switched the device or prescriber, the refill date before the earliest switch date was the censoring date. That is, for patients who made a switch, we only examined the dispensing records before the switch.

Refill adherence is one way to capture medication adherence and can be measured by medication possession ratio (MPR) [15]. We calculated MPR for each patient using the days of supply dispensed (excluding the last dispensing record), divided by the number of days between the first and last dispensing records, from the index date to the censoring date. Patients who had only 1 dispensing record were excluded from MPR calculation. Then patients were identified as adherent (MPR $\geq$ 0.8) vs. non-adherent (MPR $<$ 0.8).

To capture persistence, we measured the duration of therapy for each patient by the time gap between any 2 dispensing records, minus the days of supply dispensed, with the earlier record from the index date to censoring date. For patients who had 1 dispensing record, the duration of therapy was measured by the time gap between the dispensing record and the censoring date, minus the days of supply dispensed. In Sweden, the reimbursement regulations only allowed the dispensing of medications for up to a 90-day supply at a time and a patient could not refill the prescriptions until 60 days after the dispensing. Therefore, a patient was considered non-persistent if the time gap was greater than 180 days.

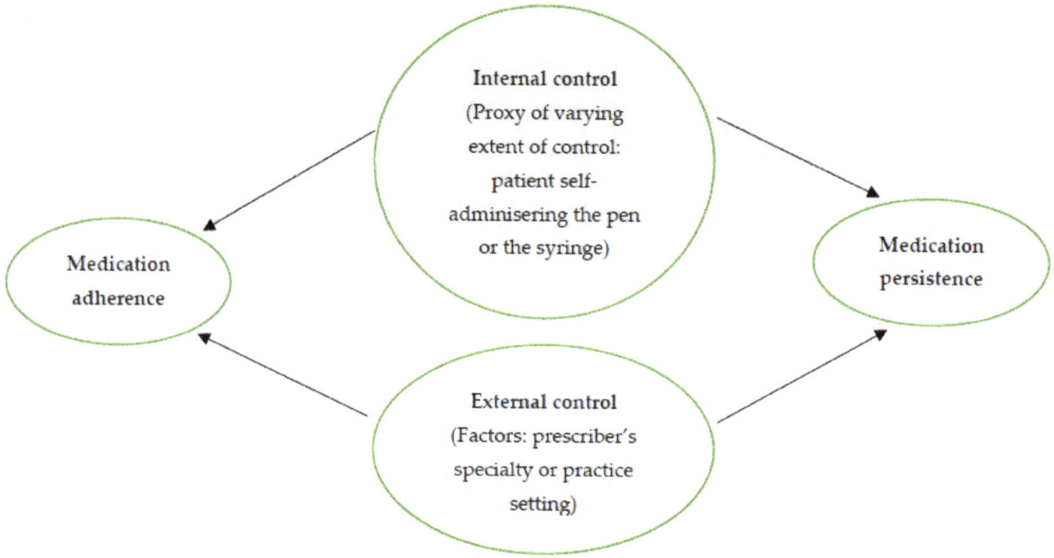

Figure 1. Proposed framework, based on health locus of control and data available.

Descriptive statistical analyses were performed for adherence (yes/no), MPR, persistence (yes/no), days of persistence, and the other variables. A logistic regression was conducted, in which the outcome variable was medication refill adherence (yes/no) and the independent variables included age group, sex, dispensing device, prescriber specialty, and prescriber practice setting. A Cox proportional hazards model was developed, in which the outcome variable was medication non-persistence (yes/no), and the independent variables were the same as in the logistic regression. We used the Statistical Analysis System (SAS Institute, Cary, NC, USA) to restructure the original data and the Statistical Package for Social Science (IBM Corporation, Armonk, NY, USA) to analyze the data after the data restructure.

3. Results

A total of 1083 patients were identified and included in the analyses, of which 52.6% were female and 61.3% used the pen (Table 1). The prescriber for most patients was a gastroenterologist, and more than half of the patients had a prescriber who worked in an internal medicine setting. The average MPR was 0.93, with 790 patients (89%) identified as medication adherent (MPR $\geq$ 0.8) and 837 patients (77%) identified as medication persistent.

The self-administration device and the prescriber practice setting were significant predictors of medication adherence in the logistic regression (Table 2). Compared with the patients using a syringe, the patients using a pen were more likely to be adherent, with an odds ratio (OR) of 1.78 (95% confidence interval [CI]: 1.14, 2.78). The patients whose prescribers worked in a gastroenterology center were more likely to be adherent than the patients whose prescribers worked in an internal medicine center, with an OR of 1.70 (95% CI: 1.04, 2.79).

In the Cox proportional hazards model of medication non-persistence, the self-administration device, the prescriber practice setting, and the sex of the patient were significant predictors (Table 3). The patients using a pen were less likely to be nonpersistent than those using a syringe, with a hazard ratio (HR) of 0.74 (95% CI: 0.56, 0.97). The patients whose prescribers worked in a gastroenterology center were less likely to be nonpersistent than the patients whose prescribers worked in an internal medicine center, with an HR of 0.64 (95% CI: 0.48, 0.86). Compared with the female patients, the male patients were less likely to be nonpersistent, with an HR of 0.75 (95% CI: 0.57, 0.97).

Table 1. Patient and prescriber characteristics.

Characteristic	Values
Adherence, *n* (%)	
Yes (MPR ≥ 0.8)	790 (88.6)
No (MPR < 0.8)	102 (11.4)
Total [a]	892 (100)
MPR	
Mean (SD)	93.47 (14.97)
Range	9.98–100
Total, N [a]	892
Persistence, *n* (%)	
Yes (gap ≤ 180 days)	837 (77.3)
No (gap > 180 days)	246 (22.7)
Total	1083 (100)
Days of persistence	
Mean (SD)	233.09 (217.12)
Range	0–1315
Total, N	1083
Age group, *n* (%)	
20–29	300 (29.0)
30–39	246 (23.8)
40–49	237 (22.9)
50+	251 (24.3)
Total, N [a]	1034 (100)
Sex, *n* (%)	
Women	570 (52.6)
Men	513 (47.4)
Total	1083 (100)
Self-administration device, *n* (%)	
Pen	664 (61.3)
Syringe	419 (38.7)
Total	1083 (100)
Prescriber specialty, *n* (%)	
Gastroenterology	994 (96.2)
Others	39 (3.8)
Total [b]	1033
Prescriber practice setting, *n* (%)	
Internal medicine center	598 (55.3)
Gastroenterology center	413 (38.2)
Others	71 (6.5)
Total [b]	1082

[a] Total numbers vary because of missing value and exclusion of cases for which MPR was not calculable. [b] Total numbers vary because of missing values. MPR = medication possession ratio; SD=standard deviation.

Table 2. Logistic regression model of medication possession ratio (N [a] = 818).

Independent Variables	Beta Coefficient	Odds Ratio (95% Confidence Interval)
Age group [b]		
30–39	−0.40	0.67 (0.37, 1.21)
40–49	−0.29	0.75 (0.41, 1.36)
50+	0.30	1.36 (0.69, 2.65)
Sex (male) [c]	−0.06	0.94 (0.61, 1.46)
Self-administration device (pen) [d]	0.58 [e]	1.78 (1.14, 2.78)
Prescriber specialty (other) [f]	0.66	1.94 (0.44, 8.54)
Prescriber practice setting [g]		
Gastroenterology	0.53 [e]	1.70 (1.04, 2.79)
Other	0.93	2.53 (0.76, 8.42)

[a] N = 818 due to missing values. [b] The reference group is 20–29 years. [c] The reference group is female. [d] The reference group is syringe. [e] Significant at the 0.05 level. [f] The reference group is gastroenterology. [g] The reference group is internal medicine.

Table 3. Cox proportional hazards model of adalimumab non-persistence.

Regression Model	Adalimumab Non-Persistence (N [a] =961)	
Chi-square	20.48 [b]	
Independent Variables	**Beta Coefficient**	**Hazard Ratio (95% Confidence Interval)**
Age group [c]		
30–39	−0.05	0.95 (0.65, 1.38)
40–49	−0.10	0.90 (0.62, 1.32)
50+	0.11	1.11 (0.78, 1.59)
Sex (Men) [d]	−0.30 [e]	0.75 (0.57, 0.97)
Dispensing device (pen) [f]	−0.30 [e]	0.74 (0.56, 0.97)
Prescriber specialty (other) [g]	−0.02	0.99 (0.46, 2.11)
Prescriber practice setting [h]		
Gastroenterology	−0.45 [b]	0.64 (0.48, 0.86)
Other	0.08	1.08 (0.59, 2.00)

[a] N = 961 due to missing values. [b] Significant at the 0.01 level. [c] The reference group is 20–29 years. [d] The reference group is female. [e] Significant at the 0.05 level. [f] The reference group is syringe. [g] The reference group is gastroenterology. [h] The reference group is internal medicine.

4. Discussion

In this retrospective cohort study, the medication adherence rate was 89%. It was consistent with a pooled adalimumab adherence rate of 83% in a systematic review of adalimumab-treated patients with IBD [16]. Knowledge of the factors associated with TNF inhibitor adherence and persistence may help health care professionals to identify patients at risk of nonadherence and non-persistence, and to modify their prescribing practices or their medication management strategies among Swedish patients with CD.

Our study shows that health locus of control helps understand medication adherence and persistence. The predictive utility of the pen supported our hypothesis. Based on the improved design of the pen [13], we hypothesized that the self-administration of the pen would give patients a larger extent of internal control than the syringe. In fact, the pen is perceived as easier to use and more convenient [17]. Moreover, patients experience less pain when using the pen as opposed to the syringe, to self-administer adalimumab therapy [18]. The literature suggests that internal control is generally associated with better medication adherence than external control [9]. What this study adds to the literature, is that within the dimension of internal control, a larger extent of control is associated with better adherence to and persistence with adalimumab therapy. Therefore, the different extent of internal control can play a role in determining health outcomes.

Between the two external factors, the prescriber's practice setting affected both the medication adherence and persistence, whereas the prescriber's specialty had no impact. Specifically, the patients treated in a gastroenterology center were 70% more likely to be adherent to adalimumab therapy and 36% more likely to be persistent with adalimumab therapy, compared with the patients treated in an internal medicine center. There may be various aspects of medication management in a specialty practice setting that positively influence patients' adherence and persistence, such as enhanced patient education and prescriber communication. Also, patients who visit a gastroenterology center may have more severe conditions, and thus may be more adherent to and persistent with the therapy.

In our analysis, the male patients with CD were less likely to be nonpersistent with adalimumab therapy than the female patients. This finding has been previously reported, though the results across the studies are inconsistent. Kane and Dixon reported that female patients with CD were less likely to be adherent to infliximab therapy [19], and Liu et al. found that women with CD were less adherent to adalimumab therapy than men [20]. However, sex has not predicted medication adherence in other studies of patients with IBD [16,21–23].

Our study had four limitations. First, the 0.8 MPR threshold used to define adherence is commonly used in medication adherence research, but whether the threshold is clinically optimal for a specific study sample is unknown [24]. Additionally, we assumed that medication refill was equivalent to medication usage. Second, because we retrospectively extracted dispensing-related information from a secondary database, we did not have any information on the baseline disease characteristics, such as the disease activity, disease duration, concomitant and prior therapies, the duration of therapy, comorbidities, surgical history, or other disease- and treatment-related factors that may have influenced the patients' medication adherence and persistence. Third, our study had limited generalizability. Our analysis included only Swedish patients with CD and may not be generalizable to other non-northern European populations. Similarly, we only included adalimumab therapy, and the results may not be generalizable to other therapies. Fourth, the study timeframe was constrained by data access. Unfortunately, we do not have access to updated data.

For future research, updated or more specific data are needed to understand the reasons underlying TNF inhibitor adherence and persistence among patients with CD. For example, further explorations of disease-related factors may allow clinicians to target patients with appropriate disease management strategies. In addition, understanding the specific factors that explain the better medication adherence and persistence in gastroenterology centers may allow health care systems to optimize their treatment paradigms for patients with CD.

5. Conclusions

In this study, among Swedish patients with CD, the medication adherence rate was 89% and the one-year medication persistence rate was 70%. Under health locus of control, the self-administration device of adalimumab therapy could be regarded as a proxy for varying internal control. In Swedish patients with CD, the pen (a proxy for a larger extent of internal control than the syringe) and treatment in a gastroenterology center (an external control factor) had a positive impact on both the adherence to and persistence with adalimumab therapy.

Author Contributions: Conceptualization, Y.L.; methodology, Y.L.; formal analysis, Y.L.; investigation, Y.L.; resources, J.S. and J.C.; data curation, Y.L., J.S. and J.C.; writing—original draft preparation, Y.L.; writing—review and editing, Y.L., J.S. and J.C.; project administration, J.C.; funding acquisition, Y.L. All authors have read and agreed to the published version of the manuscript.

Funding: The study was funded by AbbVie Inc., North Chicago, IL, USA.

Institutional Review Board Statement: An ethical review exemption was granted by the University of Missouri–Kansas City Institutional Review Board for this study, due to existing data.

Informed Consent Statement: Not applicable.

Data Availability Statement: Data sharing is not applicable to this article.

Acknowledgments: We acknowledge Parvez M. Mulani for his support with this study, and Dana L. Randall for her medical writing services.

Conflicts of Interest: At the time of study, Jingdong Chao was an employee of AbbVie Inc.

References

1. Ng, S.C.; Shi, H.Y.; Hamidi, N.; Underwood, F.E.; Tang, W.; Benchimol, E.I.; Panaccione, R.; Ghosh, S.; Wu, J.C.Y.; Chan, F.K.L.; et al. Worldwide incidence and prevalence of inflammatory bowel disease in the 21st century: A systematic review of population-based studies. *Lancet* **2017**, *390*, 2769–2778. [CrossRef]
2. Zhao, M.; Gönczi, L.; Lakatos, P.L.; Burisch, J. The Burden of Inflammatory Bowel Disease in Europe in 2020. *J. Crohn's Colitis* **2021**, *15*, 1573–1587. [CrossRef] [PubMed]
3. Shivananda, S.; Lennard-Jones, J.; Logan, R.; Fear, N.; Price, A.; Carpenter, L.; Van Blankenstein, M. Incidence of inflammatory bowel disease across Europe: Is there a difference between north and south? Results of the European Collaborative Study on Inflammatory Bowel Disease (EC-IBD). *Gut* **1996**, *39*, 690–697. [CrossRef]
4. Forss, A.; Clements, M.; Bergman, D.; Roelstraete, B.; Kaplan, G.G.; Myrelid, P.; Halfvarson, J.; Olén, O.; Ludvigsson, J.F. A nationwide cohort study of the incidence of inflammatory bowel disease in Sweden from 1990 to 2014. *Aliment. Pharmacol. Ther.* **2022**, *55*, 691–699. [CrossRef] [PubMed]
5. Büsch, K.; Ludvigsson, J.F.; Ekström-Smedby, K.; Ekbom, A.; Askling, J.; Neovius, M. Nationwide prevalence of inflammatory bowel disease in Sweden: A population-based register study. *Aliment. Pharmacol. Ther.* **2014**, *39*, 57–68. [CrossRef]
6. Cramer, J.A.; Roy, A.; Burrell, A.; Fairchild, C.J.; Fuldeore, M.J.; Ollendorf, D.A.; Wong, P.K. Medication compliance and persistence: Terminology and definitions. *Value Health* **2008**, *11*, 44–47. [CrossRef]
7. Wallston, K.A.; Wallston, B.S. Who is responsible for your health? The construct of health locus of control. In *Social Psychology of Health and Illness*; Sanders, G., Suls, J., Eds.; Lawrence Erlbaum and Associates: Hillsdale, MI, USA, 1982; pp. 65–95.
8. Luszczynska, A.; Schwarzer, R. Multidimensional health locus of control: Comments on the construct and its measurement. *J. Health Psychol.* **2005**, *10*, 633–642. [CrossRef]
9. Nazareth, M.; Richards, J.; Javalkar, K.; Haberman, C.; Zhong, Y.; Rak, E.; Jain, N.; Ferris, M.; van Tilburg, M.A.L. Relating health locus of control to health care use, adherence, and transition readiness among youths with chronic conditions, North Carolina, 2015. *Prev. Chronic Dis.* **2016**, *21*, E93. [CrossRef]
10. Gerland, H.E.; Prell, T. Association between the health locus of control and medication adherence: An observational, cross-sectional study in primary care. *Front. Med.* **2021**, *8*, 705202. [CrossRef]
11. Terdiman, J.P.; Gruss, C.B.; Heidelbaugh, J.J.; Sultan, S.; Falck-Ytter, Y.T. AGA Institute Clinical Practice and Quality Management Committee. American Gastroenterological Association Institute guideline on the use of thiopurines, methotrexate, and anti-TNF-α biologic drugs for the induction and maintenance of remission in inflammatory Crohn's disease. *Gastroenterology* **2013**, *145*, 1459–1463.
12. Gomollón, F.; Dignass, A.; Annese, V.; Tilg, H.; Van Assche, G.; Lindsay, J.O.; Peyrin-Biroulet, L.; Cullen, G.J.; Daperno, M.; Kucharzik, T.; et al. 3rd European evidence-based consensus on the diagnosis and management of Crohn's Disease 2016: Part 1: Diagnosis and medical management. *J. Crohn's Colitis* **2017**, *11*, 3–25. [CrossRef] [PubMed]
13. Kivitz, A.; Segurado, O.G. HUMIRA pen: A novel autoinjection device for subcutaneous injection of the fully human monoclonal antibody adalimumab. *Expert Rev. Med. Devices* **2007**, *4*, 109–116. [CrossRef] [PubMed]
14. Sandberg, M. . *Reinforced Nordic Collaboration on Data Resources: Challenges from Six Perspectives*; Nordic Council of Ministers: Copenhagen, Denmark, 2012.
15. Andrade, S.E.; Kahler, K.H.; Frech, F.; Chan, K.A. Methods for evaluation of medication adherence and persistence using automated databases. *Pharmacoepidemiol. Drug Saf.* **2006**, *15*, 565–574. [CrossRef] [PubMed]
16. Lopez, A.; Billioud, V.; Peyrin-Biroulet, C.; Peyrin-Biroulet, L. Adherence to anti-TNF therapy in inflammatory bowel diseases: A systematic review. *Inflamm. Bowel Dis.* **2013**, *19*, 1528–1533. [CrossRef] [PubMed]
17. Borrás-Blasco, J.; Gracia-Pérez, A.; Rosique-Robles, J.D.; Casterá, M.D.; Abad, F.J. Acceptability of switching adalimumab from a prefilled syringe to an autoinjection pen. *Expert Opin. Biol. Ther.* **2010**, *10*, 301–307. [CrossRef] [PubMed]
18. Kivitz, A.; Cohen, S.; Dowd, J.E.; Edwards, W.; Thakker, S.; Wellborne, F.R.; Renz, C.L.; Segurado, O.G. Clinical assessment of pain, tolerability, and preference of an autoinjection pen versus a prefilled syringe for patient self-administration of the fully human, monoclonal antibody adalimumab: The TOUCH trial. *Clin. Ther.* **2006**, *28*, 1619–1629. [CrossRef]
19. Kane, S.; Dixon, L. Adherence rates with infliximab therapy in Crohn's disease. *Aliment. Pharmacol. Ther.* **2006**, *24*, 1099–1103. [CrossRef]
20. Liu, Y.; Yang, M.; Chao, J.; Mulani, P.M. Greater refill adherence to adalimumab therapy for patients using specialty versus retail pharmacies. *Adv. Ther.* **2010**, *27*, 523–532. [CrossRef]

21. Nahon, S.; Lahmek, P.; Saas, C.; Durance, C.; Olympie, A.; Lesgourgues, B.; Gendre, J.P. Socioeconomic and psychological factors associated with nonadherence to treatment in inflammatory bowel disease patients: Results of the ISSEO survey. *Inflamm. Bowel Dis.* **2011**, *17*, 1270–1276. [CrossRef]
22. Selinger, C.P.; Eaden, J.; Jones, D.B.; Katelaris, P.; Chapman, G.; McDonald, C.; Smith, P.; Lal, S.; Leong, R.W.; McLaughlin, J. Modifiable factors associated with nonadherence to maintenance medication for inflammatory bowel disease. *Inflamm. Bowel Dis.* **2013**, *19*, 2199–2206. [CrossRef]
23. Pittet, V.; Rogler, G.; Mottet, C.; Froehlich, F.; Michetti, P.; de Saussure, P.; Bernard, B.; John-Paul, V. The Swiss IBD Cohort Study Group Patients' information-seeking activity is associated with treatment compliance in inflammatory bowel disease patients. *Scand. J. Gastroenterol.* **2014**, *49*, 662–673. [CrossRef] [PubMed]
24. Peterson, A.M.; Nau, D.P.; Cramer, J.A.; Benner, J.; Gwadry-Sridhar, F.; Nichol, M. A checklist for medication compliance and persistence studies using retrospective databases. *Value Health* **2007**, *10*, 3–12. [CrossRef] [PubMed]

nursing reports

MDPI

Article

Influence of Sociodemographic Factors on Level Stress and Coping Strategies of Nurses and Midwives Caring for Newborns with Lethal Defects

Katarzyna Anna Urbańska [1,*], Beata Naworska [2] and Agnieszka Drosdzol-Cop [3]

[1] Neonatology Unit, BCM The Guardian Angels Hospital of the Brothers Hospitallers of St. John of God in Katowice, Markiefki 87, 40-211 Katowice, Poland

[2] Department of Gynaecology and Obstetrics, Faculty of Health Sciences in Katowice, Medical University of Silesia in Katowice, 40-751 Katowice, Poland

[3] Chair and Department of Gynecology, Obstetrics and Oncological Gynecology, Faculty of Medical Sciences in Katowice, Medical University of Silesia in Katowice, 40-211 Katowice, Poland

* Correspondence: kasiaurbanskaaa@gmail.com

Abstract: Introduction: Nurses and midwives caring for newborns with lethal defects experience significant emotional stress. Understanding coping strategies and the factors influencing stress is crucial for improving their well-being and ensuring high-quality care. **Objectives:** The aim of this study was to identify the coping strategies used by nurses and midwives in stressful situations and to analyse the relationship between stress levels and selected sociodemographic and professional factors. **Methods:** A cross-sectional study was conducted in the second quarter of 2023 among 307 nurses and midwives working in neonatal and obstetric wards in the Silesian metropolitan area, Poland. A diagnostic survey method was applied using a standardised questionnaire. The Perceived Stress Scale (PSS-10) and the MINI-COPE Inventory were used to assess stress levels and coping mechanisms. A stratified random sampling method was employed to ensure representation from various professional backgrounds. Data analysis was conducted using descriptive statistics, chi-square tests, Spearman's correlation, and Cohen's d coefficient, with statistical significance set at $p < 0.05$. **Results:** High stress levels were associated with shorter professional experience, frequent exposure to lethal defects, and emotional discomfort in interactions with grieving families. The most commonly used coping strategies were active coping (M = 2.06, SD = 0.635) and planning (M = 1.95, SD = 0.590), whereas self-blame (M = 1.20, SD = 0.714, $p < 0.001$) and denial (M = 0.88, SD = 0.751, $p < 0.001$) were linked to higher stress levels. Positive reinterpretation ($r = -0.211$, $p < 0.001$) and seeking emotional support ($r = -0.129$, $p = 0.024$) correlated with lower stress levels. Nurses and midwives with secondary education reported higher stress levels compared to those with higher education ($\chi^2(10) = 30.651$, $p = 0.001$). Work experience played a role, with moderate stress levels most frequently observed among those with 2–5 years of professional experience ($\chi^2(14) = 24.023$, $p = 0.046$). Emotional involvement, particularly supporting parents during their farewell to the child (69.1%), was identified as the most stressful aspect of their work. **Conclusions:** Promoting adaptive coping strategies, such as positive reinterpretation and emotional support, can help reduce stress and improve the well-being of nurses and midwives. Implementing psychological support programmes and stress management training is essential for maintaining high-quality neonatal care.

Keywords: level stress; sociodemographic factors; coping strategies; nurses; midwives; lethal defects; palliative care; neonatal nursing; congenital abnormalities

1. Introduction

Nursing is an extremely demanding and stressful profession that affects both the physical and mental health of nurses and midwives. The sources of stress are emotionally challenging situations, such as caring for critically ill patients or the need to manage the emotions of patients and their families [1]. This profession is associated with high levels of emotional, psychological, and physical strain, often leading to dissatisfaction with work [2]. More than 50% of nurses experience high levels of stress, making their profession more demanding than other medical fields, due to their direct involvement in patient care [1,3].

While a key aspect of midwifery is supporting patients through natural processes such as pregnancy and childbirth, in practice, they often face difficult and stressful experiences. These include complications during pregnancy, the birth of a child with serious illness or a lethal defect, miscarriage or stillbirth, all of which can lead to significant psychological distress among medical staff [4]. Death and dying are among the most challenging aspects of nursing and midwifery work, triggering extreme emotions and stress-related symptoms [1].

Studies show that occupational stress negatively affects the health of nurses and midwives, increasing the risk of health problems, absenteeism, errors, and burnout [2,5,6]. The death of a child is a traumatic experience not only for the mother and her family but also for the nursing staff, which can reduce the quality of care provided [7].

The term "stress" is widely used in various scientific fields and everyday language, yet there is no universally accepted definition. According to Alhabri [8], stress is a state of discomfort resulting from situations perceived as excessively demanding or beyond an individual's coping abilities. Goudarzian et al. highlight that nurses encounter various types of stress, including occupational, environmental, psychological, and emotional stress [1]. Occupational stress can result from heavy workloads, excessive empathy for patients' suffering, or a sense of responsibility [9]. The National Labour Inspectorate defines occupational stress as a state in which employees experience psychological discomfort due to work conditions or demands exceeding their abilities [10].

Additional factors triggering stress for nurses and midwives include delivering distressing news to patients and their families, life-threatening situations, ethical dilemmas, and the need to provide end-of-life care information [11–14]. Long-term exposure to a stressful work environment not only affects staff health but also increases the need for stress coping strategies [15]. A strategic approach includes both physical and psychological actions aimed at mitigating the negative effects of stress [16].

In recent years, healthcare organisations have implemented various interventions to support staff in managing stress. Growing interest is being given to stress management methods and improving the mental health of nurses, such as mindfulness, meditation, psychological support, and relaxation techniques [17,18]. While some of these interventions show promising results, studies by Chesak et al. [19] and Li et al. [20] indicate their moderate effectiveness, emphasising the need for further research. According to De Diego-Cordero et al. [21], nurses use a wide range of stress-coping strategies, with one of the key methods being reliance on religious and spiritual beliefs.

The phenomenon of stress in nursing includes reactions that arise in response to demands and pressures exceeding an individual's abilities [22].

In Poland, a three-tier referral system of care for pregnant women and newborns operates, providing differentiated levels of care depending on the complexity of the pregnancy and the health status of the newborn [23,24]:

1. Level I—provides basic care for women with physiological pregnancies and healthy newborns. At this level, prenatal education, childbirth preparation, and breastfeeding

and childcare education are conducted. Care focuses on prevention and early detection of abnormalities, which is crucial in reducing the risk of perinatal complications.

2. Level II—pertains to care for pregnancies at moderate risk and treatment of newborns with mild health problems. Level II hospitals have neonatology departments that care for premature infants and those needing medical supervision but not intensive therapy. Nurses and midwives at this level often face difficult clinical decisions and provide support to families dealing with complications during pregnancy and childbirth.
3. Level III—provides highly specialised care for high-risk pregnancies and intensive therapy for newborns born with serious defects and illnesses requiring advanced treatment. At this level, neonatal intensive care units (NICUs) are equipped with the latest medical technologies, such as mechanical ventilation, ECMO therapy, and advanced surgical procedures. Nurses working at this level must demonstrate high mental resilience and expertise in caring for critically ill patients.

Each of these levels involves varying degrees of psychological and physical strain for the medical staff. Working in Level II and III departments often requires coping with emotionally challenging situations such as the birth of a child with a fatal defect, prolonged hospitalisation of a newborn, or supporting families through the grieving process.

Therefore, implementing strategies to reduce stress among nursing staff and providing appropriate psychological support is of crucial importance.

Nursing staff working in neonatal intensive care units (NICUs) make every effort to provide the best care for critically ill children and their families. The death of a newborn and the grieving process significantly impact the staff, often causing deep emotional stress for nurses and midwives. Working in a NICU, Maternity Ward, Delivery Room, neonatology department, or perinatal hospice involves constant contact with suffering newborns and their families, leading to serious consequences for the mental, emotional, and physical health of the staff. Prolonged exposure to difficult situations, such as the death of patients, helplessness in the face of newborn suffering, or the need to support grieving families, can lead to post-traumatic stress disorder (PTSD) [25], burnout, and depression. Unfortunately, nurses and midwives do not always receive appropriate support from family, colleagues, or employers, making this issue an important topic for further research. The introduction of psychological support programmes, stress management training, and regular supervision could help improve the mental health of staff and the quality of care provided to patients.

2. Objectives

1. Identifying coping strategies in stressful situations. The first aim of the study was to identify specific coping strategies used by nurses and midwives in the face of stressful situations while caring for newborns with lethal malformations. This involved examining the coping mechanisms, resilience and potential adaptive or maladaptive behaviours that healthcare workers adopt to cope with the emotional and professional challenges associated with such critical care scenarios.

2. Exploring the relationship between stress levels and socio-demographic/professional factors. The second aim was to determine how stress levels among nurses and midwives correlated with selected socio-demographic and professional factors. This involved examining variables such as age, years of experience, work environment, educational level and personal background to assess their impact on the perception and management of stress in the context of palliative neonatal care.

3. Material and Methods

The study was conducted in the second quarter of 2023 in medical centres with secondary and tertiary levels of reference within the Silesian agglomeration in Poland. In order to obtain an opinion on the necessity of ethical approval for the study, a request was submitted to the Bioethics Committee of the Medical University of Silesia in Katowice. According to the decision of the Bioethics Committee of the Medical University of Silesia in Katowice (approval number: PCN/CBN/0052/KB/33/23 dated 28 March 2023), the study was not classified as a medical experiment and did not require ethical review by the Committee. Participation in the study was voluntary, and respondent anonymity was ensured.

A request for permission to conduct the study was sent to seven hospitals with tertiary-level reference in the three-tier system of care for pregnant women and neonates operating in the Silesian Voivodeship. Due to the refusal of three tertiary-level hospitals, an additional secondary-level hospital, which includes a perinatal hospice, was included in the study. In the Silesian Voivodeship, tertiary-level reference hospitals comprise University Hospital Clinics and Provincial Specialist Hospitals, secondary-level reference hospitals include Provincial Hospitals, Municipal Hospitals, and one private hospital, while primary-level reference hospitals include District Hospitals and other private hospitals. According to the report of the Supreme Council of Nurses and Midwives in Poland [26], published in 2023, there were 39,685 registered nurses and 4905 registered midwives (a total of 44,950 nurses and midwives) in the Silesian Voivodeship.

Initially, the maximum margin of estimation error was assumed to be 5%, which resulted in a required sample size of 381 participants. However, due to the nature of the study and the target group—nurses and midwives performing their duties in centres within the level III reference system of the three-tiered care system for pregnant women and newborns—the representative sample ultimately consisted of 306 individuals.

The study was quantitative in nature, and the study group comprised nurses and midwives working in neonatal, intensive care, and neonatal pathology units, obstetric wards, delivery suites, and perinatal hospices. The questionnaire was distributed to 340 respondents, with 316 returned, of which 307 complete questionnaires were qualified for analysis.

The sample size was calculated using the formula for a finite population:

$$n = \frac{0.5(1-P)}{\frac{e^2}{Z^2} + \frac{P(1-P)}{N}} = \frac{0.5(1-0.5)}{\frac{0.05^2}{1.96^2} + \frac{0.5(1-0.5)}{44950}} = 380.87 \; n = \frac{0.5(1-P)}{\frac{e^2}{Z^2} + \frac{P(1-P)}{N}} = \frac{0.5(1-0.5)}{\frac{0.05^2}{1.96^2} + \frac{0.5(1-0.5)}{1503}} = 305.95$$

where N—population size, Z—value derived from the assumed confidence level (for 95%, $Z = 1.96$), P—estimated proportion in the population, e—acceptable estimation error.

A diagnostic survey method was applied, using a proprietary questionnaire that included questions regarding sociodemographic and occupational factors such as education, workplace, professional experience, and reasons for choosing the current workplace. Additionally, it contained questions on the frequency of care provided to patients diagnosed prenatally with a lethal foetal anomaly, exposure to neonatal death, nursing procedures related to the care of neonates with lethal anomalies, the degree of discomfort experienced, and factors contributing to psychological burden. The questionnaire was supplemented with standardised research tools: the Mini-COPE Inventory for measuring coping strategies and the Perceived Stress Scale (PSS-10).

To measure coping strategies, the shortened version of the COPE questionnaire by Carver, Scheier, and Weintraub, adapted into Polish by Juczyński and Ogińska-Bulik [27], was used. The Polish version of Mini-COPE consists of 28 statements assigned to 14 coping strategies. Respondents rated their behaviours on a four-point Likert scale (0—almost never, 1—rarely, 2—often, 3—almost always).

The Perceived Stress Scale (PSS-10) by Cohen, Kamarck, and Mermelstein, adapted into Polish by Juczyński and Ogińska-Bulik [28], comprises 10 questions assessing the intensity of stress related to life situations. Respondents rated the frequency of specific feelings on a scale from 0 (never) to 4 (very often). The total score ranged from 0 to 40 points, with values of 0–13 indicating low stress, 14–26 moderate stress, and 27 or more high stress levels.

The psychometric properties of the standardised tools used are presented below.

Mini-COPE:

- Internal consistency (reliability): Guttman's coefficient is 0.87, indicating high reliability of the tool.
- Score range: 0–3 for each strategy.
- Score distributions: Problem-focused coping strategies, such as active coping (M = 2.06, SD = 0.635) and planning (M = 1.95, SD = 0.590), have the highest mean values.
  - Less adaptive strategies, such as substance use (M = 0.66, SD = 0.712) and denial (M = 0.88, SD = 0.751), show lower means.
  - Skewness and kurtosis indicate slight deviations from a normal distribution.
- PSS-10 (Perceived Stress Scale):
- Internal consistency (reliability): Cronbach's alpha is 0.86, suggesting high reliability of the tool.
- Score range: 0–4 per question, 0–40 for the entire scale.
- Score distributions: The highest mean scores were observed for questions related to feeling nervous and tense (M = 2.70, SD = 0.883) and perceived ability to handle problems (M = 2.67, SD = 0.831). The lowest values were recorded for feeling helpless in the face of increasing difficulties (M = 1.85, SD = 0.914), which may suggest that respondents experienced extreme negative emotional states less frequently.

Statistical analysis was conducted using IBM SPSS 25.01 and Microsoft Excel. The following statistical methods were applied:

- Descriptive statistical analysis (measures of central tendency and dispersion) to characterise quantitative variables.
- Frequency analysis—percentage distributions of qualitative variables.
- Chi-square tests and contingency tables to assess relationships between nominal and ordinal variables.
- Cohen's d effect size measure to determine the magnitude of differences between groups.
- Spearman's correlation coefficient for quantitative variables deviating from normal distribution.

A significance level of $\alpha = 0.05$ was adopted (results with $p < 0.05$ were considered statistically significant), with a confidence level of 95%.

4. Results

Description of the Cross-Tabulation of PSS10 Scores with Various Demographic and Professional Variables

The cross-tabulation analysis examined the relationship between PSS10 (Perceived Stress Scale) scores and various demographic and professional variables.

The analysis revealed a significant association between education level and categorical distribution ($\chi^2(10) = 30.651$, $p = 0.001$, Cohen's $d = 0.2234$). Individuals with a secondary medical high school education (66.7%) and a bachelor's degree (56.3%) were most frequently classified in the high category, suggesting that these educational backgrounds may provide sufficient preparation for excelling in their professional roles.

Interestingly, individuals with a post-secondary vocational school education were predominantly in the medium category (83.3%), indicating that this level of education might offer a solid but not necessarily advanced foundation for professional performance. Notably, all participants with a doctoral degree fell into the medium category (100.0%), which may suggest that holding a doctorate does not directly translate to superior performance or may reflect that individuals in these roles undertake different responsibilities that do not align with the assessed criteria.

Higher levels of education generally correlate with a greater likelihood of classification in the high category. However, doctoral-level education does not appear to confer a clear advantage in this specific professional context.

A statistically significant relationship was observed between years of service and category distribution ($\chi^2(14) = 24.023$, $p = 0.046$, Cohen's $d = 0.1978$). The 11–15 years (53.7%) and 16–20 years (51.2%) groups had the highest proportion of individuals in the high category, indicating that experience contributes positively to professional performance.

Employees with the shortest tenure (up to one year) were predominantly in the medium category (63.6%), which is expected as they are still acquiring experience and adapting to their roles. In contrast, those with 21–25 years of service exhibited a more even distribution across all categories, suggesting that beyond a certain threshold, experience alone may not be a definitive factor in high performance.

Professional experience is positively associated with higher performance, particularly after six years in the department. However, after 20–25 years, the impact of additional experience appears to plateau, possibly due to factors such as routine, job fatigue, or changes in work dynamics.

No statistically significant relationship was found between workplace setting and category distribution ($\chi^2(8) = 7.984$, $p = 0.435$, Cohen's $d = 0.1140$). Nevertheless, some differences were observed. The highest proportions in the high category were found in the neonatal intensive care unit (47.1%), Maternity Ward (48.0%), and Delivery Block (46.3%), suggesting that these environments may offer greater opportunities for skill development or require higher levels of professional engagement.

Conversely, the perinatal hospice showed an unusual trend, with an even distribution between the low (40.0%) and high (40.0%) categories. This may indicate that individuals in this setting either thrive due to personal dedication or struggle due to the unique emotional and psychological challenges of the role.

While no direct correlation was found between workplace setting and performance, the nature of the department may influence individual development. Units with higher patient turnover and acute care demands (e.g., NICU) seem to foster higher performance levels.

A significant association was found between the reason for workplace choice and categorical distribution ($\chi^2(10) = 33.477$, $p < 0.001$, Cohen's $d = 0.2335$). The highest proportions in the high category were observed among individuals who chose their workplace based on the decision of superiors (83.3%), a sense of calling (55.0%), and a desire to help (51.7%). This suggests that intrinsic motivation and external expectations play a crucial role in professional effectiveness.

Conversely, those who selected their workplace due to financial conditions were predominantly in the medium category (54.5%), implying that while financial incentives may sustain motivation, they are not necessarily linked to high performance.

Employees driven by intrinsic motivation (such as a sense of calling) or external professional guidance (such as superior recommendations) are more likely to achieve high levels of performance. In contrast, financial motives alone do not appear to foster excellence. The details are in Table 1.

The study analysed various aspects of caregivers' work in the context of caring for newborns with prenatally diagnosed lethal conditions. The focus was on the frequency of contact with such newborns and the factors that may influence the psychological burden on caregivers, such as discomfort, stress, and emotional involvement. The statistical analyses (chi-square tests, χ^2) and effect size calculations using Cohen's d coefficient allowed for the drawing of significant conclusions regarding these relationships.

Table 1. Dependence of PSS 10 level on demographic variables.

Variables	Categories	Low (n, %)	Medium (n, %)	Hight (n, %)	χ^2 Test Results df p	d Cohena
Education	Secondary: Medical High School	3 (7.7%)	10 (25.6%)	26 (66.7%)	30,651 10 0.001	0.2234
	Post-secondary vocational school	0 (0.0%)	10 (83.3%)	2 (16.7%)		
	Post-secondary vocational studies	7 (21.2%)	15 (45.5%)	11 (33.3%)		
	Bachelor's degree	15 (18.8%)	20 (25.0%)	45 (56.3%)		
	Master's degree	23 (16.3%)	61 (43.3%)	57 (40.4%)		
	Doctoral degree	0 (0.0%)	2 (100.0%)	0 (0.0%)		
Years of Service in the Current Department	Up to year	2 (18.2%)	7 (63.6%)	2 (18.2%)	24,023 14 0.046	0.1978
	2–5 years	13 (20.0%)	21 (32.3%)	31 (47.7%)		
	6–10 years	3 (7.0%)	23 (53.5%)	17 (39.5%)		
	11–15 years	7 (13.0%)	18 (33.3%)	29 (53.7%)		
	16–20 years	3 (7.3%)	17 (41.5%)	21 (51.2%)		
	21–25 years	9 (36.0%)	9 (36.0%)	7 (28.0%)		
	26–30 years	8 (19.5%)	12 (29.3%)	21 (51.2%)		
	Over 30 years	3 (11.1%)	11 (40.7%)	13 (48.1%)		
Workplace	Neonatology Department	15 (17.6%)	33 (38.8%)	37 (43.5%)	7984 8 0.435	0.1140
	Neonatal Intensive Care Unit	13 (10.7%)	51 (42.1%)	57 (47.1%)		
	Maternity Ward	9 (18.0%)	17 (34.0%)	24 (48.0%)		
	Delivery Block	7 (17.1%)	15 (36.6%)	19 (46.3%)		
	Perinatal Hospice	4 (40.0%)	2 (20.0%)	4 (40.0%)		
Reason for Choosing the Current Workplace	Job availability	26 (26.3%)	33 (33.3%)	40 (40.4%)	33,477 10 <0.001	0.2335
	Desire to help	4 (6.7%)	25 (41.7%)	31 (51.7%)		
	Calling	9 (11.3%)	27 (33.8%)	44 (55.0%)		
	Financial conditions	3 (9.1%)	18 (54.5%)	12 (36.4%)		
	Decision of superiors	0 (0.0%)	2 (16.7%)	10 (83.3%)		
	Other (distance, finances, working with children, chance, health)	6 (26.1%)	13 (56.5%)	4 (17.4%)		

Frequency of Patients with Prenatally Diagnosed Lethal Conditions. The analysis revealed a significant difference in the distribution of responses to the question regarding the frequency of encounters with patients with prenatally diagnosed lethal conditions ($\chi^2(6) = 35.123$, $p < 0.001$). The majority of respondents (55.6%) encountered such patients "several times a year", and 44.4% reported care "once a quarter". The responses in the "several times a month" category amounted to 54.1%.

The high percentage of caregivers indicating frequent encounters with patients in cases of prenatal lethal diagnoses suggests that this is a frequent aspect of work in neonatal care. It is worth noting that the frequency of these cases correlates with higher emotional burdens, which may influence how staff cope with such challenging situations.

Cohen's d = 0.2392 indicates a small to medium effect, meaning that the frequency of encountering patients with lethal conditions has a moderate impact on caregivers' emotional and professional responses.

Frequency of Contact with Dying Newborns. A significant difference in the frequency of contact with dying newborns was evident in the analysis ($\chi^2(6) = 30.496$, $p < 0.001$). The most frequent responses were in the "several times a year" category (45.7%), followed by "several times a month" (65.5%). In the "once a quarter" category, responses from 57.1% of respondents were recorded.

Close contact with dying newborns is one of the most difficult experiences for a neonatologist. The frequency of such cases affects the emotional condition of caregivers, who must deal with challenging, traumatic experiences, leading to increased stress.

Cohen's d = 0.2229 indicates a moderate effect, suggesting that the frequency of contact with dying newborns significantly influences caregivers' emotions.

Frequency of Performing Nursing Tasks Related to the Care of a Newborn with a Lethal Condition. In the studied group, the most common responses were regarding performing nursing tasks "several times a month" (61.8%), followed by "several times a year" (46.7%) and "once a quarter" (48.1%). The chi-square test showed statistical significance ($\chi^2(6) = 31.510$, $p < 0.001$).

More frequent nursing tasks are associated with higher levels of responsibility and greater stress. Caregivers who more often care for newborns with lethal conditions face both technical and emotional challenges, which may cause increased discomfort and difficulty.

Cohen's d = 0.2265 suggests that the frequency of performing such tasks has a moderate impact on caregivers' stress and emotional exhaustion.

Degree of Discomfort Experienced in the Care of a Newborn with a Lethal Condition. The analysis showed that the degree of discomfort depends on the frequency of contact with newborns with lethal conditions. The majority (74.4%) experienced "very large" discomfort, particularly with frequent interactions. In the "small/minimal" and "medium" discomfort categories, people with frequent contact were clearly dominant.

The experience of working with dying children and newborns with lethal conditions is associated with significant stress and emotional burden. The more frequent the contact, the higher the level of discomfort. This indicates the need for psychological support for caregivers who regularly face such traumatic situations.

Cohen's d = 0.2212 indicates a small to medium effect, suggesting that more frequent interactions are associated with greater discomfort.

Factors Affecting Psychological Burden Considered to Cause Stress in the Care of a Newborn with a Lethal Condition.

Time Pressure: A significant relationship was observed ($\chi^2(2) = 7.326$, $p = 0.026$). The majority of respondents (69.6%) considered time pressure as a major stressor. Cohen's d = 0.1092 indicates a small effect. Close Contact with Death: A significant difference was noted ($\chi^2(2) = 13.610$, $p = 0.001$), where 76.2% of respondents identified death as a stressful factor. Cohen's d = 0.1489 indicates a medium effect. Helplessness or Limited Ability to Help: This factor also contributed to caregivers' stress ($\chi^2(2) = 6.903$, $p = 0.032$). Around 43.9% of respondents felt helpless in the face of newborns' lethal conditions. Cohen's d = 0.1060 indicates a small effect. Excessive Emotional Involvement: No significant difference was found ($\chi^2(2) = 3.205$, $p = 0.201$), with a minimal effect (Cohen's d = 0.0722). Close Contact with Parents' Suffering: No significant differences were observed ($\chi^2(2) = 2.309$, $p = 0.315$), with a minimal effect (Cohen's d = 0.0613). Close Contact with the Child's Suffering: A result close to significance was observed ($\chi^2(2) = 5.579$, $p = 0.061$), with a small effect (Cohen's d = 0.0953).

The analysis indicates that frequent exposure to caring for newborns with lethal conditions is associated with higher levels of discomfort and stress among caregivers. Factors such as time pressure, proximity to death, and helplessness in difficult situations are significant sources of stress. However, some factors, such as excessive emotional involvement or contact with the suffering of parents, did not have a large impact on stress levels. The results suggest the need for psychological and educational support for neonatal care workers to help them better cope with the difficult experiences associated with caring for dying children. The details are in Table 2.

Table 2. Dependence of PSS 10 level on professional variables.

Variables	Categories	Low (n, %)	Medium (n, %)	Hight (n, %)	χ^2 Test Results df p	d Cohena
Frequency of Patients with a Prenatally Diagnosed Lethal Condition	Once a quarter	0 (0.0%)	16 (44.4%)	20 (55.6%)	35,123 6 <0.001	0.2392
	Several times a year	22 (14.0%)	78 (49.7%)	57 (36.3%)		
	Several times a month	26 (23.9%)	24 (22.0%)	59 (54.1%)		
	Several times a week	0 (0.0%)	0 (0.0%)	5 (100.0%)		
Frequency of Contact with Death and Dying of Neonates	Several times a year	35 (16.7%)	96 (45.7%)	79 (37.6%)	30,496 6 <0.001	0.2229
	Once a quarter	1 (2.9%)	14 (40.0%)	20 (57.1%)		
	Several times a month	12 (20.7%)	8 (13.8%)	38 (65.5%)		
	Several times a week	0 (0.0%)	0 (0.0%)	4 (100.0%)		
Frequency of Performing Nursing Tasks Related to the Care of a Newborn with a Lethal Condition	Several times a year	25 (13.6%)	86 (46.7%)	73 (39.7%)	31,510 6 <0.001	0.2265
	Once a quarter	2 (7.4%)	12 (44.4%)	13 (48.1%)		
	Several times a month	6 (10.9%)	15 (27.3%)	34 (61.8%)		
	Several times a week	15 (36.6%)	5 (12.2%)	21 (51.2%)		
Degree of Discomfort Experienced in Care of a Newborn with a Lethal Condition	None	6 (21.4%)	8 (28.6%)	14 (50.0%)	30,041 8 <0.001	0.2212
	Small/Minimal	6 (13.0%)	13 (28.3%)	27 (58.7%)		
	Medium	24 (21.6%)	49 (44.1%)	38 (34.2%)		
	Large	8 (9.6%)	42 (50.6%)	33 (39.8%)		
	Very large	4 (10.3%)	6 (15.4%)	29 (74.4%)		
Factors Affecting Psychological Burden Considered to Cause Stress in the Care of a Newborn with a Lethal Condition	Time pressure	0 (0.0%)	7 (30.4%)	16 (69.6%)	7326 2 0.026	0.1092
	Close contact with death	1 (4.8%)	16 (76.2%)	4 (19.0%)	13,610 2 0.001	0.1489
	Helplessness or limited ability to help	20 (24.4%)	26 (31.7%)	36 (43.9%)	6903 2 0.032	0.1060
	Excessive emotional involvement	2 (7.1%)	9 (32.1%)	17 (60.7%)	3205 2 0.201	0.0722
	Close contact with parents' suffering	24 (17.6%)	62 (36.3%)	85 (49.7%)	2309 2 0.315	0.0613
	Close contact with the child's suffering	16 (11.1%)	63 (43.8%)	65 (45.1%)	5579 2 0.061	0.0953

The descriptive statistics from the Mini-COPE questionnaire reveal a wide range of coping strategies used by the participants in response to challenging situations.

The analysis of basic descriptive statistics for the Mini-COPE tool indicates a variation in stress-coping strategies within the studied group (N = 307). Below, the results for individual variables are discussed, taking into account their mean values (M), standard deviation (SD), median (Me), and range of scores, as well as skewness and kurtosis indices.

Most Frequently Used Strategies

Problem-focused coping strategies, such as active coping (M = 2.06, SD = 0.635) and planning (M = 1.95, SD = 0.590), obtained the highest mean values. This suggests that the respondents frequently engage in actions aimed at constructively solving problems. The negative skewness values for these strategies (−0.91 and −0.64) indicate an asymmetrical distribution with a predominance of higher values, confirming their dominance in the studied group.

Emotion-Focused Strategies

Emotion regulation strategies, such as positive reframing (M = 1.81, SD = 0.690) and acceptance (M = 1.86, SD = 0.574), also achieved relatively high scores. Their slight skewness (−0.54 and −0.34) and kurtosis values indicate a distribution close to normal.

Seeking emotional support (M = 1.79, SD = 0.716) and seeking instrumental support (M = 1.76, SD = 0.663) were also relatively frequently used, suggesting that respondents significantly rely on social support in difficult situations.

Less Adaptive Strategies

Less adaptive strategies, such as denial (M = 0.88, SD = 0.751) and substance use (M = 0.66, SD = 0.712), had lower mean values. Their positive skewness (ranging from 0.50 to 0.69) indicates a distribution shift towards lower scores, meaning that most participants rarely use these mechanisms.

Self-blame (M = 1.20, SD = 0.714) and behavioural disengagement (M = 0.95, SD = 0.689) also obtained relatively low scores, suggesting that these strategies are not predominantly employed in the studied group.

Analysis of Score Distributions

Most variables show skewness within the range of −1 to 1, indicating moderate asymmetries in distribution. The kurtosis values fluctuate around 0, suggesting slight deviations from normality. An exception is active coping, where kurtosis is 1.53, meaning that this score is more concentrated around the mean compared to a normal distribution.

Dominance of Adaptive Strategies

The studied group more frequently applies adaptive strategies, such as active coping, planning, and positive reframing. This indicates a constructive approach to problems and an ability to regulate emotions effectively.

Rare Use of Avoidant and Maladaptive Strategies

Strategies based on avoiding problems (e.g., denial, substance use) are used significantly less frequently, suggesting that the respondents do not rely heavily on escapist mechanisms when dealing with stress.

Importance of Social Support

Relatively high scores for emotional and instrumental support-seeking strategies highlight the importance of interpersonal relationships in the stress-coping process. This suggests a preference for strategies that engage social resources.

Potential Implications for Psychological Interventions

The results indicate the need to promote adaptive coping strategies and minimise maladaptive ones through appropriate psychological interventions, such as stress management training and psychological support programmes.

In summary, the psychometric analysis of the Mini-COPE tool indicates a predominant use of constructive stress-coping strategies within the studied group, which may have positive consequences for the participants' psychological well-being. Details can be seen in Table 3.

The Spearman correlation analysis between the PSS-10 score and coping strategies from the Mini-COPE questionnaire reveals significant relationships between stress levels and coping methods.

Positive correlations, indicating higher stress levels, were found with strategies like self-blame, giving up, denial, turning to religion, and substance use. The strongest positive correlation was with self-blame, suggesting that individuals who frequently use this strategy tend to experience higher stress.

Table 3. Basic descriptive statistics if stress MiniCope coping strategies.

	N	*M*	*SD*	*Me*	Min.	Max	Skewness	Kurtosis
MiniCope Active Coping	307	2.06	0.635	2.00	0.00	3.00	−0.91	1.53
MiniCope Planning	307	1.95	0.590	2.00	0.00	3.00	−0.64	1.54
MiniCope Positive Reappraisal	307	1.81	0.690	2.00	0.00	3.00	−0.54	0.26
MiniCope Acceptance	307	1.86	0.574	2.00	0.00	3.00	−0.34	0.74
MiniCope Sense of Humour	307	0.88	0.681	1.00	0.00	2.50	0.51	−0.56
MiniCope Turning to Religion	307	1.12	0.915	1.00	0.00	3.00	0.54	−0.61
MiniCope Seeking Emotional Support	307	1.79	0.716	2.00	0.00	3.00	−0.41	−0.09
MiniCope Seeking Instrumental Support	307	1.76	0.663	2.00	0.00	3.00	−0.18	−0.17
MiniCope Occupying	307	1.76	0.683	2.00	0.00	3.00	−0.34	0.16
MiniCope Denial	307	0.88	0.751	1.00	0.00	3.00	0.50	−0.53
MiniCope Venting	307	1.49	0.620	1.50	0.00	3.00	−0.29	0.02
MiniCope Substance Use Psychoactive	307	0.66	0.712	0.50	0.00	2.50	0.69	−0.56
MiniCope Desistance	307	0.95	0.689	1.00	0.00	3.00	0.42	−0.33
MiniCope Self-Blame	307	1.20	0.714	1.00	0.00	3.00	0.34	−0.26

On the other hand, negative correlations, indicating lower stress levels, were found with positive reinterpretation and seeking emotional support. These strategies may be linked to more adaptive coping, contributing to lower stress.

Other strategies, such as active coping, planning, acceptance, sense of humour, seeking instrumental support, and distraction, showed no significant correlations with stress levels, indicating that their relationship with stress was not confirmed in this sample.

In conclusion, the analysis suggests that strategies like positive reinterpretation and seeking emotional support may help reduce stress, while strategies such as self-blame, denial, and giving up are associated with higher stress levels. These findings highlight the importance of promoting more adaptive coping strategies for stress management (Table 4).

What is the Most Stressful Aspect of Caring for a Newborn with a Lethal Defect?

Table 5 illustrates the percentage of responses regarding the most stressful actions for medical staff caring for newborns with lethal defects.

The majority of respondents (69.1%) identified accompanying parents during their farewell to the child as the most stressful task. This emotionally intense interaction involves confronting the newborn's death and the parents' profound grief.

The second most commonly mentioned stressor (19.2%) was preparing keepsakes, such as footprint impressions. Despite its technical nature, the symbolic significance of this task can be emotionally taxing.

Providing palliative care without life-prolonging treatment and handling funeral documentation were cited as stressful by 13% of respondents. These activities require both medical expertise and emotional sensitivity when supporting grieving families.

Post-mortem care, including preparing the newborn's body, was stressful for 11.4% of respondents, likely due to the direct contact with the deceased, which can be emotionally challenging.

A smaller proportion of respondents found nursing tasks (3.9%) and participating in baptism ceremonies (2.9%) stressful. These actions, though less commonly cited, carry emotional weight, especially in spiritual or ritual contexts.

Additionally, 4% mentioned other factors, such as various aspects of palliative care, involving multitasking and tailored approaches in complex clinical situations.

Table 4. Correlations between PSS10 score and MiniCope coping strategies.

Correlations			
			PSS10
Spearman's rho	MiniCope Active Coping	Correlation coefficient Significance (bilateral)	−0.098 0.087
	MiniCope Planning	Correlation coefficient Significance (bilateral)	−0.046 0.421
	MiniCope Positive Reappraisal	Correlation coefficient Significance (bilateral)	−0.211 0
	MiniCope Acceptance	Correlation coefficient Significance (bilateral)	−0.055 0.335
	MiniCope Sense of Humour	Correlation coefficient Significance (bilateral)	0.065 0.258
	MiniCope Turning to Religion	Correlation coefficient Significance (bilateral)	0.15 0.008
	MiniCope Seeking Emotional Support	Correlation coefficient Significance (bilateral)	−0.129 0.024
	MiniCope Seeking Instrumental Support	Correlation coefficient Significance (bilateral)	0.061 0.285
	MiniCope Occupying	Correlation coefficient Significance (bilateral)	0.021 0.713
	MiniCope Denial	Correlation coefficient Significance (bilateral)	0.215 0
	MiniCope Venting	Correlation coefficient Significance (bilateral)	0.153 0.007
	MiniCope Substance Use Psy-choactive	Correlation coefficient Significance (bilateral)	0.122 0.032
	MiniCope Desistance	Correlation coefficient Significance (bilateral)	0.266 0
	MiniCope Self-Blame	Correlation coefficient Significance (bilateral)	0.32 0

Table 5. Activities during farewell with the child.

Activity	Percentage (%)
Accompanying parents during their farewell with the child	69.1
Preparing keepsakes for parents (e.g., footprints)	50
Providing care free of disproportionate life-prolonging treatment	40
Providing documentation for funeral arrangements	30
Performing post-mortem care	20
Carrying out nursing activities	15
Participation in baptism ceremonies	10
Other (e.g., individualised care, all mentioned to varying extents)	5

Overall, the findings indicate that the primary source of stress for medical staff is the emotional engagement with parents during their farewell. Technical and administrative duties, like preparing keepsakes and funeral documentation, also contribute to stress but to a lesser extent.

Coping Strategies for Stress in the Context of Caring for a Newborn with a Lethal Defect

Table 6 presents the most commonly used methods of coping with stress employed by staff members in relation to their work, particularly in the context of caring for newborns with a lethal congenital defect. The results are expressed as percentages and refer to various emotional support methods and stress coping techniques. More than half of the respondents (52.8%) indicated that talking to loved ones and receiving support from close individuals is a key strategy for coping with stress. This is the most popular form of emotional support, highlighting the importance of interpersonal relationships in the process of emotional tension reduction.

Table 6. Coping mechanism in stressful situations.

Coping Mechanism in Stressful Situations	Percentage (%)
Talking with loved ones/support from close people	52.8
Joking at work	32.9
Support from colleagues	28.6
Entertainment	25.7
Sport	23.4
Hobbies	22.1
Faith	17.3
Relaxation techniques	16
SPA treatments	11.7
Overeating	8.1
Using stimulants (cigarettes, alcohol)	7.8
Psychologist's help	2.3

The second most frequently indicated strategy is humour in the workplace. Almost one-third of the respondents (32.9%) use jokes as a way to ease difficult emotions, emphasising the role of distance and humour in coping with professional challenges.

Another significant strategy, used by 28.6% of respondents, is support from colleagues. A sense of community with other workers and their help in managing mental strain constitutes an important source of relief at work.

Entertainment and physical activity, such as sports, are popular methods of stress relief used by 25.7% and 23.4% of respondents, respectively. These activities can be viewed as forms of active relaxation and a way for individuals to detach themselves from professional issues.

For 22.1% of individuals, developing personal passions outside of work represents an effective stress coping strategy. This is an important way to unwind and relax, allowing for engagement in activities outside the work environment.

For 17.3% of people, faith provides support in coping with stress, which may reflect the spiritual dimension of dealing with difficult experiences. Additionally, relaxation techniques, used by 16% of respondents, may include meditation, breathing exercises, or other methods of tension reduction.

A less common, but still used strategy, is the use of spa treatments, as indicated by 11.7% of respondents. Such activities can support both physical and mental regeneration.

Less constructive ways of coping with stress, such as overeating (8.1%) and the use of substances like cigarettes or alcohol (7.8%), are chosen relatively infrequently, yet they remain present among some respondents.

The least commonly used strategy is seeking professional psychological help (2.3%). This result may suggest that these individuals rarely seek specialist support, possibly due to personal beliefs or barriers to accessing such help.

The findings show that medical staff most frequently rely on emotional support from loved ones and colleagues, as well as humour and recreational strategies. Fewer individuals turn to professional psychological help or engage in less constructive methods like overeating or substance use.

5. Discussion

The results of the study conducted on a group of 307 nurses and midwives provide valuable insights into the relationships between perceived stress levels and sociodemographic, professional, and coping strategies factors in the context of working with newborns with lethal congenital conditions. The primary aim of the study was to identify the coping strategies used by individuals working in this specific environment and to determine the impact of selected variables on perceived stress levels. The discussion of the results not only allows for the analysis of the obtained data in comparison with the existing literature but also highlights potential interventions aimed at reducing the psychological burden on medical staff.

The study revealed that stress levels were significantly dependent on the respondents' education. Nurses and midwives with secondary education (obtained from a medical high school) more frequently reported high levels of stress (66.7%) compared to those with post-secondary education, among whom no cases of high stress were recorded. These findings can be interpreted as the result of differences in professional preparation, expectations, and attitudes toward work. Individuals with post-secondary education may adopt a more pragmatic approach to their professional duties, which reduces their susceptibility to stress. However, international literature shows some discrepancies—Chatzigiani and colleagues [29] demonstrated that nurse assistants, who undergo shorter professional training, experience higher stress levels. These differences may arise from diverse educational structures and specific approaches to work in different countries.

Work experience turned out to be another factor significantly influencing perceived stress levels. In this study, individuals with 2–5 years of professional experience more frequently reported medium levels of stress (47.7%), which may align with the adaptive curve model, where this period is characterised by the highest professional productivity but also by increased emotional burden. High stress levels were evenly distributed across all other experience categories, indicating that longer work experience may be associated with the development of adaptive mechanisms. According to Harris and Tao [30], nurses with shorter work experience (2–5 years) exhibit the highest levels of burnout, which correlates with the findings presented in this paper. In contrast, Chatzigiani and colleagues [29] argue that older nurses (over 50 years old) more frequently report high stress levels, which could result from the accumulation of difficult experiences and decreased psychological resilience.

Data analysis also showed that the workplace did not have a direct correlation with stress levels, suggesting that factors specific to the department, rather than the work environment itself, determine the psychological burden. The highest percentage of individuals with high stress levels worked in neonatal intensive care units (47.1%), which is consistent with the literature. McMeekin and colleagues [31] confirm that nurses working in these units experience higher stress levels compared to those in other specialties. In different cultural conditions, such as in Saudi Arabia, studies have shown moderate or low stress levels among nurses working in intensive care units [8], which may indicate differences in organisational structures and professional support across healthcare systems.

Motivational factors also turned out to be significant in the analysis of stress levels. Respondents who chose the profession for ideological reasons ("calling") more often reported high levels of stress (55.0%). Such motivation may be linked to greater emotional involvement and the pressure of high moral standards. As Zbyrad [32] points out, idealists often dominate in service professions, which is confirmed by the findings of this study. In contrast, individuals driven by pragmatic motives showed lower stress levels, suggesting a more detached approach to professional duties.

Contact with newborns with lethal congenital conditions and their families was one of the most stress-inducing factors. The results indicate that the frequency of contact with patients who gave birth to a child with a lethal congenital condition had a significant impact on the stress levels of the participants. Nurses and midwives who encountered such cases several times a month or once a quarter more often reported high stress levels. This result aligns with the studies of Baranauskas and colleagues [33], who observed moderate to high stress levels among nurses after the death of a patient. Similar results were obtained in studies conducted in Greece [33] and Iran [2], where patient death was one of the main sources of stress in nurses' work.

High stress levels were also correlated with experiencing psychological discomfort. Respondents reporting strong emotional discomfort made up as much as 74.4% of the group with high stress levels. This finding underscores the importance of psychological support when working with newborns with lethal congenital conditions. McAndrew and colleagues [34] found that intensive care nurses experience significant discomfort when professional tasks conflict with their ability to provide holistic care. Vincent and colleagues [35] highlighted the phenomenon of "moral distress", which occurs when there is a conflict between knowledge of ethically correct behaviour and the procedures in place at a given workplace.

The study revealed that coping strategies had a significant impact on the professional functioning of nurses and midwives. The most commonly used strategies, such as active coping and planning, were adaptive and associated with lower stress levels. Avoidant strategies, such as denial, self-blame, or using psychoactive substances, were correlated with higher levels of psychological burden. These findings are consistent with research by Tesfaye [36] and Zhang and colleagues [37], who also emphasised the importance of active coping in stress reduction. An interesting strategy found was the empathetic approach to patients, which, according to Rivaldi and colleagues [38], helps reduce burnout levels.

Conversations with close ones (52.8%) and support from colleagues (28.6%) were the most commonly used coping methods in the study group. These results highlight the crucial role of interpersonal relationships in reducing psychological burdens. Similar conclusions were drawn by Andre and colleagues [39] and Laing and colleagues [40], who emphasised the importance of sharing professional experiences as a preventive measure against burnout.

The study results showed that the greatest stress in working with newborns with lethal congenital conditions comes from the need to accompany parents in their farewell to their child (69.1%). These experiences are not only emotionally burdensome but also require significant interpersonal skills. Research by Christoffersen et al. [41] indicates that an emotional approach to such situations, including "emotional release" (e.g., crying, journaling), can help in coping with difficulties. At the same time, a task-oriented approach, such as participating in farewell ceremonies with the family, also appears to be an essential element of psychological adaptation. Such an approach allows for closure of a difficult stage and reduces the risk of long-term emotional strain.

Another challenge in the work of neonatal staff was preparing keepsakes and providing palliative care for families. Christoffersen et al. [41] emphasise that confronting the emotions of parents when they lose their child is one of the most stressful aspects of working in neonatology. These studies align with the results of earlier authors who also pointed to the psychological burden associated with assisting families during the most difficult moments [42].

Patterson [43] in her research demonstrated that while traumatic experiences related to caring for dying patients often result in negative consequences, they can also contribute to personal and professional growth. According to the researcher, difficult experiences at work can lead to increased self-confidence, appreciation of life, and spiritual development. Similar conclusions were presented by authors of studies on stress in the nursing and midwifery profession in the context of their functioning after experiencing traumatic events [44]. Midwives involved in these studies reported increased inner strength, existential changes, and a sense of deeper meaning in life, which may have acted as an adaptive mechanism to working in challenging conditions.

In conclusion, the results of the study highlight the complexity of factors influencing stress levels among nurses and midwives working with newborns with lethal congenital conditions. They also emphasise the need for psychological and systemic interventions that could support medical staff in coping with professional challenges. Education on effective stress coping strategies, strengthening social support, and access to professional psychological help are key areas to consider when improving the well-being of this professional group.

An analysis of the study results in the context of contemporary health behaviour theories provides a better understanding of stress-coping mechanisms among nurses and midwives. One of the key concepts is the Coping with Stress Model developed by Endler and Parker, which distinguishes three coping styles: task-oriented, emotion-oriented, and avoidance-oriented. Research indicates that task-focused strategies, such as active problem-solving and planning, are more adaptive and effectively reduce occupational stress levels [45,46]. Furthermore, the Concept of Psychological Resilience highlights the role of individual resources, such as self-efficacy and flexibility in coping with stress. Strengthening these traits through training and support programmes can contribute to better management of professional demands [47,48].

Additionally, the Social Support Theory suggests that support from colleagues, family, and friends plays a crucial role in mitigating the effects of stress. Creating a work environment that encourages experience-sharing and emotional support can significantly improve the well-being of medical staff [49,50].

6. Practical Implications

The findings highlight the necessity of implementing psychological support programmes and stress management training for medical staff. It is particularly important to promote adaptive strategies, such as positive reappraisal and active coping, which can effectively reduce stress levels. Furthermore, healthcare institutions should consider introducing rotation systems to decrease the frequency of employees' exposure to challenging clinical situations. The study underscores the need for further research to better understand the mechanisms of occupational stress and to develop effective support programmes.

Our study has certain limitations. It focuses on nurses and midwives providing care for newborns with lethal defects and their families exclusively in the Silesian agglomeration in Poland. As a result, its findings cannot be considered representative of the entire professional group of nurses working in perinatal palliative care across the country.

However, a key strength of this study is that its findings may serve as a foundation for many essential initiatives aimed at providing psychological and interventional support for nurses and midwives in perinatal palliative care in Poland, which is currently not institutionally available.

7. Conclusions

The study revealed that individuals with secondary education experienced higher levels of stress compared to those with higher education, possibly due to differences in professional preparation. Employees with 2–5 years of experience reported moderate stress, linked to the growing demands at this stage of their careers. Longer work experience did not significantly affect stress levels, suggesting the development of adaptive mechanisms. Neonatal intensive care units (NICUs) emerged as major stress factors, particularly in the care of critically ill newborns.

Motivation also played a significant role—those motivated ideologically experienced higher stress, while pragmatic approaches were associated with lower levels of stress. High stress levels were linked to emotional discomfort, and coping mechanisms such as talking to loved ones or receiving support from colleagues helped reduce stress. In the context of NICU work, interpersonal skills were crucial, especially when preparing keepsakes or providing palliative care. Therefore, it is important to provide appropriate emotional and psychological support to help employees effectively manage occupational stress.

Author Contributions: Conceptualization—K.A.U., B.N. and A.D.-C.; data curation—K.A.U.; formal analysis—K.A.U., B.N. and A.D.-C.; funding acquisition—K.A.U. and A.D.-C.; investigation—K.A.U., B.N. and A.D.-C.; methodology—K.A.U., B.N. and A.D.-C.; project administration—K.A.U., B.N. and A.D.-C.; resources—K.A.U.; software—A.D.-C. and B.N.; supervision—A.D.-C. and B.N.; validation—K.A.U., B.N. and A.D.-C.; visualisation—K.A.U., B.N. and A.D.-C.; writing—original draft—K.A.U., B.N. and A.D.-C.; writing—review and editing—K.A.U., B.N. and A.D.-C. All authors have read and agreed to the published version of the manuscript.

Funding: This research received no external funding.

Institutional Review Board Statement: In accordance with the decision of the Bioethics Committee of the Medical University of Silesia in Katowice (approval number: PCN/CBN/0052/KB/33/23, dated 28 March 2023) the survey is not a medical experiment and does not require an assessment by the Bioethics Committee of the Medical University of Silesia. The study was voluntary and was conducted with the anonymity of the persons participating in the survey.

Informed Consent Statement: Informed consent was obtained from all the participants.

Data Availability Statement: The data generated during and analysed during the current study are available from the corresponding author on reasonable request.

Public Involvement Statement: No public involvement in any aspect of this research.

Guidelines and Standards Statement: All methods were carried out in accordance with relevant guidelines and regulations.

Use of Artificial Intelligence: AI or AI-assisted tools were not used in drafting any aspect of this manuscript.

Acknowledgments: The authors would like to thank the directors of the participating institutions for their support and cooperation in conducting this research. Special thanks to the nurses and midwives who participated in the study. Additionally, we appreciate the assistance provided by the Bioethics Committee of the Medical University of Silesia in Katowice for their approval and guidance.

Conflicts of Interest: The authors declare no conflicts of interest.

References

1. Goudarzian, A.H.; Nasrabadi, A.N.; Sharif-Nia, H.; Farhadi, B.; Navab, E. Exploring the concept and management strategies of caring stress among clinical nurses: A scoping review. *Front. Psychiatry* **2024**, *15*, 1337938. [CrossRef]
2. Babapour, A.-R.; Gahassab-Mozaffari, N.; Fathnezhad-Kazemi, A. Nurses' job stress and its impact on quality of life and caring behaviors: A cross-sectional study. *BMC Nurs.* **2022**, *21*, 1–10. [CrossRef] [PubMed]
3. Kramer, V.; Papazova, I.; Thoma, A.; Kunz, M.; Falkai, P.; Schneider-Axmann, T.; Hierundar, A.; Wagner, E.; Hasan, A. Subjective burden and perspectives of German healthcare workers during the COVID-19 pandemic. *Eur. Arch. Psychiatry Clin. Neurosci.* **2021**, *271*, 271–281. [CrossRef] [PubMed]
4. Zhong, Y.; Black, B.P.; Kain, V.J.; Song, Y. Facilitators and Barriers Affecting Implementation of Neonatal Palliative Care by Nurses in Mainland China. *Front. Pediatr.* **2022**, *10*, 887711. [CrossRef]
5. Zhang, X.-J.; Song, Y.; Jiang, T.; Ding, N.; Shi, T.-Y. Interventions to reduce burnout of physicians and nurses: An overview of systematic reviews and meta-analyses. *Medicine* **2020**, *99*, e20992. [CrossRef]
6. Zhang, M.; Murphy, B.; Cabanilla, A.; Yidi, C. Physical relaxation for occupational stress in healthcare workers: A systematic review and network meta-analysis of randomized controlled trials. *J. Occup. Health* **2021**, *63*, e12243. [CrossRef]
7. Van Horne, S.; Downing, V.; Farley, H.M. Supporting Well-being Through the Implementation of Education and a Relaxing Retreat Space. *Jona J. Nurs. Adm.* **2020**, *50*, 655–662. [CrossRef]
8. Alharbi, H.; Alshehry, A. Perceived stress and coping strategies among ICU nurses in government tertiary hospitals in Saudi Arabia: A cross-sectional study. *Ann. Saudi Med.* **2019**, *39*, 48–55. [CrossRef] [PubMed] [PubMed Central]
9. Huang, Y.; Yu, L. Sources of care stress of nursing staff for patients with infectious diseases during the prevalence of COVID-19: A case study of some regional teaching hospitals in southern Taiwan. *Healthcare* **2021**, *9*, 462. [CrossRef]
10. Kaszubska, A. Stres w Środowisku Pracy. Stres w Pracy. In *Poradnik Dla Pracodawcy*; Państwowa Inspekcja Pracy Główny Inspektorat Pracy: Warszawa, Poland, 2023; pp. 5–6. Available online: www.pip.gov.pl (accessed on 13 October 2024).
11. Vahedian-Azimi, A.; Hajiesmaeili, M.; Kangasniemi, M.; Fornés-Vives, J.; Hunsucker, R.L.; Rahimibashar, F.; Pourhoseingholi, M.A.; Farrokhvar, L.; Miller, A.C. Effects of Stress on Critical Care Nurses: A National Cross-Sectional Study. *J. Intensiv. Care Med.* **2019**, *34*, 311–322. [CrossRef]
12. Ibrahim, M.A.; Isa, K.Q.; Haji-Idris, H.-A.; Nawi, S.-H.; Teo, Y.C.; Rahman, H.A.; Abdul-Mumin, K.H. Spiritual Coping with Stress Among Emergency and Critical Care Nurses: A Cross-Sectional Study. *Community Ment. Health J.* **2020**, *56*, 287–293. [CrossRef] [PubMed]
13. Yliluoma, P.; Palonen, M. Telenurses' experiences of interaction with patients and family members: Nurse–caller interaction via telephone. *Scand. J. Caring Sci.* **2020**, *34*, 675–683. [CrossRef] [PubMed]
14. Yao, X.; Shao, J.; Wang, L.; Zhang, J.; Zhang, C.; Lin, Y. Does workplace violence, empathy, and communication influence occupational stress among mental health nurses? *Int. J. Ment. Health Nurs.* **2021**, *30*, 177–188. [CrossRef]
15. Betke, K.; Basińska, M.A.; Andruszkiewicz, A. Sense of coherence and strategies for coping with stress among nurses. *BMC Nurs.* **2021**, *20*, 1–10. [CrossRef]
16. Akbar, R.E.; Elahi, N.; Mohammadi, E.; Khoshknab, M.F. What Strategies Do the Nurses Apply to Cope With Job Stress?: A Qualitative Study. *Glob. J. Health Sci.* **2015**, *8*, 55–64. [CrossRef]
17. Delgado, C.; Upton, D.; Ranse, K.; Furness, T.; Foster, K. Nurses' resilience and the emotional labour of nursing work: An integrative review of empirical literature. *Int. J. Nurs. Stud.* **2017**, *70*, 71–88. [CrossRef]
18. Ghawadra, S.F.; Abdullah, K.L.; Choo, W.Y.; Phang, C.K. Mindfulness-based stress reduction for psychological distress among nurses: A systematic review. *J. Clin. Nurs.* **2019**, *28*, 3747–3758. [CrossRef]
19. Chesak, S.S.; Cutshall, S.M.; Bowe, C.L.; Montanari, K.M.; Bhagra, A. Stress Management Interventions for Nurses: Critical Literature Review. *J. Holist. Nurs.* **2019**, *37*, 288–295. [CrossRef]
20. Li, H.; Zhao, M.; Shi, Y.; Xing, Z.; Li, Y.; Wang, S.; Ying, J.; Zhang, M.; Sun, J. The effectiveness of aromatherapy and massage on stress management in nurses: A systematic review. *J. Clin. Nurs.* **2019**, *28*, 372–385. [CrossRef]
21. De Diego-Cordero, R.; Iglesias-Romo, M.; Badanta, B.; Lucchetti, G.; Vega-Escaño, J. Burnout and spirituality among nurses: A scoping review. *Explore* **2022**, *18*, 612–620. [CrossRef] [PubMed]
22. Peter, K.A.; Schols, J.M.G.A.; Halfens, R.J.G.; Hahn, S. Investigating work-related stress among health professionals at different hierarchical levels: A cross-sectional study. *Nurs. Open* **2020**, *7*, 969–979. [CrossRef] [PubMed] [PubMed Central]
23. Helwich, E. Chenges inthe organization of the newborn care in Poland from 80s of the 20th century until today. *Stand. Med. Pediatr.* **2017**, 149–154.
24. Zielińska, A.; Kluczny, A. Noworodek Urodzony Przedwcześnie-Wcześniak. In *Neonatologia Praktyczna*; Kozłowska_Rup, D., Gabryel, E., Świetliński, J., Eds.; PZWL Wydawnictwo Lekarskie: Warszawa, Poland, 2023; pp. 6–7.
25. Maslach, C.; Leiter, M.P. Understanding the burnout experience: Recent research and its implications for psychiatry. *World Psychiatry* **2016**, *15*, 103–111. [CrossRef]

26. Available online: https://nipip.pl/wp-content/uploads/2023/12/RAPORT-O-STANIE-PIELEGNIARSTWA-I-P-OLOZNICTWA-W-POLSCE-MAJ-2023.pdf (accessed on 25 February 2025).
27. Juszczyński, Z.; Ogińska-Bulik, N. Inwentarz do pomiaru radzenia sobie ze stresem—Mini-COPE. In *Narzędzia Do Pomiaru Stresu i Radzenia Sobie Ze Stresem*; Pracownia Testów Psychologicznych Polskiego Towarzystwa Psychologicznego: Warszawa, Poland, 2012; Volume rozdział 3, pp. 45–58.
28. Juszczyński, Z.; Ogińska-Bulik, N. Skala odczuwanego stresu—PSS-10. In *Narzędzia Do Pomiaru Stresu i Radzenia Sobie Ze Stresem*; Pracownia Testów Psychologicznych Polskiego Towarzystwa Psychologicznego: Warszawa, Poland, 2012; Volume rozdział 1, pp. 11–22.
29. Sarafis, P.; Chatzigianni, D.; Chatzigianni, D.; Tsounis, A.; Tsounis, A.; Markopoulos, N.; Markopoulos, N. Occupational Stress Experienced by Nurses Working in a Greek Regional Hospital: A Cross-Sectional Study. *Iran. J. Nurs. Midwifery Res.* **2018**, *23*, 450–457. [CrossRef]
30. Harris, S.; Tao, H. The Impact of US Nurses' Personal Religious and Spiritual Beliefs on Their Mental Well-Being and Burnout: A Path Analysis. *J. Relig. Health* **2022**, *61*, 1772–1791. [CrossRef]
31. McMeekin, D.E.; Hickman, R.L., Jr.; Douglas, S.L.; Kelley, C.G. Stress and Coping of Critical Care Nurses After Unsuccessful Cardiopulmonary Resuscitation. *Am. J. Crit. Care* **2017**, *26*, 128–135. [CrossRef] [PubMed]
32. Zbyrad, T. Ryzyko wypalenia zawodowego pracowników służb społecznych. *Ann. Univ. Mariae Curie-Skłodowska Sect. J-Paedagog.-Psychol.* **2017**, *30*, 87–105. [CrossRef]
33. Baranauskas, M.; Kalpokas, M.; Kupčiūnaitė, I.; Lieponienė, J.; Stukas, R. Self-Perceived Stress in Association with Emotional Experiences Following Patient Death and Coping Adequacy among Clinical Nurses in Lithuania: A Cross-Sectional Study. *J. Clin. Med.* **2024**, *13*, 2533. [CrossRef] [PubMed]
34. McAndrew, N.S.; Leske, J.; Schroeter, K. Moral distress in critical care nursing: The state of the science. *Nurs. Ethic.* **2018**, *25*, 552–570. [CrossRef]
35. Vincent, H.; Jones, D.J.; Engebretson, J. Moral distress perspectives among interprofessional intensive care unit team members. *Nurs. Ethic-* **2020**, *27*, 1450–1460. [CrossRef]
36. Tesfaye, T.D. Coping strategies among nurses in South-west Ethiopia: Descriptive, institution-based cross-sectional study. *BMC Res. Notes* **2018**, *11*, 421. [CrossRef] [PubMed]
37. Zhang, Y.; Wang, C.; Pan, W.; Zheng, J.; Gao, J.; Huang, X.; Cai, S.; Zhai, Y.; Latour, J.M.; Zhu, C. Stress, Burnout, and Coping Strategies of Frontline Nurses During the COVID-19 Epidemic in Wuhan and Shanghai, China. *Front. Psychiatry* **2020**, *11*, 565520. [CrossRef]
38. Ravaldi, C.; Levi, M.; Angeli, E.; Romeo, G.; Biffino, M.; Bonaiuti, R.; Vannacci, A. Stillbirth and perinatal care: Are professionals trained to address parents' needs? *Midwifery* **2018**, *64*, 53–59. [CrossRef] [PubMed]
39. André, B.; Dahlø, R.; Eilertsen, T.; Shorey, S.; Ringdal, G.I. Experiences with perinatal death among midwives, obstetricians, and assistant nurses: Results from a qualitative study in Norway/Erfahrungen von Hebammen, Geburtshelfern und Kinderpflegern mit perinatalem Tod: Ergebnisse einer qualitativen Studie in Norwegen. *Int. J. Health Prof.* **2020**, *7*, 24–32. [CrossRef]
40. Laing, R.E.; Fetherston, C.M.; Morrison, P. Responding to catastrophe: A case study of learning from perinatal death in midwifery practice. *Women Birth* **2020**, *33*, 556–565. [CrossRef]
41. Christoffersen, L.; Teigen, J.; Rønningstad, C. Following-up midwives after adverse incidents: How front-line management practices help second victims. *Midwifery* **2020**, *85*, 102669. [CrossRef] [PubMed]
42. Martos-López, I.M.; Sánchez-Guisado, M.d.M.; Guedes-Arbelo, C. Duelo por muerte perinatal, un duelo desautorizado = Bereavement for perinatal death, unauthorized bereavement. *Rev. Espanola De Comun. En Salud* **2016**, *7*, 300–309. [CrossRef]
43. Patterson, J. Traumatised Midwives Traumatised Women. *Aims J. When Birth Becomes Trauma.* **2019**, *30*. Available online: https://www.aims.org.uk/assets/media/996/aimsjournal2018v30n4whenbirthbecomestrauma.pdf#page=8 (accessed on 3 January 2025).
44. Beck, C.T.; Rivera, J.; Gable, R.K. A Mixed-Methods Study of Vicarious Posttraumatic Growth In Certified Nurse-Midwives. *J. Midwifery Women's Health* **2017**, *62*, 80–87. [CrossRef]
45. Piernikowska, E.; Podsiadły, J. Strategie Radzenia Sobie ze Stresem w opinii Pielęgniarek. *Innow. W Pielęgniarstwie I Nauk. O. Zdrowiu* **2019**, *1*, 15–26. Available online: https://wyd.edu.pl/images/Czasopisma_naukowe/PPA/IwP2018/IwP_2019_1_4/IwP_2019_1_4_Piernikowska_Podsiadly.pdf?utm_source=chatgpt.com (accessed on 17 March 2025).
46. Parker, J.D.A.; Sheinin, G. Coping. In *The Wiley Encyclopedia of Personality and Individual Differences*; Carducci, B.J., Nave, C.S., Fabio, A., Saklofske, D.H., Stough, C., Eds.; Wiley: Hoboken, NJ, USA, 2020. [CrossRef]
47. Uczak, A.; Najmiec, A. Wybrane Metody Profilaktyki Stresu Wśród Personelu Medycznego Psychiatrycznej Opieki Zdrowotnej. Bezpieczeństwo Pracy. *Nauka I Praktyka* **2019**, *6*, 16–20. Available online: https://www.umb.edu.pl/photo/pliki/WNoZ_jednostki/wnoz-z-zintegrowanej-opieki-medycznej/monografie/mierc_pacjenta_jako_obciazenie_w_grupie_zawodowej_pielegniarek.pdf?utm_source=chatgpt.com (accessed on 17 March 2025).

48. Kosirnik, C.; Philippe, R.A.; Pomini, V. Investigating the Links Between Performers' Self-Compassion, Mental Toughness and Their Social Environment: A Semi-Systematic Review. *Front. Psychol.* **2022**, *13*, 887099. [CrossRef] [PubMed]
49. CIOP-PIB. Profilaktyka Stresu Personelu Medycznego Psychiatrycznej Opieki Zdrowotnej. *Centralny Instytut Ochrony Pracy—Państwowy Instytut Badawczy.* 2019. Available online: https://www.ciop.pl/CIOPPortalWAR/appmanager/ciop/pl?_nfpb=true&_pageLabel=P53400446641589386203555&html_klucz=77777&html_klucz_spis=&html_tresc_id=3001338&html_tresc_root_id=11502&utm_source=chatgpt.com (accessed on 17 March 2025).
50. Dall'ora, C.; Ball, J.; Reinius, M.; Griffiths, P. Burnout in nursing: A theoretical review. *Hum. Resour. Health* **2020**, *18*, 1–17. [CrossRef] [PubMed]

nursing reports

MDPI

Correction

Correction: Urbańska et al. Influence of Sociodemographic Factors on Level Stress and Coping Strategies of Nurses and Midwives Caring for Newborns with Lethal Defects. *Nurs. Rep.* 2025, *15*, 116

Katarzyna Anna Urbańska [1,*], Beata Naworska [2] and Agnieszka Drosdzol-Cop [3]

[1] Neonatology Unit, BCM The Guardian Angels Hospital of the Brothers Hospitallers of St. John of God in Katowice, Markiefki 87, 40-211 Katowice, Poland
[2] Department of Gynaecology and Obstetrics, Faculty of Health Sciences in Katowice, Medical University of Silesia in Katowice, 40-751 Katowice, Poland; bnaworska@sum.edu.pl
[3] Chair and Department of Gynecology, Obstetrics and Oncological Gynecology, Faculty of Medical Sciences in Katowice, Medical University of Silesia in Katowice, 40-211 Katowice, Poland; adrosdzol@sum.edu.pl
* Correspondence: kasiaurbanskaaa@gmail.com

There was an error in the original publication [1]. The version posted on the Nursing Reports website contains the same description of the results in Table 5 and Table 6.

A correction has been made to Section 4, Paragraph 67–70 (Description of Table 6).

Table 6 presents the most commonly used methods of coping with stress employed by staff members in relation to their work, particularly in the context of caring for newborns with a lethal congenital defect. The results are expressed as percentages and refer to various emotional support methods and stress coping techniques. More than half of the respondents (52.8%) indicated that talking to loved ones and receiving support from close individuals is a key strategy for coping with stress. This is the most popular form of emotional support, highlighting the importance of interpersonal relationships in the process of emotional tension reduction.

The second most frequently indicated strategy is humour in the workplace. Almost one-third of the respondents (32.9%) use jokes as a way to ease difficult emotions, emphasising the role of distance and humour in coping with professional challenges.

Another significant strategy, used by 28.6% of respondents, is support from colleagues. A sense of community with other workers and their help in managing mental strain constitutes an important source of relief at work.

Entertainment and physical activity, such as sports, are popular methods of stress relief used by 25.7% and 23.4% of respondents, respectively. These activities can be viewed as forms of active relaxation and a way for individuals to detach themselves from professional issues.

For 22.1% of individuals, developing personal passions outside of work represents an effective stress coping strategy. This is an important way to unwind and relax, allowing for engagement in activities outside the work environment.

For 17.3% of people, faith provides support in coping with stress, which may reflect the spiritual dimension of dealing with difficult experiences. Additionally, relaxation techniques, used by 16% of respondents, may include meditation, breathing exercises, or other methods of tension reduction.

A less common, but still used strategy, is the use of spa treatments, as indicated by 11.7% of respondents. Such activities can support both physical and mental regeneration.

Less constructive ways of coping with stress, such as overeating (8.1%) and the use of substances like cigarettes or alcohol (7.8%), are chosen relatively infrequently, yet they remain present among some respondents.

The least commonly used strategy is seeking professional psychological help (2.3%). This result may suggest that these individuals rarely seek specialist support, possibly due to personal beliefs or barriers to accessing such help.

The findings show that medical staff most frequently rely on emotional support from loved ones and colleagues, as well as humour and recreational strategies. Fewer individuals turn to professional psychological help or engage in less constructive methods like overeating or substance use.

The authors state that the scientific conclusions are unaffected. This correction was approved by the Academic Editor. The original publication has also been updated.

Reference

1. Urbańska, K.A.; Naworska, B.; Drosdzol-Cop, A. Influence of Sociodemographic Factors on Level Stress and Coping Strategies of Nurses and Midwives Caring for Newborns with Lethal Defects. *Nurs. Rep.* **2025**, *15*, 116. [CrossRef] [PubMed]

MDPI AG
Grosspeteranlage 5
4052 Basel
Switzerland
Tel.: +41 61 683 77 34

MDPI Books Editorial Office
E-mail: books@mdpi.com
www.mdpi.com/books

www.ingramcontent.com/pod-product-compliance
Lightning Source LLC
LaVergne TN
LVHW070450061126
851858LV00011B/198